OXFORD MEDICAL PUBLICATIONS

Poverty, inequality, and health

Poverty, inequality, and health

An International Perspective

Edited by

David A. Leon

and

Gill Walt

London School of Hygiene
& Tropical Medicine
London, UK

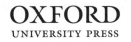

OXFORD

UNIVERSITY PRESS

OXFORD

UNIVERSITY PRESS

Great Clarendon Street, Oxford OX2 6DP

Oxford University Press is a department of the University of Oxford.
It furthers the University's objective of excellence in research, scholarship,
and education by publishing worldwide in

Oxford New York

Athens Auckland Bangkok Bogotá Buenos Aires Calcutta
Cape Town Chennai Dar es Salaam Delhi Florence Hong Kong Istanbul
Karachi Kuala Lumpur Madrid Melbourne Mexico City Mumbai
Nairobi Paris São Paulo Shanghai Singapore Taipei Tokyo Toronto Warsaw
with associated companies in Berlin Ibadan

Oxford is a registered trade mark of Oxford University Press
in the UK and in certain other countries

Published in the United States
by Oxford University Press, Inc., New York

© Oxford University Press, 2001

The moral rights of the authors have been asserted

Database right Oxford University Press (maker)

First published 2001

Reprinted 2001

A catalogue record for this title is available from the British Library

Library of Congress Cataloging in Publication Data
Poverty, inequality and health: an international perspective/edited by
David A. Leon and Gill Walt.
Includes bibliographical references and index.
1. Poor–Medical care–Cross cultural studies. 2. Poor–Diseases–
Cross-cultural studies. 3. Poor–Medical care–Developing
countries–Cross-cultural studies. 4. Poor–Developing countries–Health
aspects–Cross-cultural studies. I. Leon, David A. II. Walt, Gill.
RA418.5.P6 P685 2000 362.1'09172'4–dc21 00–058883

1 3 5 7 9 10 8 6 4 2
ISBN 0 19 263196 9

Printed in Great Britain
on acid free paper by
T.J. International Ltd, Padstow, Cornwall

Preface & Acknowledgements

In April 1999 the London School of Hygiene & Tropical Medicine held its ninth Public Health Forum entitled 'Poverty, Inequality, and Health'. This three-day meeting attracted over 150 participants from all over the world. It was successful in bringing together people working on poverty, inequality, and health from a wide range of perspectives from the developing and the developed world. The papers reflected this diversity, ranging from the micro to the macro level and from aetiology to intervention. With the exception of Chapter 1, the contributions to this book are based on presentations given at the Forum. However, it is important to emphasize that the book is not a conference proceeding. The content of the chapters has in most cases been extended and developed from the verbal presentation, links made between chapters, and the format modified to be suitable for publication as a book, thus producing what is a more integrated whole.

We would like to acknowledge the financial support given by the UK Department for International Development and the Rockefeller Foundation for the core costs of the Forum and assistance with expenses of participants from around the world. The Forum meeting was organized by a steering group chaired by David Leon with Richard Hayes, Martin McKee, and Carolyn Stephens. Satellite workshops were organized by Virginia Berridge, Elizabeth Dowler, and Kelley Lee.

With respect to this book we would like to thank the authors, who all showed great willingness to respond to our suggestions and comments. We would also like to thank Mark Haines from the LSHTM Library for undertaking the important but onerous task of checking the references in each chapter. Helen Liepman, our editor at OUP, has always been very encouraging and helpful. Finally, we would like to thank Alice Dickens for all her work, shouldering the dual task of being the administrator of the Forum and our in-house editor for the book.

David A. Leon and Gill Walt
February 2000

Contents

List of contributors   ix

1 Poverty, inequality, and health in international
perspective: a divided world?   01
David A. Leon and Gill Walt

2 The health consequences of the collapse of the
Soviet Union   17
Martin McKee

3 Industrialization and health in historical perspective   37
Richard H. Steckel

4 Common threads: underlying components of
inequalities in mortality between and within countries   58
David A. Leon

5 Life-course approaches to socio-economic differentials
in cause-specific adult mortality   88
George Davey Smith, David Gunnell, and Yoav Ben-Shlomo

6 The impact of health interventions on inequalities:
infant and child health in Brazil   125
Cesar G. Victora, Fernando C. Barros, and J. Patrick Vaughan

7 Children's health in developing countries: issues of
coping, child neglect, and marginalization   137
Claudio F. Lanata

8 Accounts of social capital: the mixed health effects of
personal communities and voluntary groups   159
Stephen J. Kunitz

9 Do health care systems contribute to inequalities?   175
Maureen Mackintosh

10 Measuring health inequality: challenges and
new directions   194
Christopher J. L. Murray, Julio Frenk, and Emmanuela E. Gakidou

11 Poverty and inequalities in health within developing
    countries: filling the information gap   217
    Davidson R. Gwatkin

12 Poverty, inequality, and mental health in developing
    countries   247
    Vikram Patel

13 Injuries, inequalities, and health: from policy vacuum
    to policy action   263
    Anthony Zwi

14 Inequalities in health: is research gender blind?   283
    Sally Macintyre

15 From science to policy: options for reducing health
    inequalities   294
    Hilary Graham

16 Do poverty alleviation programmes reduce inequities
    in health? The Bangladesh experience   312
    A. Mushtaque R. Chowdhury and Abbas Bhuiya

17 Economic progress and health   333
    Amartya Sen

    Index   346

List of contributors

Dr Fernando C. Barros, Latin American Center for Perinatology, Pan American Health Organization, Uruguay

Dr Yoav Ben-Shlomo, University of Bristol, Department of Social Medicine, Canynge Hall, Whiteladies Road, Bristol BS8 2PR, UK

Dr Abbas Bhuiya, Head, Social and Behavioural Sciences Programme, ICDDR,B, GPO Box 128, Dhaka, Bangladesh

Dr A. Mushtaque R. Chowdhury, Director of Research, BRAC, 75 Mohakhali, Dhaka 1212, Bangladesh

Professor George Davey Smith, University of Bristol, Department of Social Medicine, Canynge Hall, Whiteladies Road, Bristol BS8 2PR, UK

Dr Julio Frenk, Executive Director, Evidence and Information for Policy, World Health Organization, 1211 Geneva 27, Switzerland

Ms Emmanuela E. Gakidou, World Health Organization, 1211 Geneva 27, Switzerland

Professor Hilary Graham, Department of Applied Social Science, Cartmel College, Lancaster University, Lancaster LA1 4YL, UK

Dr David Gunnell, University of Bristol, Department of Social Medicine, Canynge Hall, Whiteladies Road, Bristol BS8 2PR, UK

Dr Davidson R. Gwatkin, Director, International Health Policy Program, The World Bank, Washington DC, USA

Dr Stephen J. Kunitz, Department of Community and Preventive Medicine, University of Rochester Medical Center, Box 644, 601 Elmwood Avenue, Rochester, NY 14642, USA

Dr Claudio Lanata, Instituto de Investigacion Nutricional, Av. La Universidad No 685, La Molina, Lima, Peru

Professor David Leon, Epidemiology Unit, London School of Hygiene & Tropical Medicine, Keppel Street, London WC1E 7HT, UK

Professor Sally Macintyre, MRC Social and Public Health Sciences Unit, University of Glasgow, Glasgow G12 8RZ, UK

Professor Martin McKee, European Centre on Health of Societies in Transition, London School of Hygiene & Tropical Medicine, Keppel Street, London WC1E 7HT, UK

Professor Maureen Mackintosh, The Open University, Faculty of Social Sciences, Walton Hall, Milton Keynes MK7 6AA, UK

Dr Christopher J. L. Murray, World Health Organization, 1211 Geneva 27, Switzerland

Dr Vikram Patel, Section of Epidemiology and General Practice, Institute of Psychiatry, London and Sangath Centre, 841/1 Porvorim, Goa 403521, India.

Professor Amartya Sen, Master, Trinity College, Cambridge, UK and Lamont University Professor Emeritus, Harvard University, USA

Dr Richard H. Steckel, Economics and Anthropology Departments, Ohio State University, Columbus, OH 43210, USA and US National Bureau of Economic Research

Professor J. Patrick Vaughan, Health Policy Unit, London School of Hygiene & Tropical Medicine, Keppel Street, London WC1E 7HT, UK

Professor Cesar G. Victora, Universidade Federal de Pelotas, CP 464, 96001–970 Pelotas, Brazil

Dr Gill Walt, Health Policy Unit, London School of Hygiene & Tropical Medicine, Keppel Street, London WC1E 7HT, UK

Dr Anthony Zwi, Health Policy Unit, London School of Hygiene & Tropical Medicine, Keppel Street, London WC1E 7HT, UK

1 Poverty, inequality, and health in international perspective: a divided world?

David A. Leon and Gill Walt

There has been a remarkable improvement in health status in most countries of the world over the past few decades. Infant and child survival in developing countries has increased dramatically while in many developed countries mortality rates from major causes such as coronary heart disease (CHD) have been falling. However, despite these general improvements, there remain substantial inequalities in health between countries, regions, socio-economic groups, and individuals. Indeed, some inequalities are widening. Many African countries are bearing the full brunt of the HIV epidemic, and have sharply declining life expectancy, while the collapse of communism has been associated with major mortality increases in the mid-1990s in parts of the former Soviet Union. Within a number of high-income countries, including the UK, there is evidence that relative inequalities in health have also been widening over the past few decades.

While concern about these contradictions has been expressed in a number of publications and meetings, at both national and international levels, there have been only limited attempts to provide an international overview of the problems of inequalities in health. This book sets out to raise issues around health inequities and inequalities in a global context. As well as documenting new facets of the global health divide, it also explores how far there are common global themes in science and policy that may shed new light on inequalities in health, and strategies to reduce them.

This introductory chapter has two aims. Firstly to identify and reflect on some of the main issues dealt with in the book and to explore their interconnections. Secondly to look at some important questions that, although implicit in much of the book, are not directly addressed by any particular chapter. For clarity we have organized the chapters around four main themes. The first chapters are concerned with the health consequences of social and economic change. The next address conceptual issues around health and wealth; differing perceptions; conceptual problems of measurement; explanatory approaches; and the role of health services. Following these are the chapters focusing on emerging and neglected priorities, and the final chapters look at evidence for policy and interventions. Inevitably, these themes do not capture all dimensions of poverty, inequality, and health, and there are other, cross-cutting issues that recur in different parts of the book. We start by considering two issues which underlie many chapters: the relationship between ethics, policy, and science, and how far these impact on the way inequalities are understood and acted upon.

Ethics, policy, and science

There are many arguments that may be made in favour of reducing inequalities in health and producing more equitable health care systems.[1] For example, as discussed later in this introduction, there is a resurgence of interest in the economic argument that improving the health of the poor helps them extract themselves from poverty. However, our view is that health inequalities and inequities are ultimately ethical issues: a perspective that is implicit throughout this book. Working towards the elimination of absolute poverty and the adverse health consequences that accompany it, is essentially to be justified on moral grounds, not in terms of economic return.

We believe that inequalities and inequities can be reduced through appropriate policies in public health, in the health system, and in other areas. How far they may be eliminated altogether is debatable—but speculation about this ultimate objective should not distract attention from the many obvious steps that may be taken to improve the current situation. However, we are aware that there is still much to be learnt about the processes generating inequalities in health and about devising appropriate policy responses. Indeed, the widely ranging perspectives on this problem provided by this book illustrate the complexity of the subject. Different chapters explore the difficulties in establishing relationships between cause and effect (between societal, economic, psychological, biological, and other factors); in taking time into account (understanding factors spanning a lifetime); in huge obstacles (both conceptual and logistical) in measurement; and in knowing what public policies will be most effective. Drawing on experiences in high-, middle-, and low-income countries, the chapters provide a rich array of ideas and practice from which to learn and progress our understanding of, and ability to address, inequalities in health.

Are poverty and health inequalities on the policy agenda?

Global inequalities in health are just one facet of the enormous disparities between rich and poor. Falling aid budgets in the 1990s[2] and the increasing burden of international debt suffered by the poorest countries are leading to a more inequitable world. Other trends, such as the rapid pace and spread of information technologies, also carry a risk of increasing global division, with the poorest countries unable to take advantage of these new areas of economic growth. These trends do not provide a sound basis for reducing international health inequalities.

International agencies and donor countries have responded by focusing policies on the 'poor'. In 1996, the Development Assistance Committee of the OECD proposed that 'a global development partnership' should aim for a reduction of one-half in the proportion of the world's population living in extreme poverty by 2015 (OECD, 1996). The first objective of the World Bank's recently revised mission statement is 'to fight poverty with passion and professionalism'. The UK's aid strategy is being increasingly formulated in terms of 'pro-poor' policies, while in 1999 the Rockefeller Foundation announced a new global mission that focuses on 'the challenges faced by poor people around the world who have been excluded from the benefits of globalization'. How far these various international initiatives will translate into programmes that will actually help to alleviate poverty and reduce inequalities in health between countries is uncertain. On the positive side, international action to write off the debts of the highly indebted poor countries, in part catalysed by international organizations such as Jubilee 2000, may go some way to helping poor countries cope in extremely constrained economic environments.

With respect to health inequalities, however, part of the problem lies in the fact that in many countries these are not perceived to be an important issue, or ones which governments can, or should, address. Nevertheless, in the 1990s there has been increased international concern about health inequalities within low-income countries, as witnessed by a number of new World Bank country studies, and collaborative research actions such as the Rockefeller Foundation's Global Health Equity Initiative (Whitehead *et al.*, in press). There has also been clear government interest, in Europe and elsewhere, in health inequalities within national borders. In the UK, for example, a new Labour Government showed its commitment to addressing health inequalities by appointing a Minister for Public Health in 1997, whose brief explicitly included an independent inquiry into inequalities in health (Acheson, 1998). Echoing once more the theme of targeting the poor, the inquiry highlighted the importance of improving the living standards of the poor, although its brief precluded advocacy of broader macro-economic policies such as redistribution of income and wealth. Hilary Graham, a member of the Inquiry, draws on this exercise in her discussion of strategies to reduce inequalities in health in chapter 15.

The health consequences of social and economic change

One of the central tenets of this book is that the way in which a society is organized, where resources are invested, and in whose interests they are deployed, has a profound impact on the health of individuals within it. What can be seen at the national level also has a corollary at the global level. The growing interconnectedness of the world means that the nature of the global society and economy also influences people's health, for example through global environmental change or through the effects of chronic indebtedness suffered by many of the world's poorest nations.

Most significant differences in health between countries or populations are not a consequence of genetic differences, nor are they in any other sense biologically inevitable. However, not all inequalities in health are equally susceptible to reduction. Working towards a health care system that is based on principles of equity may be easier than changing health-related behaviours that are embedded in a particular world view developed and sustained through experience of personal adversity and deprivation. More fundamentally, some inequalities in risk of disease between populations may reflect profound long-term differences in the way in which societies have grown and developed; they are not just an expression of concurrent differences in circumstances. An example of this is given by Leon in chapter 4. Rates of stomach cancer mortality today (the world's second most common cancer cause of death) seem to reflect levels of hygiene and household crowding found many years ago: an effect driven by infection contracted in childhood.

The history of nineteenth-century sanitary reforms in Europe continues to provide inspiration for those working to improve population health. In the middle of the nineteenth century, there was a gradual recognition and then acceptance that the health of nations was susceptible to considerable improvement if adequate steps were taken to deal with poor sanitation, overcrowding, absence of clean water, and so on. This was by no means obvious to all at the start, and was disputed by many.[3]

The health crisis confronting the nineteenth-century reformers was one that was driven by a massive process of social and economic change. The rapid urbanization that characterized industrialization in many European countries in the first part of the nineteenth century brought with it increased rates of diseases and mortality from communicable diseases that spread easily in the bad environmental conditions characteristic of most cities. Recognition of the importance of specific poor environmental circumstances in the aetiology of these and other diseases was in fact inextricably linked to uncovering their strong connection with poverty. Thus, the nineteenth-century experience is also one that underlines how our insights into the links between social organization and health are inextricably bound up with understanding socio-economic inequalities in health.

There still remains much to be understood about the way in which the health of populations changes as part of the broader social and economic changes that societies undergo. In chapter 3, Steckel looks at the complex link between industrialization and height used as a measure of health and general welfare. As we start the twenty-first century, the records and data of the twentieth century will provide a critical base from which to observe and measure new, emerging, or continuing inequalities. These are not simply academic points about history, but bear on central issues of development strategy. In the book's final chapter, Sen contrasts the benefits of 'support led' development, in which priority is given to social welfare, education, and health even in poor societies, with the 'growth-mediated' view that such investments can only be justified and 'afforded' once a country has reached a certain basic level of affluence (Sen, this volume, chapter 17). His powerful argument is one that sees investment in welfare, education, and health as ensuring successful development in its broadest sense, which requires the removal of impediments to people's capability, including illness and disease.

The most striking contemporary evidence for massive and rapid changes in the social and economic fabric having an overwhelming impact on the health of nations, lies in the health crisis that overtook Russia, and other parts of the former Soviet Union, in the 1990s, as McKee illustrates in chapter 2. The mechanisms involved in the catastrophic decline of six years in male life expectancy that occurred in Russia between 1990 and 1994 have still to be firmly established. However, there is no dispute that this mortality reversal was intimately connected to the social and economic chaos that followed the collapse of the Soviet Union. While there have been reductions in mortality in more recent years, the continuing very poor health status of the Russian population constitutes one of the major priorities that should be addressed in terms of international inequalities in health within the industrialized world.

Broadening the conceptual base

There are many conceptual problems in establishing why inequalities occur, and the causal links between different factors. We have identified five general areas, each considered below.

Health and wealth

In much of what is written about the link between health and wealth, it is often implicitly assumed that the direction of causality is from wealth (or poverty) to health (or disease). However, the possibility that either at the individual or population level, there can also be a causal link running from health to wealth needs to be considered. The view that poor health contributes to impoverishment is not new: it was a central part of the outlook of Edwin Chadwick, the nineteenth-century public health pioneer. Having originally believed that the Poor Laws in Britain should make poverty as unattractive a proposition as possible, through the workhouse system, Roy Porter (1997) describes Chadwick's change in perspective:

> The New Poor Law was meant to cut claimants and hence costs. Chadwick monitored its operation, and to his chagrin found that his brainchild wasn't working. Why did pauperism not decrease under this expertly designed system? He concluded that it was because much poverty was due not to fecklessness but to disease. Many of those entering the workhouses were the chronic sick and

disabled, so much so that it was necessary to build special workhouse infirmaries at public expense. sickness bred poverty...

A modern-day version of this perspective is now being given striking prominence by the World Health Organization (WHO). In the 1999 World Health Report, a whole section is devoted to 'Health and Economic Productivity'. Although the evidence looking at this issue is problematic (and deserves further critical examination), WHO considers it firm enough to suggest that:

> Because ill-health traps people in poverty, sustained investment in the health of the poor could provide a policy lever for alleviating persistent poverty (WHO, 1999)

This perspective, emphasizing ill-health as an obstacle to economic progress, is being used by Gro Harlem Brundtland, the Director General of the WHO, to take forward her central commitment to moving health up the agenda of governments and politicians. She argues as follows: if a nation invests in the health of its citizens, it improves productivity and wealth-creating potential. Using this argument then places advocates for health in a position where they will no longer be relegated to dealing solely with Ministries of Health (traditionally weak compared to many others) but will be able to capture the direct attention of Prime Ministers and Ministers of Finance. The issue of health will be transformed from one that is perceived as a net drain on the public purse, to one that is central to the whole strategy of wealth creation.

As we noted at the outset of this introduction, these sorts of utilitarian/human capital arguments need to be kept in perspective, and should not overshadow the ethical imperatives concerning inequalities in health.[4] Nevertheless, acknowledging that there may be an important sense in which ill-health leads to or perpetuates poverty (whether absolute or relative in definition) does not mean that the conditions of poverty do not lead to disease and ill-health. Causality almost certainly runs in both directions—generating a mutually reinforcing vicious or virtuous cycle. Strategies aimed at reducing inequalities in health need to take account of this complexity.

Differing perceptions

There are considerable conceptual difficulties around the competing understandings of the nature and mechanisms that drive and perpetuate inequalities in health. Surveying the literature and debates reveals that there is no consensus as to what are the core issues involved. In countries such as the UK, Sweden, and the Netherlands, over the past few decades, there has been much research on inequalities in health that has been overwhelmingly preoccupied with understanding why there are socio-economic gradients in ill-health and mortality. From this perspective, inequality in health is principally about disease aetiology, and the policy issues that arise are around primary prevention.

In contrast, in low- and middle-income countries, those working on inequalities in health over the same period more usually understand the problem as one of inequitable access to health care, with the related policy questions being around ways of devising more equitable health care provision. Much of the discussion about low-income countries has therefore focused on 'equity' as an issue of fairness and justice, rather than differences in health inequalities between groups. A strong concern about equity of access, however, is also found in the US, with its privatized health care system leaving many poorer people without adequate medical care.[5] Interestingly, this coexists with a separate but strong interest in inequalities in health status, and the aetiological mechanisms that drive them.

The contrast between developed and developing country perceptions of the problem of 'inequalities in health' is an oversimplification, but it contains an important element of truth, as there are good reasons why this division should exist. In many Western European countries, access to health services is *relatively* universal, and not strongly dependent upon socio-economic circumstances or geography. Added to this is a particularly strong tradition among public health researchers in these countries, influenced by such thinkers as Thomas McKeown, that the health sector and medical advances have played very little part in explaining the improvements of health of populations in the long term.[6]

In developing countries, the shadow of structural adjustment and the pressure to reduce government expenditure on health, and to reorganize the health sector to bring in private provision and payments for service, has been seen by many as a major threat to equity (Stott, 1999). Awareness of the serious equity problems in the funding of the private health care system in the US may also have sensitized people to these issues. Beyond this, it is abundantly clear that a large proportion of the world's population does not have access to anything approaching an adequate level and standard of health care provision, and is denied treatments and medical care that are of undoubted efficacy. Focusing on equity of health care provision in the developing world therefore has a compelling logic.

There is another reason why the issue of inequalities in health in developing countries tends to be focused on questions of equity of access, and largely ignores the issue of socio-economic inequalities in disease occurrence. To investigate inequalities in disease occurrence, and certainly to provide population-based data on these differences, presupposes the existence of a relatively elaborate routine data collection system. However, such an information infrastructure tends only to exist in developed, high-income countries. In many developing countries, reliable population estimates are often difficult to obtain, and there is no reliable medical certification of cause of death. It should be noted that the existence of a tradition of routine data collection does not in itself ensure the production of data on socio-economic inequalities in health, there being substantial variation between developed counties in the extent to which such data has generally been collected, analysed, and results disseminated.

As Gwatkin describes (chapter 11), considerable efforts are going into the development of survey methods for measurement of inequalities within low- and middle-income countries that will go some way towards redressing the imbalance in the way inequalities in health are perceived around the world. Nevertheless, there remains the question as to whether enough work is being done in developing countries to study the underlying determinants of socio-economic differences in health. This question will become increasingly pressing as the epidemiological profile of diseases shifts away from communicable to non-communicable diseases.

From the other side, however, there needs to be more attention given to the issue of health service access in developed countries. There is mounting evidence, for example, that socio-economic differences in access to health care may be influencing survival from cancer in countries such as the UK (Coleman *et al.*, 1999). Beyond this, as argued in chapter 9 by Mackintosh, there is a compelling case to assess critically the extent to which the values of health care systems, whether in developed or developing countries, are contributing to social inequalities and inequities in the broadest sense. This issue may be all the more pressing given reforms to the organization and financing of health care systems which are being undertaken or considered in many countries. This reform process is very often driven from a technocratic perspective of efficiency and effectiveness, with little consideration given to core values of equity of care.

Problems in measuring inequalities in health

The first studies of socio-economic differences in health go back to the nineteenth century. Many of the early investigations involved comparison of mortality and disease rates between geographic areas that differed according to their socio-economic characteristics, an approach that is still used today, albeit using much more sophisticated methods. There is also a strong tradition of analysing mortality and ill-health according to socio-economic groups created as aggregations of individuals based on characteristics such as occupation, education, or income. The occupational social class schemas, first used in analyses of mortality around the 1921 Census of England and Wales, present particularly serious problems when attempts are made to compare across time or between countries.[7] Alternative methods of defining social groups have also been employed. Educational level has been particularly favoured, being equally applicable to men and women and to people in developing and developed countries.

In the 1990s, a series of Europe-wide studies was conducted with the aim of producing the most internationally comparable data on inequalities in morbidity and mortality. The project took great care with many of the basic methodological problems inherent in such exercises. However, the interpretation of the socio-economic differentials has been controversial. For example, Sweden was found to have one of the largest relative socio-economic differences in mortality of any Western European country (Kunst *et al.*, 1998*b*). This was regarded as extraordinary, given the fact that Sweden is well known for having pursued social and economic policies with the explicit aim of creating a more equitable society, and does have in fact one of the most equitable income distributions in the world.[8]

On closer examination, this result highlighted an important problem in how we measure the size of inequalities in health, rather than casting doubt upon Sweden's achievements. The problem is this. In this analysis, and in many others, the size of the socio-economic effect was measured as a *ratio* of mortality in one group compared to another. If instead, the measure of inequality is taken as the simple *difference* in mortality rates, a very different picture emerges (Leon, 1998). In the case of Sweden, because rates in both the high and low socio-economic group are very low, so is the difference between them in absolute terms—in fact it is the lowest of any country included. Thus, the answer to the question as to whether in one population or moment in time inequalities are greater or lesser than in another, partly depends upon whether we choose to measure the inequality in relative or absolute terms.

The problems of comparability of socio-economic classifications are regarded as sufficiently serious by some to require abandoning this approach altogether. The challenge of developing a consistent and valid way to measure inequalities in health for any population in the world has recently led to the suggestion that it is necessary to go beyond 'social group' analysis. Murray and colleagues (1999) argue in chapter 10 that, rather than look at the way in which health or disease rates vary between socio-economic groups, an approach which is based on measuring the distribution of health across all individuals in a population is preferable. Such a measure is meant to be analogous to measures of income inequality, and would be estimated from the spread of health (at an individual or household level) across the population.

There are a number of difficulties with this proposed new approach. Some are technical. Health is not like income. It is not possible to assign to each individual in a population an objective 'health' index akin to their income. Survival is not a simple substitute because at the individual level it takes only two values—dead or alive. However, beyond these technical issues there is a fundamental problem with any proposal to replace the 'social group' approach with the distributional one. Despite the attractions of such a 'pure' measure of health inequality, such a measure ignores the reality that health is socially patterned (Braveman et al., 2000).

Regardless of the problems of comparability, the tradition of analysing socio-economic differences in health will always retain a central relevance. It calls attention to the manifold ways in which disadvantage is a multi-dimensional phenomenon—a crucial observation if we are to be successful in developing strategies for reduction of inequities within and between countries. In contrast, the distributional approach to inequalities in health provides in itself no substantive information about the likely social and biological mechanisms which generate differences in health within a population. Nevertheless, this challenge to the conventional approach is welcome, particularly as it will require a far more critical assessment of how we measure and compare inequalities in health.

Finally, conceptual and methodological difficulties in the measurement of inequalities in health are compounded by logistical ones. As has already been said, reliable and long-term data is often missing, especially in middle- and low-income countries. In chapter 11, Gwatkin draws attention to the fact that, while inter-country comparisons exist, much comparative data that does exist is so aggregated, that it gives little indication of distributional aspects of health status intra-country—specifically, how the poorest groups fare in relation to inequalities. There is also an almost complete lack of information about recent time trends in health inequalities. However, this is beginning to change, and the same chapter provides some interesting early analysis of intra-group inequalities, based on economic quintiles (defined in terms of consumption). These are important steps in gathering information for policy makers, especially in meeting development objectives: for example, by reformulating health improvement targets more in terms of reductions in inequalities within countries, and not just in terms of average levels for countries as a whole. However, in those low-income countries where almost half the child population is under the poverty line, such refinements may need to come later.

Explanatory approaches

Socio-economic inequalities in health and disease are ubiquitous. They have been observed in populations throughout the world that are at varying levels of social and economic development. Moreover, they are as obvious today as they were 100 years ago, despite the fact that absolute poverty and deprivation are largely a thing of the past in high-income countries, and that the profile of life-threatening diseases has moved decisively from communicable to non-communicable diseases.[9] It is this persistence of socio-economic differences in health across such changing contexts that provides such a challenge to our understanding, indicating that a single, unifying explanation is unlikely to be found.

Many of the links between absolute poverty and ill-health are relatively straightforward to understand in terms of disease aetiology, with poor housing, sanitation, and hygiene leading to increased exposure to communicable diseases, and malnourishment reducing individual resistance to infection. However, even here there are complexities. In chapter 7, Lanata considers evidence that shows that, despite living in absolute poverty, the extent to which parents have the (psychological) capacity to use their scant resources in a constructive way can have an important influence on morbidity and mortality from childhood infection. This is an important insight that underlines the need to develop people's capacities and resourcefulness as an important component of strategies to reduce the effects of absolute deprivation on health.

Inequalities in the occurrence of non-communicable diseases such as cancer and heart disease are more challenging to understand. For conditions such as lung cancer there is overwhelming evidence that the greater risk observed among people today who are in manual compared to non-manual social classes in

Britain may be explained by differences in tobacco smoking. Attempts to explain socio-economic gradients for other non-communicable diseases have not been as straightforward. In a classic paper, Marmot and colleagues (1984) reported that they were unable to explain the pronounced gradient in mortality from CHD among Whitehall civil servants in terms of known risk factors such as smoking, cholesterol, and blood pressure. This, together with the observation that many of the major causes of death in countries such as Britain all show an inverse association with socio-economic position (i.e. risk increases as one goes down the socio-economic scale), has led Marmot and others to suggest that there may be a mechanism of general susceptibility involved that is driven by psycho-social stress rather than conventional risk factors.

The full psycho-social explanation for inequalities in conditions such as CHD hypothesizes that there are direct, adverse physiological consequences of stress that in themselves lead to increased risk of disease. Wilkinson (1996) has integrated this hypothesis into his account of the link between disease risk and income inequality. This intriguing idea proposes that in high-income countries, it is the degree of income inequity that is positively associated with mortality rather than level of absolute national wealth (such as GDP per capita). In other words it is income inequity *per se* and its correlates (such as level of social capital and cohesion) that generate ill-health, operating, in part at least, through a psycho-social stress mechanism. It should be noted, however, that the empirical basis for a general link between income inequality and mortality has been disputed. Moreover, as Kunitz discusses later in chapter 8, social capital is a difficult and ambiguous concept that is not invariably associated with progressive approaches to society and better health.

The psycho-social stress explanation for inequalities in health within and between countries is, nevertheless, an appealing one. It provides a basis for explaining how inequalities in health can persist in the absence of absolute deprivation, and appears to offer a common class of mechanisms to explain the observation that many common causes of death show an inverse socio-economic gradient. There are, however, problems with these approaches, not least that one of the basic planks of the argument—that of general susceptibility—is weak. Davey Smith and colleagues suggest in chapter 5 that there is in fact considerable heterogeneity among causes of death in terms of the associations they show with socio-economic position. Some show inverse associations, others (such as breast cancer) direct associations.

To account for the failure of conventional risk factors to explain inequalities in health within and between countries may not require resort to a psycho-social theory of general susceptibility. An alternative approach advanced in several chapters of this book (chapters 4, 5, 6, and 15), is to conceptualize inequalities in health as being generated by influences operating across the life course (Kuh and Ben-Shlomo, 1997). The imprint of these influences will not all be equally visible in adult life and middle age (depending upon the aetiological specificities of each disease), and hence will be missed by studies that only have information about individuals at these older ages. However, it is important to note that the life-course approach is in its infancy, and much further work needs to be undertaken before a definitive judgement can be made as to whether it really does provide a substantially improved framework for understanding inequalities in health.

The role of the health care system

Finally, in terms of mechanisms that may generate or contribute to inequalities in health we need to look briefly at the role of the health sector. As already discussed, there is, in developed countries at least, a strong element of scepticism about the potential contribution of health services to population health, and thus to inequalities in health. This scepticism may well be overstated. Certainly it is increasingly plausible that differences in availability of anti-hypertensive medication (Kiivet *et al.*, 1998) may account for a component of East–West differences in mortality from stroke. Equitable access to good quality neonatal services may account for the absence of socio-economic differences in neonatal mortality in Sweden (Leon *et al.*, 1992), while differential access to such services may account for the widening of infant mortality differences in the Czech Republic (Koupilová *et al.*, 1998). Striking evidence that the introduction of effective medical interventions into society can in fact exacerbate socio-economic inequalities in health outcomes is provided in a series of studies from Brazil presented by Victora and colleagues in chapter 6. This chapter suggests that, in many countries, those who are socio-economically advantaged are most likely to be the first beneficiaries of new treatments, even if in the longer term they are made available to all. This gradual diffusion of the intervention through different strata of society will leave a characteristic trace on inequalities in outcomes, which may be expected to widen before they are diminished.

Emerging and neglected priorities

Within the general problems related to health inequalities and poverty, some issues have not been given the attention they deserve. Globally and nationally, both mental health and injuries are famously low on government policy agendas. Indeed, in chapter 12, Patel suggests that many believe that mental illness is a 'luxury' the poor cannot afford in developing countries. Yet he shows that depression, anxiety, and alcohol abuse are common disorders, especially among the poor, and suggests a bi-directional relationship—where the state of being poor may lead to mental illness, which in itself may then result in further impoverishment. Likewise, Zwi demonstrates in chapter 13 that injuries account for a significant burden of mortality and morbidity, with the poorest suffering the most, in both high- and low-income countries. Exposure and vulnerability are important aspects of both injuries and mental illness, reflecting biologically as well as socially-mediated precepts, and it seems there is considerable work to be done in trying to capture these elusive concepts in order to test cause and effect in health experiences. In chapter 14, Macintyre attempts to disentangle biological differences between males and females from those which are created by the social construct of gender. She supports the view that inequalities in health may be due to differential exposure or vulnerability, and suggests that gender differences may not be as constant over time, cultural context, and health measure as has often been assumed.

It should be noted that these chapters touch on neglected areas, but do not cover them all: as populations grow older, so health inequalities in the aged will need to be marked out, measured, tested, and policies devised to ameliorate inequalities. Likewise, issues around ethnicity, and the way health inequalities are mediated through different ethnic experience and culture, are likely to demand greater attention as people move around the world. Finally, as genetic advances accelerate this century, there are real concerns that these may exacerbate socio-economic inequalities in health—through unequal access to expensive technologies or treatments for particular diseases.

Evidence for policy and interventions

Recognizing neglected problems is a necessary, but not sufficient condition for doing something about them. Many of the chapters in this book suggest ways forward, or what needs to be done, ranging from the global and general to the local and specific. At the broadest international level, suggestions include commitment to specifically targeting aid for the poorest countries, and within them the poorest groups; or mobilizing global interest in meeting the shortcomings in current data, and finding better ways of measuring and comparing intra-country differences.

At the national level, policies (social, economic, and fiscal) form an integral part of public health strategies to reduce inequalities, but there are policy choices to be made—in chapter 15, Graham outlines three: re-distribution of income to protect the living standards of the poor; improving employment opportunities; and publicly-funded welfare services, including health care and education. Policies in these areas struggled to find advocates in the post-welfare, neo-liberal environment of the last decades of the twentieth century. However, there are signs that increasing concern about growing inequalities both within and between countries is leading to a search for alternative policies—for example, the notion that relationships based on 'duties', not only 'rights', can strengthen the position of the poor in access to health care; legitimizing the claim by the poor to good services and treatment. Thus, Mackintosh argues in chapter 9 that policies should focus on ways of strengthening the capacity of the poor to make claims (a point reflected in Lanata's chapter 7 about the need to build capacity and confidence among the poor). Policies should also seek to associate middle-class reliance on privilege with middle-class acceptance of duty to others—and not encourage the better off to segregate themselves institutionally by, for example, leaving public health services only for the very poor.

Even in very poor countries, there are encouraging signs. As Chowdhury and Bhuiya show in chapter 16, one of the poorest and most populated countries in the world, Bangladesh, provides an example to others, of what can be done through specific, targeted programmes. But the last word belongs to Sen (chapter 17), who concludes that although economic growth will lead to improvements in health, the extent to which such improvements are reflected in greater or lesser differences in health inequalities will be mediated through the way income generated by economic growth is used. Like Graham (chapter 15), he places emphasis on the state's ability to address inequalities through reducing the burden of poverty by judicious public policies. Further, he argues that even if economic growth is minimal, 'intelligent and equitable social policies' can play a role in improving health.

A divided world?

The issues raised in this book reflect the complexity of the scientific, conceptual, and policy issues inherent in addressing the issue of poverty, inequality, and health. Major inequalities in health status remain within and between countries. There are also substantial differences in the way the problem is perceived, the priority given to it, and the solutions advanced according to country and region. Nevertheless, the international perspective taken by this book allows one to discern a number of important common axes or themes, which cast new light upon the way in which this problem is dealt with in different countries. One common theme that appears to be emerging everywhere is a move towards focusing upon the poor within each country. Another is the issue of focus: are inequalities principally a matter of inequitable access to health services or of determinants of socio-economic differences in health status and disease? Seeing the way in which this focus varies around the world provides a stimulus to review whether in any one place the balance is correct. The problems of measurement and comparison of inequalities is another common problem—with great scope for exchange of approaches in order that the wheel is not reinvented once more. A common lesson that emerges from this book and that applies across the globe is that inequalities in health are not static or inevitable phenomena. They have a dynamic, driven by the interplay of biology, social organization, and health systems. This is a cause for optimism. Things can change and do change. We hope that the diversity of this book stimulates people to take a fresh look at the problems of poverty, inequality, and health that they are most familiar with, and in so doing contributes in a small way to tackling this major problem.

Notes

1. See, for example, Gilson, 1998.
2. The 1999 *World Bank Global Development Finance Report* found that net flows of

overseas aid to developing countries have fallen to their lowest level in real terms since 1981, with little significant recovery in prospect.

3. For a succinct account of these issues concerning the development of public health in the nineteenth century, see Porter, 1997, chapter 13.

4. Amartya Sen's approach to human capability (laid out most recently in his book *Development as freedom*, Knopf/OUP, 1999) provides one solution to the tension between the human capital argument and one that says that such an approach is morally unsound. In it, ill-health (along with education, poverty, etc.) is seen as a dimension of capability deprivation—meaning an obstacle that gets in the way of individual's being able to achieve or attain those things that they have reason to value. The crucial distinction between the human capital and capability approach is that while in the former everything is ultimately measured against the yardstick of economic activity, the capability approach places at the centre the individual and their capacity to achieve their own goals.

5. Paul Farmer (1999) makes an explicit link between the plight of the poor in countries such as Haiti and those living in the inner cities of the USA. He sees a shared exclusion from access to effective treatments (particularly for communicable diseases) that are available to the affluent.

6. It should be noted that this tradition has not gone unchallenged. See for example various papers by Stephen Kunitz (1991), Johan Mackenbach and colleagues (1988), and John Bunker *et al.* (1994).

7. See, for example, Kunst *et al.*, 1998*a*.

8. In the World Bank's *World Development Report 1999/2000*, Sweden is shown to have almost the lowest Gini coefficient for income of any country in the world. See Table 5, pp. 238–239.

9. For a provocative analysis of the current state of the inequalities in health debate informed by this historical background, see Illsley and Baker, 1997.

REFERENCES

Acheson ED. Report of the Independent Inquiry into Inequalities in Health. London: The Stationery Office, 1998

Braveman P, Krieger N, Lynch J. Health inequalities and social inequalities in health. *Bulletin of the World Health Organization*, 2000; **78**:232–4

Bunker JP, Frazier HS, Mosteller F. Improving health: measuring effects of medical care. *Milbank Quarterly*, 1994; **72**:225–58

Coleman MP, Babb P, Damiecki P *et al.* Cancer survival trends in England and Wales 1971–1995: deprivation and NHS region. Series SMPS No. 61. London: The Stationery Office, 1999

Farmer P. *Infections and inequalities: the modern plagues.* Los Angeles: University of California Press, 1999

Gilson L. In defence and pursuit of equity. *Social Science and Medicine*, 1998; **47**:1891–6

Illsley R, Baker D. Inequalities in health: adapting the theory to fit the facts. Bath
    Social Policy Paper No. 26. Bath: University of Bath Centre for the Analysis of
    Social Policy, July 1997
Kiivet RA, Bergman U, Rootslane L, Rago L, Sjoqvist F. Drug use in Estonia in
    1994–1995: a follow-up from 1989 and comparison with two Nordic countries.
    European Journal of Clinical Pharmacology, 1998; **54**:119–24
Koupilová I, Bobák M, Holcik J, Pikhart H, Leon DA. Increasing social variation in
    birth outcomes in the Czech Republic after 1989. *American Journal of Public Health*,
    1998; **88**:1343–7
Kuh D, Ben-Shlomo Y. *A life course approach to chronic disease epidemiology*. Oxford:
    Oxford University Press, 1997
Kunitz SJ. The personal physician and the decline of mortality. In: Schofield R, Reher
    D, Bideau A (eds) *The decline of mortality in Europe*. Oxford: Oxford University
    Press, 1991, pp 248–62
Kunst AE , Groenhof F, Borgan JK *et al.* Socio-economic inequalities in mortality.
    Methodological problems illustrated with three examples from Europe. *Revue
    d'Epidemiologie et de Santé Publique*, 1998a; **46**:467–79
Kunst AE, Groenhof F, Mackenbach JP, Health EW. Occupational class and cause
    specific mortality in middle aged men in 11 European countries: comparison of pop-
    ulation based studies. EU Working Group on Socioeconomic Inequalities in Health.
    British Medical Journal, 1998b; **316**:1636–42
Leon DA, Vågerö D, Olausson PO. Social class differences in infant mortality in
    Sweden : comparison with England and Wales. *British Medical Journal*, 1992;
    305:687–91
Leon DA. Unequal inequalities across Europe. *British. Medical Journal*, 1998; **316**:1642
Mackenbach JP, Looman CW, Kunst AE, Habbema JD, van der Maas PJ. Post-1950
    mortality trends and medical care: gains in life expectancy due to declines in mortal-
    ity from conditions amenable to medical intervention in The Netherlands. *Social
    Science and Medicine*, 1988; **27**:889–94
Marmot MG, Shipley MJ, Rose G. Inequalities in death—specific explanations of a
    general pattern? *Lancet*, 1984; **i**:1003–06
Murray CJ, Gakidou EE, Frenk J. Health inequalities and social group differences:
    what should we measure? *Bulletin of the World Health Organization*, 1999; **77**:537–43
OECD Development Assistance Committee. Shaping the 21st Century: The
    Contribution of Development Co-operation. Paris: OECD, 1996
Porter R. *The greatest benefit to mankind*. London: Fontana Press, 1997, chapter 13
Sen A. *Development as freedom*. Oxford: Oxford University Press, 1999
Stott R. The World Bank. *British Medical Journal*, 1999; **318**:822–3
Whitehead M, Evans T, Diderichsen F, Bhuiya A (eds). *Inequities in health: a global
    perspective*. Oxford: Oxford University Press, forthcoming 2000
Wilkinson RG. *Unhealthy societies: the afflictions of inequality*. London: Routledge,
    1996
World Bank. *Global Development Finance 1999*. Washington DC: World Bank, 1999a
World Bank. *World Development Report 1999/2000. Entering the 21st century: the
    changing development landscape*. Washington DC: World Bank, 1999b
World Health Organization. *The World Health Report 1999. Making a difference*.
    Geneva: WHO, 1999

2 The health consequences of the collapse of the Soviet Union

Martin McKee

A brief history

The events leading up to the collapse of the Soviet Union are well known. The introduction, by Gorbachev, of the philosophy of glasnost had created an environment in which issues that had been simmering beneath the surface could emerge (Gorbachev, 1996). Vast nationalist rallies began in the Baltic States in 1988 and 1989. In 1990, nationalist parties won elections in the Baltic Republics. On 19 August 1991, a coup was mounted against Gorbachev. The following day Estonia and Latvia joined Lithuania in declaring independence. A few days later they were joined by Ukraine, Belarus, and Moldova. In December 1991, the presidents of Russia, Ukraine, and Belarus declared that the Soviet Union had ceased to exist.

The economic circumstances in which the new countries found themselves were far from encouraging. The Soviet Union had suffered greatly from the very high levels of military expenditure during the arms race in the 1980s. Investment in agriculture and in civilian industry was minimal, and inefficiencies in the distribution system meant that much of what was produced was wasted (Davies, 1996). This situation was exacerbated by the collapse of established trading links. The newly emerging countries had been locked into a highly complex system in which raw materials and components from all over the Soviet Union were brought together in a final manufacturing location. The removal of one element by, for example, the closing of borders, brought the entire process to a halt. The economic crisis was also exacerbated by the effects of conflict (Goldenberg, 1994).

The rapid and unplanned process of what can only be described as de-colonization provided very little preparation for self government, and laid down an inheritance of a number of features that, in some countries, mitigated strongly against the development of effective policy responses to major challenges to health.

These events coincided with major changes in mortality. In the Soviet Union, life expectancy at birth had been declining steadily from the mid 1960s. A striking improvement in 1985–7, associated with Secretary General Gorbachev's anti-alcohol campaign (White, 1996), was short-lived, and there was a steady decline until 1991. In the subsequent three years, the decline accelerated markedly, only to reverse in 1995. Between 1991 and 1994, taking all the former Soviet republics together, life expectancy at birth for males fell by 4 years and for females by 2.3 years.

A measure such as life expectancy at birth does not, however, provide a measure of the absolute scale of the crisis. In 1995, the mortality rate among men aged 35–44 was four times that in Western Europe. It has been estimated that Russia experienced between 1.3 and 1.6 million premature deaths between 1990 and 1995 (Bennett *et al.*, 1998), which is approximately ten times that lost by the 55,000 Americans dying during the Vietnam war or three times that of the 240,000 Americans who died from AIDS in the same period.

If one is to understand the determinants of health at a population level, it is essential that one understands what happened in the former Soviet Union. The scale and pace of change were, to many commentators, simply unbelievable. A central issue is whether the lessons from these events are generalizable or whether there was something unique about the Soviet Union. Specifically, why should mortality have changed so rapidly there and not in countries in other parts of the world that have experienced comparable political and economic shocks?

The same but different

Although the republics became independent in 1991, and subsequently followed somewhat different political and economic pathways, for many, the general pattern of mortality was similar (Figs 2.1 and 2.2). While in the interests of brevity, only life expectancy at birth is shown, it is important to note that this is a poor indicator of mortality in this region, as it conceals differing trends in certain age groups. For example, between the 1960s and 1980s, throughout Central and Eastern Europe and the former Soviet Union, improving infant mortality obscures the rising death rate among young and middle-aged men (Chenet *et al.*, 1996).

For clarity, the fifteen republics have been divided into regional groupings. Certain features require comment. Turning first to the Caucasus, the most striking finding is that life expectancy has consistently been higher than in other parts of the former Soviet Union, so that, even in 1980, male life expectancy at birth in Armenia was over eight years longer than in Russia. Unfortunately, available data from Georgia are fragmentary, limited to the period until 1991 and the single year of 1994. This is due largely to the impact of the civil war and the effective cessation of significant parts of Georgian territory. For reasons to be discussed later, it is important to note that, in Armenia, the improvement following the 1985 anti-alcohol campaign was much less steep than elsewhere and it did not experience to anything like the same extent as elsewhere the

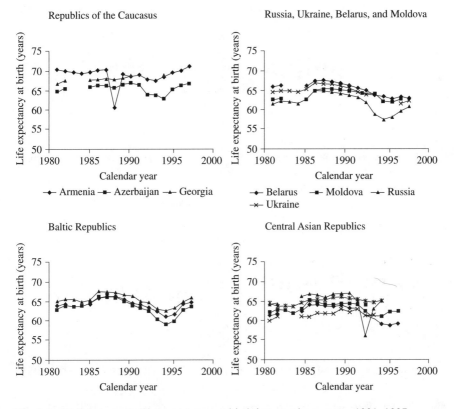

Fig. 2.1 Trends in male life expectancy at birth in years by country 1981–1997

decline after 1990, although this must be interpreted with caution because of the effects of war and migration.

The republics of the European part of the former Soviet Union have experienced the largest changes, both in 1985–6 and in the early 1990s. The patterns are strikingly similar, although the pace and magnitude of change has been greater in Russia than elsewhere. Belarus, a country that has essentially retained the Soviet system of government, did not experience either the acceleration in the decline in life expectancy or the later improvement seen in Russia in the 1990s, instead following a steady downward course.

The Baltic Republics, although quite different in cultural and economic terms, from each other and from Russia, have behaved remarkably similarly. The central Asian republics display a mixed picture. At the risk of oversimplification, those republics with the highest proportions of ethnic Russians in the population show a pattern similar to that seen in Russia, whereas those that are rather less Russified, such as Uzbekistan, exhibited much less change. The decline in Tajikistan in 1993 can be attributed largely to the effects of civil war affecting

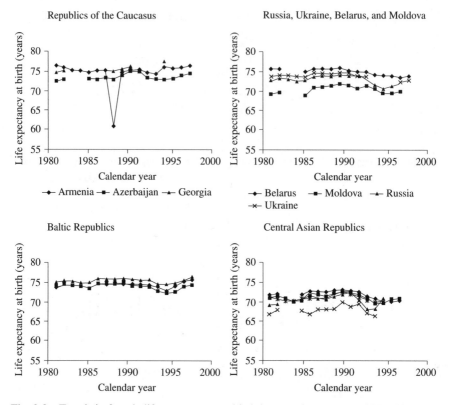

Fig. 2.2   Trends in female life expectancy at birth in years by country 1981–1997

both mortality and data completeness. Turkmenistan deserves special mention, with female life expectancy at birth substantially lower than that in other republics.

An examination of the health consequences is incomplete if limited to broad measures of mortality. Although space does not permit a detailed discussion, it is necessary to note the impact of the collapse of the Soviet Union on levels of communicable diseases. The rate of increase in some diseases has been extremely alarming. For example, the number of new cases testing positive for HIV in Kaliningrad, a Russian territory between Lithuania and Poland (the former German Konigsberg) rose from 1 to 100 per month in a four-month period in 1996, with intravenous drug use as the most important risk factor (Liitsola *et al.*, 1998). Rates of tuberculosis (Zalesky *et al.*, 1997) and, most worrying, multi-drug resistant disease (Hoffner, 1995; Viljanen *et al.*, 1998), have also risen markedly.

Methodological issues

Before going further, it is necessary to consider whether the data on which any analysis of the crisis is based are valid. There is an inevitable suspicion about data from the former Soviet Union because of the long-standing culture of secrecy. Mortality data ceased to be supplied to the World Health Organization in the early 1980s and, even when data were available, certain causes, such as homicide and some infectious diseases, were hidden (Shkolnikov *et al.*, 1995). Despite this secrecy, it is now clear that there was continuing high-level political concern about trends in mortality (Gorbachev, 1996), and Goskomstat undertook regular evaluations of the quality of coding, which suggested that, at least in urban centres, there were no major distortions affecting the main causes of death (Meslé *et al.*, 1995).

The issue of secrecy has, largely, been overcome, and a team of Russian and French demographers have brought together a continuous series of mortality data from 1965 (Meslé *et al.*, 1992). Similar projects are underway in Ukraine and the Baltic Republics. There are, however, problems in some central Asian republics, with suggestions of political involvement to ensure that headline figures such as maternal and infant mortality appear lower than they actually are by, for example, reclassifying deaths in the late post-neonatal period into the category of one-year-olds or excluding deaths following abortion from maternal mortality rates.

In some countries there are also obvious problems with data because of war. For example, the *de facto* boundaries of the republics in the Caucasus have been unclear throughout this period and some regions have experienced massive movement of population. Accurate mortality data ceases to be a governmental priority in such situations.

The validity of the data has received extensive attention in Russia. In response to concerns that the fluctuations in mortality could be due to artefact, either because of simply erroneous data or errors in the numerator or denominator such as an influx of migrants to Russia who would appear in the numbers of deaths but not in the population, which was estimated on the basis of the 1989 census, a detailed study of trends in age- and cause-specific death rates was undertaken. In brief, this confirmed that both the decline in mortality in 1985–7 and the increase after 1989 had affected the same age groups and causes (Leon *et al.*, 1997). Changes were most marked for alcohol-related disorders, injuries and violence, heart disease, and pneumonia. Importantly, there was virtually no change in deaths from neoplasms. There were no sudden discontinuities in the data. These findings were inconsistent with any major flaws in the population denominators or in mortality data when considered by broad categories of cause of death. This view is also consistent with evidence from detailed analysis of reconstructed life tables by Anderson and Silver (1997).

These findings cannot, however, be generalized. In some republics, the data may be of higher quality than in Russia. During the Soviet period, all republics, with the exception of Lithuania, used the Soviet mortality classification. Although this mapped to the International Classification of Disease (ICD), it was somewhat less precise and the match was not perfect. In Lithuania, data were initially coded using ICD-8 and later ICD-9, but were recoded into the less precise Soviet system before dispatch to Moscow and hence to WHO. The ICD is now in use in the Baltic Republics but the Soviet system remains in force elsewhere. Historical data from Lithuania have tended to have a lower frequency of non-specific codes than elsewhere. Consequently, comparisons between Lithuania and other republics in trends of cause of death must be treated with care. This may, for example explain the very much lower death rate from cerebro-vascular disease recorded in Lithuania than in its neighbours.

In contrast, there are major concerns about the quality of data in the central Asian republics and the Caucasus. As noted above, there is some evidence that data continue to be falsified but, in addition, analyses based on reconstructed life tables indicate that reported death rates at different ages cannot be accurate (Anderson and Silver, 1997). The potential reasons are multiple, including errors due to erroneous reporting of age, with heaping at five-year intervals; biases introduced by differential rural and urban access to medical care and thus to a precise diagnosis; and simple non-recording.

Some additional problems have arisen since the transition. The role played by Goskomstat in ensuring some degree of validity of cause-of-death recording outside Russia has been removed. This can explain changes in, for example, recorded deaths from cancer among the elderly in rural areas (Shkolnikov et al., 1999a). During the 1990s, there has been a steep rise in codes relating to undetermined or poorly-specified causes of death, especially where violence is involved. These deaths are due either to homicide or to suicide, but the increasing use of this category means that both causes are likely to be significantly underestimated in many countries.

The immediate causes

Although space does not permit a detailed examination, the health effects of war must be considered. The break up of the Soviet Union left many unresolved territorial disputes. Sporadic violence had broken out even before the collapse of the Soviet Union, but the collapse of central authority in 1991 led to almost immediate conflict in the Caucasus, Tajikistan, and Moldova. However, overall, the most important factor has been the rise and subsequent fall in mortality among the young and middle-aged. Other than in those areas affected by conflict, the pattern has been similar in all republics. Deaths from cardiovascular disease, cerebro-vascular disease, injuries and violence, and suicide increased until about 1994 and then began to fall. Deaths from neoplasms have remained relatively constant, some countries exhibiting a slow downward trend, while in others the reverse.

These changes have been examined in detail in a study of the change in mortality in the European regions of the Russian Federation between 1990 and 1994 (Walberg et al., 1998). Approximately half of the decline in male life expectancy at birth was accounted for by deaths of those aged 35–64. In terms of causes, injuries and violence accounted for about a third of the overall decline and cardiovascular diseases accounted for a further quarter. The next largest category was alcohol-related disorders, accounting for approximately 15% of the decline.

Even in this restricted sample, which excluded the relatively well performing, predominantly Muslim regions in the north Caucasus and some especially poorly performing regions in Siberia, there was marked diversity. To facilitate analysis, regions were divided into quartiles by change in male life expectancy at birth between 1990 and 1994, which varied from a fall of 8.6 years in the worst performing quartile to 5 years in the best. The corresponding figures for females were rather smaller, at 4.1 and 2.6 years respectively.

Consistent with the now familiar pattern, deaths between 35 and 64 made the greatest contribution to the gap between the best and worst performing regions. Of the 3.6 years greater decline in life expectancy among men in the worst compared with the best regions, most (1.7 years) could be explained by injuries and violence, followed by alcohol-related disorders (0.8 years), and then cardiovascular disease (0.5 years). For women, the results were similar with the 1.6-year difference largely accounted for by deaths from injuries and violence (0.7 years), alcohol-related disorders (0.4 years), and cardiovascular disease (0.4 years).

Risk factors

Examination of the changing pattern of deaths from different causes and the age groups most affected immediately focuses attention on one risk factor— alcohol (Ryan, 1995). The case for alcohol playing a major role in the fluctuating mortality in the former Soviet republics is greatly strengthened by the observation that death rates from certain causes fell substantially between 1985 and 1986, coinciding with what is now recognized as, at least initially, a strikingly successful anti-alcohol campaign. Importantly, it is from the same causes, and in the same age groups that benefited most from the anti-alcohol campaign, that the increase in mortality has occurred (Leon et al., 1997).

If alcohol is responsible, some of the changes in mortality are extremely plausible. Disorders associated directly with alcohol were responsible for about one-sixth of the decline in life expectancy in European Russia. A role for alcohol in deaths from injuries and violence is also likely. However, a difficulty emerges with cardiovascular disease.

Conventional wisdom, based on many large studies in the West, is that alcohol, at least when consumed regularly and in moderate amounts, is cardio-protective (Renaud et al., 1993). Thus it is difficult to see how a reduction in alcohol consumption could lead at first sight to a fall in cardiovascular deaths, or a rise in consumption to an increase in deaths.

However, a few studies have failed to find a cardio-protective effect of increasing levels of consumption, including a study of Russians (Deev et al., 1998) and of people who had low intakes of micro-nutrients (Rimm et al., 1998). Given the low level of micro-nutrients, such as folic acid, in the diet in this region, this suggests that, even without invoking an adverse effect of alcohol on the heart, the beneficial effects of moderate drinking seen in the West may not be being achieved.

The apparent adverse effect of alcohol consumption on cardiovascular disease mortality in Russia may, however, be explained by reference to patterns of drinking rather than the amount *per se*. In Russia, there is a drinking culture that is quite different to countries such as France, and which is characterized by irregular, binge drinking of vodka, with 31% of men and 3% of women drinking at least 25 cl of vodka at one go at least once a month (Bobák *et al.*, 1999). Studies from elsewhere, in which people are classified in terms of adverse effects of drinking, such as frequent hangovers or alcohol-related difficulties with the police or at work, have consistently found an associated increased risk of cardiovascular death, frequently occurring suddenly (Britton *et al.*, 1998). One key study that specifically looked at the amount drunk at one time found a six-fold increase in the risk of cardiac death in those drinking six or more bottles of beer at a time (Kauhanen *et al.*, 1997).

The epidemiological findings are supported by evidence that the physiological effects of regular, moderate drinking and binge drinking are quite different (McKee and Britton, 1998). Binge drinking in animal models does not produce the beneficial effects in lipids seen with moderate regular drinking, and it also leads to adverse changes in lipid levels that are not seen with moderate drinking. Binge drinking is associated with an increased risk of thrombosis during the period of withdrawal. It also predisposes both to structural changes in heart muscle and to an increased risk of fatal rhythm disturbances.

Other causes of death that have fluctuated markedly over this period can also be linked to alcohol, such as stroke (van Gijn *et al.*, 1993; Hart *et al.*, 1999) and pneumonia (Schmidt and Popham, 1981).

In summary, there is compelling evidence that alcohol, while not the only factor, has been an extremely important major proximate cause of the changes in mortality in the 1980s and early 1990s.

Social and economic determinants

Even if alcohol is as important as it appears to be, it is equally important to understand why people drink in the way that they do. At the outset, it should be emphasized that, in both Czarist Russia and the Soviet Union, production of alcohol was an explicit tool of state policy designed to provide one of the few consumer goods that the regime could provide, with the aim of replenishing state coffers and ensuring the recirculation of money (White, 1996). Thus, with the exception of brief periods in the 1920s, and the early 1990s, the Soviet state can be considered to have actively encouraged alcoholism.

However, not all groups in the population have been affected to the same extent. The increase in mortality between 1988–9 and 1993–4 was substantially greater among those with lower levels of education (Shkolnikov, 1999). In

Moscow, between 1993 and 1995, a study using proportional mortality analysis also found large socio-demographic differences in the probability of dying from alcohol-related causes, with those who were of low education, unemployed, and widowed or divorced having the greatest risk (Chenet *et al.*, 1998*a*). A similar pattern was observed for deaths from non-traffic injuries (falls, fires, drowning, and choking) and for violence. However, injuries from traffic accidents displayed a much less steep gradient, possibly due to the social stratification of car ownership.

Further clues come from the analysis of regional diversity in mortality in Russia (Walberg *et al.*, 1998) mentioned earlier. The decline in life expectancy between 1990 and 1994 showed a clear geographical pattern, with the greatest increases in the large cities of Moscow and St Petersburg and the primary production regions of the north and Siberia, and the smallest in the south of Russia and in the regions along the Volga, many of which have substantial non-Russian populations, such as the Mordvins (who are distant relatives of the Finns), the Chuvash (who have historical ties with the Bulgarians), and Tartars.

In a multivariate analysis, labour force turnover in large and medium enterprises explained 42% of the regional variation in the decline in life expectancy, with the 1990 crime rate explaining a further 9% and mean household income in 1990 explaining a further 5%. These variables were all highly correlated with the percentage of people living in urban settlements. Thus, the greatest declines had taken place in urban areas, characterized by a rapid pace of economic transition, high crime rates, and relatively higher income. This interpretation is consistent with the argument that the Russian population has been subject to massive psycho-social stress in which many people were left disorientated and confused (Cornia and Pannicià, 1995; Shapiro, 1995).

Crime rates are increasingly seen as a measure of social capital, which is emerging, in several studies, as an important determinant of health at a population level. A subsequent study, using a smaller number of Russian regions but with additional survey data, has examined the relationship between social capital and mortality (Kennedy *et al.*, 1998). Importantly, they were able to examine levels of trust in local and regional government, civic engagement (measured by interest in politics and participation in voting), social cohesion (measured as strain in work relations), and perceived economic hardship. In a multivariate model, distrust in local, but not regional government, economic hardship, low social cohesion, lack of civic engagement, and high crime rates were all significantly associated with a low male life expectancy at birth. The associations were similar, although weaker, for female life expectancy. When examined by broad causes of death the associations were strongest for cardiovascular diseases, closely followed by external causes, with death rates from neoplasms associated only with crime rates and economic hardship. The authors conclude that those regions where there is relatively strong social capital, with more effective support networks for dealing with everyday problems, have done rather better than those where such networks are weak.

Although the evidence reviewed here is almost exclusively from Russia, the consistency in the decline in life expectancy in the early 1990s suggests that the mechanisms underlying the decline may be similar in each republic. These findings are consistent with a model in which rapid pace of change, in societies characterized by low levels of social capital and traditionally very high levels of alcohol consumption, has led to high levels of psycho-social stress and a substantial further increase in alcohol consumption, especially among those with the weakest social and emotional support, such as those with low educational attainment or occupational status or who have no family links. This, in turn, has led to a large rise in mortality, in particular from injuries, violence, cardiovascular disease, and alcohol-related disorders, which was most marked in those aged 20 to 60.

While correlations of data from entities as diverse as the former Soviet Republics must be interpreted with great care, it is of interest to note that those republics that experienced the greatest declines in life expectancy in the 1990s were those where life expectancy was already lowest in 1985 and which experienced the greatest improvements during the anti-alcohol campaign (Fig. 2.3). A plausible explanation is that both life expectancy in 1985 and the improvement during the anti-alcohol campaign are indirect measures of the underlying contribution that alcohol made to overall mortality in the republic concerned. In a multiple regression, these two variables explained 40% of the variation in the decline in life expectancy in the 1990s. Interpretation is constrained by concerns about data quality in the central Asian republics but it is also noteworthy that, in the Russian Federation, where such concerns are less, the levels of both of these measures in the predominantly Muslim republics in the north Caucasus and on the Volga are also consistent with this hypothesis.

Alternative theories

Other explanations have been suggested. Feshbach (1999) and colleagues have argued that the health crisis can be attributed to massive environmental degradation, coining the term 'ecocide'. It is likely that damage on this scale has had some impact on health but it cannot explain the observed changes in cause of deaths, in particular in injuries and violence. Furthermore, in the early 1990s, death rates rose at a time when industrial pollution was falling dramatically with the collapse of heavy industry.

Collapse of the Soviet system of health care, which provided universal coverage, has also been proposed (Poliakov and Seleznev, 1995; Shchepin, 1995). The most obvious evidence against this explanation is that the changes have affected most those groups who use the system least, young and middle-aged males, whereas those that are most dependent on it, the young and the very old, have been least affected.

Weaknesses in the medical care system have undoubtedly existed for many years in the Soviet Union, at least as judged by comparisons of levels of mortality amenable to medical care (Gaizauskiene and Gurevicius, 1995) but they

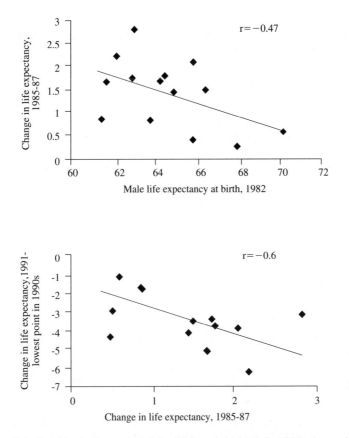

Fig. 2.3 Relationships between male life expectancy at birth in 1985, change between 1985 and 1987, and change from 1990 to lowest point in 1990s, former Soviet Republics (excluding Tajikistan)

appear not to have played a major part in the immediate aftermath of transition. However, they should not be dismissed entirely when considering the latter part of the 1990s. There has been a marked increase in deaths from diabetes among young people, with anecdotal evidence of difficulty obtaining insulin in many areas. Deaths from cerebro-vascular disease with mention of hypertension have also increased in Ukraine, which has been particularly adversely affected by economic change.

Nutrition and tobacco have also been suggested (Shchepin, 1995; Kharchenko, 1996; Lopez, 1997). These are obviously important in explaining the high underlying mortality rates in many parts of the former Soviet Union but, again, cannot explain the fluctuations. Indeed, death rates from lung cancer in Russia have actually experienced a slight decrease when overall mortality has been rising rapidly. This is due to a cohort effect, reflecting access to tobacco during and after the Second World War (Shkolnikov *et al.*, 1999*b*). Further-more, in Russia at least, nutritional intakes do not appear to have changed markedly (Popkin *et al.*, 1996).

Explaining the upturn

So far, this paper has concentrated on the increase in mortality between the late 1980s and 1994. However, it is also necessary to explain the upturn in the mid-1990s, which occurred in countries experiencing quite different economic situations (Fig. 2.4).

One of the few analyses of the changes after 1994 has been undertaken by Shkolnikov (1999), using data from Russia. This shows that the improvement in mortality is due almost entirely to a reduction towards their 1991 levels of

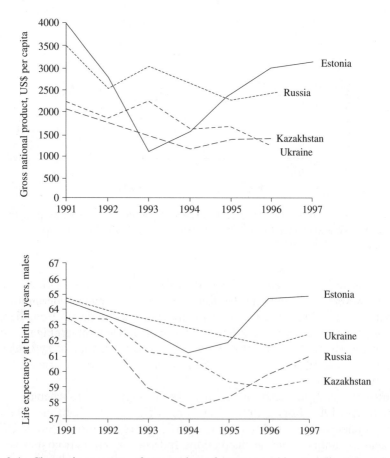

Fig. 2.4   Change in measures of economic performance and in mortality, selected former Soviet Republics

deaths at ages between 25 and 60. However, by 1997, death rates at these ages still remained about 30% higher than in 1991. There has also been a steady decline in mortality among children, although this is the continuation of a trend that was already established in the early 1990s, at a time when adult mortality was rising. In contrast, the increase that occurred in death rates at between 15 and 24 has not declined significantly. This is attributable largely to the rising death rate from tuberculosis, which counteracts the effect of a decline in other causes in this age group.

The improvement is difficult to explain. The age groups and causes involved are essentially the same as those in which death rates improved during the anti-alcohol campaign in the 1980s and then declined in the early 1990s, when alcohol was shown to have played a major role. This suggests strongly that changes in alcohol consumption are again, involved. There is some other evidence to support this. A detailed analysis of monthly trends in deaths in Moscow between 1993 and 1995 showed that, after seasonal effects were removed, the mortality turn around was seen most clearly in chronic diseases associated with alcohol consumption (McKee *et al.*, 1998a). Data from the Russian Longitudinal Monitoring Survey (RLMS) show that alcohol consumption began to fall shortly before the improvement in mortality (Zohoori *et al.*, 1998). This co-incided with trends in the price of alcohol relative to basic foodstuffs, which was falling between 1992 and 1994 and then rose through 1995 and 1996. In contrast, however, the RLMS data show that most measures of socio-economic status continued to decline. The percentage of households below the poverty line increased from 11% to 36%. Real household income fell by 23%. Income inequality rose markedly, with the ratio of income in the top 20% of households to those in the bottom 20% growing by 68%. Finally, unpaid employment increased considerably in all age groups.

The observation that mortality improved while socio-economic conditions continued to worsen is counter-intuitive. One possibility is that the most margin-alized groups, at greatest risk from alcohol, had died in the early 1990s so that their relative contribution to overall mortality became less. This requires further exploration but, in view of the scale of the changes, seems unlikely to provide a complete explanation. An alternative possibility is that these changes indicate a process of adaptation, in which individuals adopt a range of strategies to ameliorate the impact of the steadily worsening economic situation. If the development of such changes represents, in some way, an innate human capacity, it could explain why countries that have been independent since the break up of the Soviet Union, and which have pursued quite different political and economic trajectories, have experienced very similar trends in health to those seen in Russia.

A synthesis

Churchill (1939) once described Russia as 'a riddle wrapped in a mystery inside an enigma'. Although in a different context, this description could equally apply to the changing pattern of in mortality in the former Soviet Union in recent years. Research on the determinants of mortality in the West provides few clues to a single explanation for the large and rapid fluctuations in mortality. However, the observation that the changes have, to some extent, affected fifteen diverse, independent countries suggests that some common explanations must exist (Brainerd, 1998).

One problem is that, while the overall trends in life expectancy are similar, once one moves beyond the broad brush picture the situation becomes extremely complex. There are a range of specific factors at work in some countries and regions, such as the consequences of war or the social position of women in some parts of central Asia (Kadyrov, 1993; Tohidi, 1994) which, in the space available, it has been impossible to explore fully. For example, in Turkmenistan, female life expectancy at birth in rural areas is 10 years less than in the capital. Furthermore, while many causes of death are moving in parallel, others are not and, specifically, several important communicable diseases are continuing to increase at a time when mortality overall is improving.

There are, however, three issues that are important in seeking to interpret what has happened. The first is that, before the fluctuations in mortality in the 1980s, the underlying mortality rate was much higher than in the West, especially for men. In 1984, male life expectancy at birth in the Soviet Union was 9.4 years less than in the European Union. The death rate from ischaemic heart disease was 2.6 times higher and that from external causes was three times higher, despite very much less dense road traffic.

Second, in contrast to the situation in Western countries, a much higher proportion of deaths in the former Soviet Union were due to conditions such as injuries and violence where there were very short lag times between the antecedent factors and death. Furthermore, while cardiovascular death is normally seen in the West as the final event in a process that may have its origins in childhood (Kuh and Ben-Shlomo, 1997), it is now clear that binge drinking, with its much more immediate effect, is a much more important risk factor for cardiovascular death in the East than is the case in the West. This is graphically illustrated by the observation that such deaths, and especially those that are sudden, increase significantly at weekends in Moscow (Chenet et al., 1998b).

Finally, this situation arose in a population that had been exposed to several decades of policies which had the effect of creating distrust and insecurity and thus reducing those individual and societal strategies that might have ameliorated the effects of rapid social change (Wilkinson, 1996). A comparison of Swedish and Lithuanian men found that the latter had significantly higher job strain but lower social and emotional support and self-esteem, and poorer coping strategies (Kristensen et al., 1998). Similarly, data from the Kaunas–Rotterdam study suggest that the lower sense of control among Lithuanians explained a substantial proportion of the difference in subsequent cardiovascular mortality (Bosma, 1994).

It is for these reasons that the large and extremely rapid changes in mortality observed at the time of the 1985 anti-alcohol campaign become plausible. That unique experiment demonstrated just how important alcohol was as a determinant of premature mortality in the Soviet Union. The collapse of the anti-alcohol campaign in the late 1980s, while reflecting some specific political events (McKee, 1999), was also a manifestation of a more general loss of the means of social control, as shown by rising rates of crime and of inter-ethnic violence. This allowed dangerous patterns of alcohol consumption, and corresponding levels of mortality, to rise above their previous levels. The subsequent collapse of the Soviet Union led to a marked increase in insecurity and stress, among a population with limited coping mechanisms. Those affected most were those exposed to the fastest pace of change and who had the least well developed strategies for coping, whether because of a lack of education, employment, family support or, more generally, social capital. By the mid 1990s, however, the health situation began to change. The consistency with the earlier fluctuations, in terms of causes of death and age groups affected, as well as the evidence that it was preceded by a fall in alcohol consumption, argues strongly that alcohol again played a major role. However, as the change occurred at the same time in countries pursuing as diverse policies as Estonia and Russia, it seems unlikely that this was due, entirely, to any specific measure of government policy. Instead, most people were experiencing a continuing decline in their economic circumstances, new methods of coping with the changing situation were slowly emerging, so that it is now considered by many that official data on income are less valid measures of an individual's circumstances than was the case previously.

Understanding this process of adaptation remains one of the major research questions in the former Soviet Union. How this came about, what it meant in practice, and what it means for the future is still far from clear.

Although this chapter has focused entirely on the former Soviet Union, at this point it is necessary to say something about the other former communist countries of Central and Eastern Europe. They have undergone major social and economic shocks—though mostly not as great as those seen in the former Soviet Union—with immediate economic recessions, rapid increases in inflation and unemployment and, as judged by the effect on birth rates, a similar increase in insecurity and stress. There were some increases in mortality, but these were transient, largely due to short-lived increases in external causes. Indeed, in Poland, the Czech Republic, and, after a short interval, Hungary, the transition was accompanied by marked improvements in mortality. During the 1980s, these countries exhibited mortality rates that, while much higher than in Western Europe, were substantially lower than in the Soviet Union. In particular, those causes of death that, in the Soviet Union, have been linked with alcohol consumption were much lower in central Europe and, while there were some attempts to reduce consumption in the 1980s (Varvasovszky *et al.*, 1997; Varvasovszky and McKee, 1998), these had nothing like the effect of the 1985 campaign in the Soviet Union. Thus, by the late 1980s they were not starting from what, in the Soviet Union, was an artificially low level of mortality in historical terms.

The central role of alcohol in this interpretation does not preclude other risk factors as determinants of mortality in Russia. As noted earlier, there are many unresolved questions about the impact of health care, including both failures to provide effective care and the consequences of iatrogenesis and, in particular, the very high rates of hospital acquired infection (Valinteliene *et al.*, 1996). Furthermore, as noted above, there is some evidence that reduced access to care for some groups is beginning to have an impact on mortality. There must also be concern about the increase in smoking rates in young women (McKee *et al.*, 1998*b*).

Conclusion

The consequences of the collapse of the Soviet Union for the health of the peoples who inhabit its constituent countries can be characterized by elements of similarity and diversity. In the space available, it has only been possible to explore the diversity in the most superficial way. Like Sherlock Holmes' dog that did not bark, there is much to be learnt, not only from those countries that have suffered most, but also from those where the effects of transition appear to have been much less.

The areas of similarity are also instructive, given the differences in economic and social policies pursued in the 1990s. There is compelling evidence that alcohol has played a major role in the fluctuations since the 1980s. That it was able to do so is a reflection of the pattern of dangerous drinking that existed previously. The health impact of the political transition was worsened because, when it occurred, levels of mortality in Russia were unusually low but were already on an upward trend towards their previous level. In a situation where alcohol was cheap and easily available, and where there was a culture of heavy drinking, the imposition of a huge social and economic shock had consequences that, arguably, could have been considered as inevitable. The effects were exacerbated by the low level of coping mechanisms among most of the population. However, not all were affected to the same extent, and those with strong social support seem to have been relatively protected. As time has passed, there has been a progressive adaptation to the new reality and, while economic conditions have continued to deteriorate, alcohol consumption has fallen, with a corresponding improvement in health.

So was the Soviet Union different or are there generalizable findings? Perhaps chaos theory may offer a lead? A key feature of chaos theory is that much depends on the system's starting conditions. A small difference in starting conditions can have huge repercussions. The Soviet Union, in 1991, had many features that were at the least, very unusual. Perhaps not unique, as there may be parallels in some marginalized societies with high levels of alcohol consumption, such as some groups of native Americans, Inuit, and Pacific islanders. In circumstances such as those in the Soviet Union, it becomes more plausible that the consequences of a political and economic shock would be different from those following, for example, the American depression of the 1930s, the Latin American debt crisis of the 1970s, or current events in Southeast Asia.

It is impossible to predict what the future will hold but, on the basis of what is now known about the determinants of health in the former Soviet Union, there is an enormous public health agenda to be tackled.

Acknowledgements

This work is supported by the UK Department for International Development, although DFID can accept no responsibility for the views expressed. I am grateful for valuable comments from Laurent Chenet, Vladimir Shkolnikov, and David Leon.

REFERENCES

Anderson BA, Silver BD. Issues of data quality in assessing mortality trends and levels in the New Independent States. In: Bobadilla JL, Costello CA, Mitchell F (eds) *Premature death in the New Independent States*. Washington DC: National Academy Press, 1997, pp 120–55

Bennett NG, Bloom DE, Ivanov SF. Demographic implications of the Russian mortality crisis. *World Development*, 1998; **26**:1921–37

Bobák M, McKee M, Rose R, Marmot M. Alcohol consumption in a national sample of the Russian population. *Addiction*, 1999; **94**:857–66

Bosma JHA. *A cross-cultural comparison of the role of some psychosocial factors in the etiology of coronary heart disease*. Follow-up to the Kaunas-Rotterdam Intervention Study (KRIS). Maastricht: Universitaire Pres Maastricht, 1994

Brainerd E. Market reform and mortality in transition economies. *World Development*, 1998; **26**:2013–27

Britton A, McKee M, Leon DA. *Cardiovascular disease and heavy drinking: a systematic review*. Public Health and Policy Departmental Publications No. 28. London: London School of Hygiene & Tropical Medicine, 1998

Chenet L, McKee M, Fulop N et al. Changing life expectancy in central Europe: is there a single reason? *Journal of Public Health Medicine*, 1996; **18**:329–36

Chenet L, Leon D, McKee M, Vassin S. Deaths from alcohol and violence in Moscow: socio-economic determinants. *European Journal of Population*, 1998a; **14**:19–37

Chenet L, McKee M, Leon D, Shkolnikov V, Vassin S. Alcohol and cardiovascular mortality in Moscow, new evidence of a causal association. *Journal of Epidemiology and Community Health*, 1998b; **52**:772–4

Churchill WL. Radio broadcast, 1 Oct 1939

Cornia GA, Paniccià R. *The demographic impact of sudden impoverishment: Eastern Europe during the 1989–94 transition*. UNICEF Innocenti Occasional Papers, Economic Policy Studies, No. 49. Paris: UNICEF, 1995

Davies N. *Europe: a history*. Oxford: Oxford University Press, 1996

Deev A, Shestov D, Abernathy J, Kapustina A, Mahina N, Irving S. Association of alcohol consumption to mortality in middle-aged US and Russian men and women. *Annals of Epidemiology*, 1998; **8**:147–53

Feshbach M. Dying souls of Russia. *Moscow Times*, 21 January 1999

Gaizauskiene A, Gurevicius R. Avoidable mortality in Lithuania. *Journal of Epidemiology and Community Health*, 1995; **49**:281–4

Goldenberg S. *Pride of small nations: the Caucasus and post-Soviet disorder*. London: Zed, 1994

Gorbachev MS. *Memoirs*. London: Doubleday, 1996

Hart CL, Smith GD, Hole DJ, Hawthorne VM. Alcohol consumption and mortality from all causes, coronary heart disease, and stroke: results from a prospective cohort study of Scottish men with 21 years of follow up. *British Medical Journal*, 1999; **318**:1725–9

Hoffner SE. Drug resistant mycobacterium tuberculosis: some data from Sweden, Estonia and Ethiopia. *Scandinavian Journal of Infectious Diseases (Supplements)*, 1995; **98**:17–8

Kadyrov S. Some questions on the study of the Turkmen family. *Central Asian Survey*, 1993; **12**:393–400

Kauhanen J, Kaplan GA, Goldberg DE, Salonen JT. Beer binging and mortality: results from the Kuopio ischaemic heart disease risk factor study, a prospective population based study. *British Medical Journal*, 1997; **315**:846–51

Kennedy BP, Kawachi I, Brainerd E. The role of social capital in the Russian mortality crisis. *World Development*, 1998; **26**:2029–43

Kharchenko VI, Kuperberg EB, Osipov NI. The main approaches to reducing cardio-vascular morbidity and mortality in Russia. *Problemi Sotsialnoi Gigieny I Istoriia Meditsiny*, 1996; **3**:3–7

Kristenson M, Kucinskiene Z, Bergdahl B, Calkauskas H, Urmonas V, Orth-Gomer K. Increased psychosocial strain in Lithuanian versus Swedish men: the LiVicordia study. *Psychosomatic Medicine*, 1998; **60**:277–82

Kuh D, Ben-Shlomo Y. *A life course approach to chronic disease epidemiology*. Oxford: Oxford University Press, 1997

Leon DA, Chenet L, Shkolnikov V *et al.* Huge variation in Russian mortality rates 1984–1994: artefact, alcohol, or what? *Lancet*, 1997; **350**:383–8

Liitsola K, Tashnikova I, Laukkanen T *et al.* HIV1 genetic subtype A/B recombinant strain causing an explosive epidemic in injecting drug users in Kaliningrad. *AIDS*, 1998; **12**:1907–19

Lopez AD. Mortality from tobacco in the New Independent States. In: Bobadilla JL, Costello CA, Mitchell F (eds) *Premature death in the New Independent States*. Washington DC: National Academy Press, 1997, pp 262–74

McKee M. Alcohol in Russia. *Alcohol and Alcoholism*, 1999; **34**:824–9

McKee M, Britton A. The positive relationship between alcohol and heart disease in eastern Europe: potential physiological mechanisms. *Journal of the Royal Society of Medicine*, 1998; **91**:402–7

McKee M, Sanderson C, Chenet L, Vassin S, Shkolnikov V. Seasonal variation in mortality in Moscow. *Journal of Public Health Medicine*, 1998a; **20**:268–74

McKee M, Bobák M, Rose R, Shkolnikov V, Chenet L, Leon D. Patterns of smoking in Russia. *Tobacco Control*, 1998b; **7**:22–6

Meslé F, Shkolnikov V, Vallin J. Mortality by cause in the USSR in 1970–87: the reconstruction of time series. *European Journal of Population*, 1992; **8**:281–308

Meslé F, Shkolnikov V, Vallin J. A sudden increase in violent deaths in Russia. *Population*, 1995; **49**:780–90

Poliakov IV, Seleznev VD. Public health under conditions of transition to market economics. *Problemy Sotsialnoi Gigieny I Istoriia Meditsiny*, 1995; **6**:41–4

Popkin BM, Zohoori N, Baturin A. The nutritional status of the elderly in Russia, 1992 through 1994. *American Journal of Public Health*, 1996; **86**:355–60

Renaud S, Crigui MH, Farchi F, Veenstra J. Alcohol drinking and coronary heart disease. In: Vershuren PM (ed) *Health issues related to alcohol consumption*. Washington DC: ILSI Press, 1993

Rimm EB, Willett WC, Hu FB *et al.* Folate and vitamin B6 from diet and supplements in relation to risk of coronary heart disease among women. *Journal of the American Medical Association*, 1998; **279**:359–64

Ryan M. Alcoholism and rising mortality in the Russian Federation. *British Medical Journal*, 1995; **310**:646–8

Schmidt W, Popham RE. The role of drinking and smoking in mortality from cancer and other causes in male alcoholics. *Cancer*, 1981; **47**:1031–41

Shapiro J. The Russian mortality crisis and its causes. In: Aslund A (ed) *Russian Economic Reform at Risk*. Pinter: London, 1995

Shchepin OP. Current problems and the development of public health in Russia. *Problemy Sotsialnoi Gigieny I Istoriia Meditsiny*, 1995; **1**:3–8

Shkolnikov V. Smertnost i prodoljitelnost jizni. [Mortality and life expectancy]. In: Vishnevski A (ed) *Naseleniye Rossii 1998. Ejegodniy demografitcheski doklad* [Population of Russia. Annual Demographic Report]. Moscow: Centre for Demography and Human Ecology, 1999

Shkolnikov VM, Meslé F, Vallin J. Health crisis in Russia I. Recent trends in life expectancy and causes of death from 1970 to 1993. *Population*, 1995; **50**:907–43

Shkolnikov VM, Leon D, Adamets S, Andreev E, Deev A. Educational level and adult mortality in Russia: an analysis of routine data 1979 to 1994. *Social Science and Medicine*, 1998; **47**:357–69

Shkolnikov VM, McKee M, Vallin J *et al.*. Cancer mortality in Russia and Ukraine: validity, competing risks, and cohort effects. *International Journal of Epidemiology*, 1999a; **28**:19–29

Shkolnikov V, McKee M, Leon D, Chenet L. Why is the death rate from lung cancer falling in the Russian Federation? *European Journal of Epidemiology*, 1999b; **15**:203–6

Tohidi N. Gender, identity and restructuring in the Muslim countries of the former Soviet Union. Los Angeles: International Sociological Association, 1994

Valinteliene R, Jurkuvenas V, Jepsen OB. Prevalence of hospital acquired infection in a Lithuanian hospital. *Journal of Hospital Infection*, 1996; **34**:321–9

van Gijn J, Stampfer MJ, Wolfe C, Algra A. The association between alcohol and stroke. In: Vershuren PM (ed) *Health issues related to alcohol consumption*. Brussels: International Life Sciences Institute Europe, 1993, pp 43–79

Varvasovszky Z, Bain C, McKee M. Deaths from cirrhosis in Poland and Hungary: the impact of different alcohol policies during the 1980s. *Journal of Epidemiology and Community Health*, 1997; **51**:167–71

Varvasovszky Z, McKee M. An analysis of alcohol policy in Hungary. Who is in charge? *Addiction*, 1998; **93**:1815–27

Viljanen MK, Vyshnevskiy BI, Otten TF *et al.* Survey of drug resistant tuberculosis in northwestern Russia from 1984 through 1994. *European Journal of Clinical Microbiology and Infectious Diseases*, 1998; **17**:177–83

Walberg P, McKee M, Shkolnikov V, Chenet L, Leon DA. Economic change, crime, and mortality crisis in Russia: a regional analysis. *British Medical Journal*, 1998; **317**:312–8

White S. *Russia goes dry. Alcohol, state and society*. Cambridge: Cambridge University Press, 1996

Wilkinson RG. Health and civic society in eastern Europe before 1989. In: Hertzman C, Kelly S, Bobák M (eds) *East–West life expectancy gap in Europe: environmental and non-environmental determinants*. Dordrecht: Kluwer, 1996, pp 195–209

Zalesky R, Leimans J, Pavlovska I. The epidemiology of tuberculosis in Latvia. *Monaldi Archives for Chest Disease*, 1997; **52**:142–6

Zohoori N, Mroz TA, Popkin B *et al.*. Monitoring the economic transition in the Russian Federation and its implications for the demographic crisis—the Russian Longitudinal Monitoring Survey. *World Development*, 1998; **26**:1977–93

3 Industrialization and health in historical perspective

Richard H. Steckel

Generations of social observers, health policy workers, economists, historians, demographers, and other social scientists have pondered on the relationship between industrialization and health in the past. Because industrialization eventually led to generally higher incomes, one might suppose the answer to be straightforward: rising living standards associated with industrialization increased the chances that families consumed basic needs and acquired medical care that improved health. While this was true in the long run, much discussion has focused on how various groups fared during the decades that industrialization actually unfolded. Scholars of the subject have asked who gained and who lost in the process (and why), and whether industrialization was accompanied by events that adversely affected health and human welfare. Debate persists because evidence about the past is often meagre and, in any event, health and human welfare are complex and difficult to assess under the best circumstances of data availability.

This chapter draws attention to recent progress in the field made by several scholars in comparative studies of eight countries: the UK, the US, the Netherlands, France, Sweden, Germany, Australia, and Japan (Steckel and Floud, 1997). This work focuses mainly on the nineteenth century, but the process in some countries, such as Japan, continued into the next century. While using traditional measures such as per capita Gross National Product and, where available, life expectancy (or mortality rates), the authors also make extensive use of a newly forged data source: anthropometric measures, particularly human stature gathered from military records. The height data furnish important insights into nutritional status and health during childhood and adolescence.

On the supposition that some readers may be unfamiliar with the methodology of anthropometric history, the next section examines patterns of human growth and their relationship to more traditional measures of human well-being, including per capita GDP and life expectancy at birth. Following a brief discussion of the characteristics of industrialization, the chapter examines the connection between health and industrial change in the past.

Methodology

There is a long tradition among human biologists and nutritionists of using stature to assess health aspects of human welfare (Tanner, 1981). The realization that environmental conditions influenced growth stimulated interest in human growth studies in the 1820s. Auxological epidemiology (auxology is the study of human growth) arose in France, where Villermé studied the stature of soldiers; in Belgium, where Quetelet measured children and formulated mathematical representations of the human growth curve; and in England, where Edwin Chadwick inquired into the health of factory children. Charles Roberts judged the fitness of children for factory employment by using frequency distributions of stature and other measurements, such as weight-for-height and chest circumference. Franz Boas identified salient relationships between the tempo of growth and height distributions, and in 1891 co-ordinated a national growth study, which he used to develop national standards for height and weight. The twentieth century has witnessed a world-wide explosion of growth studies (Eveleth and Tanner, 1976; 1990).

These studies have shown that two periods of intense activity characterize the growth process following birth (Tanner, 1978). Figure 3.1 shows that the increase in height, or velocity, is greatest during infancy, falls sharply, and then declines irregularly into the pre-adolescent years. During adolescence, velocity rises sharply to a peak that equals approximately one-half of the velocity during infancy, then declines rapidly and reaches zero at maturity. The adolescent growth spurt begins about two years earlier in girls than in boys and during their

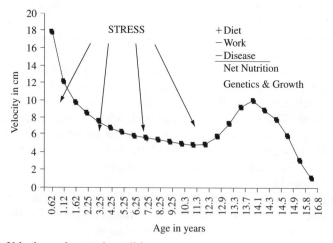

Fig. 3.1 Velocity under good conditions
Source: Tabulated from data for males in US National Center for Health Statistics (1977)

spurt girls temporarily overtake boys in average height. As adults, males are taller than females, primarily because they have approximately two additional years of growth prior to adolescence.

The height of an individual reflects the interaction of genetic and environmental influences during the period of growth (Waterlow and Schürch, 1994). According to Eveleth and Tanner (1976):

> Such interaction may be complex. Two genotypes which produce the same adult height under optimal environmental circumstances may produce different heights under circumstances of privation. Thus two children who would be the same height in a well-off community may not only be smaller under poor economic conditions, but one may be significantly smaller than the other . . . If a particular environmental stimulus is lacking at a time when it is essential for the child (times known as 'sensitive periods') then the child's development may be shunted as it were, from one line to another.

Although genes are important determinants of individual height, studies of genetically similar and dissimilar populations under various environmental conditions suggest that differences in average height across most populations are largely attributable to environmental factors. In a review of studies covering populations in Europe, New Guinea, and Mexico, Malcolm (1974) concludes that differences in average height between populations are almost entirely the product of the environment. Using data from well-nourished populations in several developed and developing countries, Martorell and Habicht (1986) report that children from Europe or European descent, Africa or African descent, and from India or the Middle East have similar growth profiles. Far-Eastern children or adults are an exception that may have a genetic basis. About two decades ago, well-off Japanese, for example, reached the fifteenth height percentile of the well-off in Britain (Tanner et al., 1982). But recent height gains in Japan suggest that the portion of the height differential that can be attributed to genetic influences is shrinking. Important for interpreting stature in the US is the fact that Europeans and people of European descent, and Africans and people of African descent who grew under good nutritional circumstances, have nearly identical stature (Eveleth and Tanner, 1976).[1]

Height at a particular age reflects an individual's history of *net* nutrition, or diet minus claims on the diet made by work (or physical activity) and disease. Metabolic requirements for basic functions such as breathing and blood circulation while at rest also make claims on the diet. The synergy between malnutrition and illness may further reduce the nutrition left over for growth (Scrimshaw et al., 1968). Poorly nourished children are more susceptible to infection, which reduces the body's absorption of nutrients. The interaction implies that analyses of stature must recognize not only inputs to health, such as diet and medical care, but also work effort and related phenomena, such as methods of labour organization. Similarly, researchers must attempt to understand ways that exposure to infectious disease may have placed claims on the diet.[2]

The sensitivity of growth to deprivation depends upon the age at which it occurs. For a given degree of deprivation, the adverse effects may be proportional to the velocity of growth under optimal conditions (Tanner, 1966). Thus, young children and adolescents are particularly susceptible to environmental insults. The return of adequate nutrition following a relatively short period of deprivation may restore normal height through catch-up growth.[3] If conditions are inadequate for catch-up, individuals may still approach normal adult height by an extension of the growing period by as long as several years. Prolonged and severe deprivation results in stunting, or a reduction in adult size.

Figure 3.2 is a useful organizing device for exploring the relationship of height to living standards. Stature is a function of proximate determinants such as diet, disease, and work intensity during the growing years, and as such it is a measure of the consumption of basic necessities that incorporates demands placed on one's biological system. Because family income heavily influences purchases of basic necessities such as food and medical care, stature is ultimately a function of access to resources and environmental sanitation. It is noteworthy that stature may be diminished by consumption of products, such as alcohol or

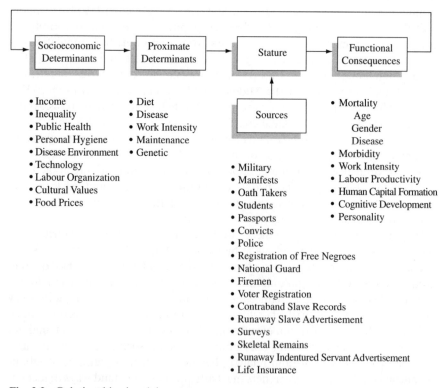

Fig. 3.2   Relationships involving stature
Source: Steckel, 1997

drugs that are harmful to health, but excessive consumption of food, while leading to rapid growth, may impair health in later life. Public health measures, personal hygiene, and the disease environment affect the incidence of disease that places claims on nutrition. In addition, human growth may have functional consequences for health, labour productivity, mental development, and personality, which in turn may influence socio-economic conditions.

Comparisons with other measures

Because real GNP per capita is the most widely used indicator of living standards, it is particularly useful to compare and contrast this measure with stature (Steckel, 1983; 1995; Floud, 1994). Income is a potent determinant of stature that operates through diet, disease, and work intensity, but one must recognize that other factors, such as personal hygiene, public health measures, and the disease environment, affect illness, while work intensity is a function of technology, culture, and methods of labour organization.[4] In addition, the relative price of food, cultural values such as the pattern of food distribution within the family, methods of preparation, and tastes and preferences for foods may also be relevant for net nutrition. Yet influential policy-makers view higher incomes for the poor as the most effective means of alleviating protein–energy malnutrition in developing countries (World Bank, 1993).[5] Extremely poor families may spend two-thirds or more of their income on food, but even a large share of their very low incomes purchases inadequate calories. Malnutrition associated with extreme poverty has a major impact on height, but at the other end of the income spectrum, expenditures beyond those needed to satisfy calorie requirements purchase largely variety, palatability, and convenience.

Gains in stature associated with higher income are not limited to developing countries. Within industrialized countries, height rises with socio-economic class (Eveleth and Tanner, 1990). These differences in height are related to improvements in the diet, reductions in physical work loads, reduced exposure to pathogens (through sewage disposal, a cleaner water supply, and improved housing), and better health care. Expenditures on health services rise with income and there is a positive relationship between health services and health (Fuchs, 1972).

At the individual level, extreme poverty results in malnutrition, retarded growth, and stunting. Higher incomes enable the parents of growing children to purchase a better diet, and height increases correspondingly, but once income is sufficient to satisfy caloric requirements, individuals often consume foods that also satisfy many vitamin and mineral requirements. Height may continue to rise with income because a more complete diet or better housing and medical care are available. As income increases, consumption patterns change to realize a larger share of genetic potential, but environmental variables are powerless after individuals attain the maximum capacity for growth.[6] The limits to this process are clear from the fact that people who grew up in very wealthy families are not physical giants.

While the relationship between height and income is non-linear at the individual level, the relationship at the aggregate level depends upon the distribution of income. Average height may differ for a given per capita income depending upon the fraction of people with insufficient income to purchase an adequate diet or to afford medical care. Because the gain in height at the individual level increases at a decreasing rate as a function of income, one would expect average height at the aggregate level to rise, for a given per capita income, with the degree of equality of the income distribution (assuming there are people who have not reached their genetic potential).

The empirical relationship between average height and per capita income has been studied by linking data from mid- or late-twentieth-century national height studies, found in Eveleth and Tanner (1976; 1990), with estimates of per capita Gross Domestic Product (in 1985 $), obtained in Summers and Heston (1991). The height studies were done on national populations in the mid and late-twentieth century. The scatter diagram in Fig. 3.3 confirms the relationship between average height and per capita income discussed above.[7] The relationship is clearly non-linear and is readily fit by a log function using regression analysis. The diagram depicts the heights of boys, but the equations below show that a similar pattern applies to girls (t-values in parentheses):

Boys aged 12: Height = 107.61   +   4.48 ln (GDP per capita), N = 18, R^2 = 0.70
$\qquad\qquad\qquad\qquad$ (t = 17.07)   (t = 6.18)

Girls aged 12: Height = 108.00   +   4.66 ln (GDP per capita), N = 17, R^2 = 0.68
$\qquad\qquad\qquad\qquad$ (t = 15.13)   (t = 5.65)

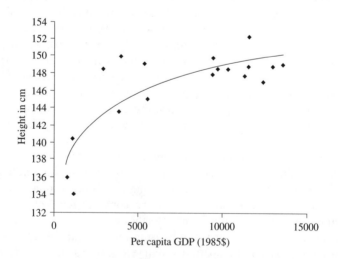

Fig. 3.3   Per capita GDP and height at age 12, boys
Source: Calculated from data in Eveleth and Tanner (1976; 1990) and Summers and Heston (1991)

Scatter around the average relationship may be explained by variation across countries in the degree of income inequality, by differences in public health policies, by food prices, and by cultural factors that affect the distribution of resources within families. These conditions affect the number and the degree to which basic needs are being met within the population. Despite the large number of factors that may influence average height at a given level of per capita income, however, the simple correlations between a country's average height and the log of its per capita GDP are in the range of 0.82 to 0.88 (Steckel, 1983; 1995).[8]

A strong association between stature and per capita income also existed a century earlier. In a study of European countries in the late nineteenth and early twentieth centuries, Floud (1994) found a height–income relationship similar to that observed in more recent data. Although the height–income relationship has been less well studied in eras before the late nineteenth century, the available evidence points to diverse outcomes, including a strong association in France, the Netherlands, and Japan, and a weak relationship in the US. Certainly counterexamples (countries with populations taller than their income alone would suggest) can be found, including Ireland in the early nineteenth century and America in the late Colonial and early National periods (Mokyr and Ó Gráda, 1988; Nicholas and Steckel, 1992; Costa and Steckel, 1997). It has also been noted that taller populations of the eighteenth and nineteenth centuries tended to live in rural, isolated, and less commercial regions (Margo and Steckel, 1983; Sandberg and Steckel, 1988; Komlos, 1989; Shay, 1994). Given that a non-linear relationship exists between height and income, and that the height–income relationship could shift over time (due to changes in medical technology, for example), it can be concluded that heights and income measure different but related aspects of the standard of living.

Figure 3.4 shows the connection between average height and life expectancy at birth for the same countries as depicted in Fig. 3.3. Unlike the height-per-capita-GDP relationship, which was clearly non-linear, the pattern in Fig. 3.4 is approximately linear, and the average trade-off may be estimated using linear regression analysis (t-values in parentheses):

Boys aged 12: Height = 106.57   +   0.601 (life expectancy), $N = 18$, $R^2 = 0.80$
                    ($t = 21.53$)   ($t = 8.09$)

Girls aged 12: Height = 110.99   +   0.521 (life expectancy), $N = 17$, $R^2 = 0.84$
                    ($t = 26.30$)   ($t = 8.87$)

The slopes range from 0.52 to 0.60, depending upon sex, which implies that a one year increase in life expectancy is associated with an increase in stature of about 0.56 cm (average of the sexes).

Unfortunately, empirical work on the association between life expectancy and average stature is thin for the nineteenth century, but there are good biological reasons for believing that a strong relationship existed. Human growth and

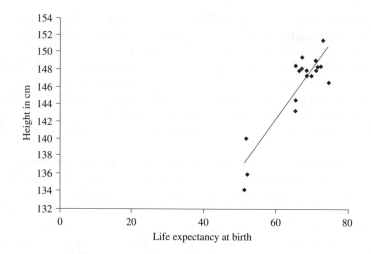

Fig. 3.4   Life expectancy and height at age 12, boys
Source: Calculated from data in Eveleth and Tanner (1976; 1990) and World Bank, *World Development Report* (various years)

health are opposite sides of the same coin, because children are at greater risk of death if they grow poorly from bad diets, hard work, or exposure to disease.

The connection between average height and life expectancy in a historical setting is most reliably calculated for the late industrial period, when better estimates of life expectancy are available. Because children's heights (and those of females) are generally unavailable for this time period, only adult males are available for study. Figure 3.5 shows the scatter diagram for the US, the UK, the Netherlands, France, Sweden, Germany, Japan, and Australia. The estimated regression line is (*t*-values in parentheses):

$$\text{Height} = 152.48 + 0.330 \text{ (life expectancy)}, \ N = 8, \ R^2 = 0.40$$
$$(t = 18.03) \qquad (t = 1.98)$$

The R^2 is substantially below that for the children aged 12 primarily because Japan is an outlier. If Japan is omitted, the R^2 rises to 0.79 and the regression coefficient is statistically significant at 0.01. Japan's stature is too low given its life expectancy, possibly because the time-frames of the observations do not agree. Conditions in the 1930s, when the young adults of mid-century were growing children, were conceivably much worse than those measured by life expectancy in 1950, a few years following the end of the Second World War. It is also possible that the height–life expectancy relationship is somewhat non-linear at low levels of health.

Whatever the explanation (i.e. whether Japan is included or excluded), the slope of the relationship is lower in Fig. 3.5 than in Figs 3.3 and 3.4. Among adult males of the late nineteenth and early twentieth centuries, a year of life expectancy was worth only 0.33 cm of stature, as opposed to 0.56 cm among

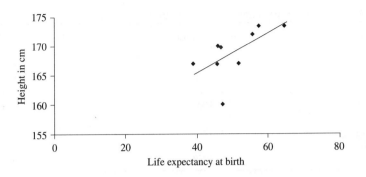

Fig. 3.5 Life expectancy and adult height, late industrial period
Source: Steckel and Floud, 1997

children aged 12. This might result from the vast gap in time periods being compared, during which medical knowledge and practice changed significantly, differentially affecting growth and mortality. It is also likely that individuals measured as adults simply had more time during their growing years to recover from environmental insults (catch-up growth), which would lessen the slope of the relationship.

Urbanization and health

Scholars do not know the extent to which human welfare during industrialization was governed by general tendencies and similar causal structures or by idiosyncratic factors and the cumulative influences of historical accidents that affected countries unequally—such as major wars or the acquisition of and settlement of new territories. Aligning the results for individual countries by stage of industrialization establishes a common framework for study, and suggests that some general tendencies prevailed.

Several decades ago, economic historians abandoned the idea that industrialization proceeded in a rigid sequence of events. They agree, however, that some order prevailed. England was clearly the first industrial country, and the process of industrialization spread across Europe from west to east. Significant industrial activity began in the US sometime in the early nineteenth century, and economic growth accelerated in Australia near the middle of the century. The transformation did not begin in Japan until the 1880s.

Table 3.1 arrays countries by the timing of their most intense period of industrial change, when mechanization and factory methods of production penetrated numerous industries and spread geographically. It should be noted that some countries never developed large industrial sectors. Australia relied extensively on agriculture and mining, while the Netherlands (lacking coal and waterpower), developed banking, shipping, and services.

Table 3.1 Height and percentage urban at mid-phase of industrialization

Country	Middle Industrial Period	Average Male Height	% Urban
United Kingdom	1800–1830	170.7	38.7
United States	1850–1880	170.6	22.3
France	1850–1880	165.4	31.0
The Netherlands	1870–1900	168.6	46.0
Sweden	1870–1900	171.4	17.2
Germany	1870–1900	167.5	43.6
Australia	1890–1920	172.0	53.0
Japan	1900–1920	158.8	60.0

Source: Steckel and Floud, 1997 (Table 11.2)

The table also shows that average male height and per cent urban (towns or cities of 2,500 population or more) varied widely across the countries during the period of most intense change. With regard to stature, the extremes were established by the Australians (172 cm) and the Japanese who fell more than 13 cm behind. In urban development, the Swedes had the smallest share living in towns or cities (only 17.2%) while the Japanese were the most urban (60%).

It was not accidental that the Japanese were both the shortest and the most urban. In an era before widespread, effective investments in public health and personal hygiene, the congestion and turnover associated with urban living increased the chances of exposure to pathogens. Other features detrimental to health are often found in cities, such as a large number of poor people who lacked the access to food, clothing, and shelter that would have increased resistance to disease.

The scatter diagram in Fig. 3.6 confirms the adverse effect of urbanization on health. The estimated regression equation is (t-values in parentheses):

Height = 174.07   –   0.153 (per cent urban), $N = 8$, $R^2 = 0.27$
          $(t = 40.69)$ $(t = -1.47)$

For every percentage point increase in the degree of urbanization, average male height fell by about 0.15 cm. This magnitude is significant in a practical sense because the transition from a low (say, 20%) level of urbanization to a moderately high level (say 50%) would have decreased average height by 4.5 cm. The notable outlier to the inverse relationship was Australia, which had the tallest population and the second highest level of urbanization. If Australia is dropped from the regression, the t-value rises to –2.60, R^2 increases to 0.57, and the regression coefficient increases (in absolute value) by 50%.

What factors explain the exceptional nature of health and urbanization in Australia? One was the relative geographic isolation of the country from major disease currents that affected cities in Europe and in North America. Another is the remoteness of the major cities within Australia from each other, which

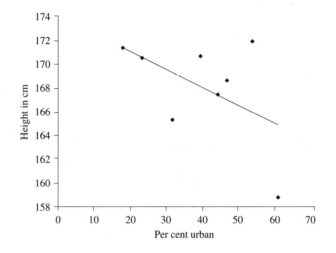

Fig. 3.6 Per cent urban and average male height
Source: Steckel and Floud, 1997

helped to reduce the spread of infectious disease. Moreover, Australia's indus-trialization (or modernization) occurred late enough to benefit from significant investments in public health. This last feature distinguishes Australia from Japan, which was also a late industrializer within this group.

Temporal patterns

Additional factors that influenced health during industrialization can be dis-cerned from study of temporal patterns within countries. The patterns can be placed into three categories of (a) important declines in health during a large phase of industrialization; (b) sustained, but not necessarily monotonic, improvement; and (c) a mixture that featured a series of short cycles.

Figures 3.7 and 3.8 show that the US and the UK fit the first pattern. Americans were very tall by global standards in the early nineteenth century as a result of their rich and varied diets, low population density, and relative equality of wealth. Between 1830 and roughly 1880, however, the average height of American men fell by about 3 cm, a reversal that was not offset until the 1920s. Consistent with this height decline, life expectancies tabulated from genealogies also show a deterioration near the middle of the century (Pope, 1992). Researchers in the field have suggested numerous possible causal factors for the decline, including the spread of disease affiliated with the development of railroads, canals, and steamboats (for discussions see Steckel, 1995 and Komlos, 1998). Also mentioned are higher food prices, growing inequality, the emergence of business cycles that led to malnutrition during contractions,

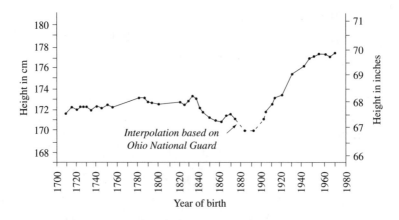

Fig. 3.7   Height of American-born white males, 1710–1974
Source: Costa and Steckel, 1997

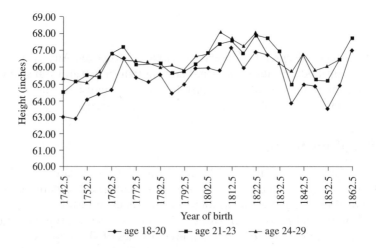

Fig. 3.8   Mean heights of British military recruits
Source: Floud and Harris, 1997

urbanization, and the rise of public schools that exposed children to major
diseases. Unfortunately, research has not advanced to the point of assigning
plausible weights to these factors.

Although health deterioration also occurred in Britain during the early to mid
nineteenth century, the timing is probably more coincidental than emblematic of
similar causal factors at work. While it is possible that growing trade and com-
merce spread disease, as in the US, it is more likely that a major culprit was rapid
urbanization and associated increases in exposure to diseases. This conclusion
is reached by noting that urban-born men were substantially shorter than the

rural-born, and between the periods of 1800–30 and 1830–70 the share of the British population living in urban areas leapt from 38.7 to 54.1%.

The UK is the only country to date for which a large database has been assembled for women in the eighteenth and nineteenth centuries, in this case from convict and prison records. Comparisons with heights of men from the same sources provide insights into resource allocation within the family, a phenomenon difficult to study from traditional sources such as wages or income. Johnson and Nicholas (1997) report that the gap between male and female heights widened during the late eighteenth and early nineteenth centuries but were substantially correlated after 1815, including the period of height decline after 1830. The relative height decline of women in the earlier period may have resulted from declining labour market opportunities for women, which led to a deterioration in diet and possibly harder work for young women.

Sweden realized the most sustained increase in health during the most intense period of industrialization (late nineteenth century), but France, the Netherlands, and Japan also posted significant, if somewhat interrupted, gains. Figure 3.9 shows that average adult male heights in Sweden rose from 168 to 172.5 cm between 1860 and 1900. The only down turn was the small reversal that occurred during the crop failures of the late 1860s, which had little to do with industrialization (Sandberg and Steckel, 1997). Paralleling the growth in stature were declines in childhood mortality rates of roughly 50%. It is notable that Sweden had the least urbanized population among the eight countries studied, and it also benefited from public health measures such as vaccination, and from relatively low food prices created by the spread of potato cultivation and imports of food from America.

Most noticeable in the Dutch experience (Fig. 3.10) was the large pre-industrial

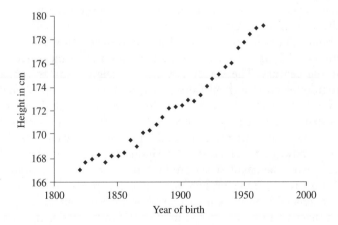

Fig. 3.9   Heights of conscripts in Sweden, 1820–1965
Source: Sandberg and Steckel, 1997

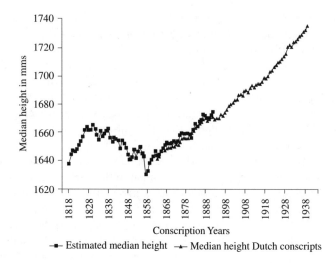

Fig. 3.10   Median heights of Dutch conscripts, 1818–1940
Source: Drukker and Tassenaar, 1997

height decline that was caused in part by rising food prices and stagnating nominal wages (i.e. a decline in purchasing power). This trend was not reversed until the conscription years of the late 1850s (birth years of the late 1830s). Thereafter, average heights increased more or less continuously into the twentieth century with the exception of the reversal and stagnation of those measured from the late 1880s through the late 1890s. The latter was associated with the income decline of the 1860s and the economic depression of the 1870s (Drukker and Tassenaar, 1997).

The French experience (Fig. 3.11) of the late nineteenth century is similar to that of the Netherlands. On the eve of industrialization, both populations attained about 164 cm and both realized slow and steady growth in heights with the exception of the slight reversal and stagnation for those measured in the last decade of the century. The steady advance in heights was accompanied by steady progress in economic measures, such as GDP per capita, and by life expectancy. Like the Netherlands, France also experienced a decline in economic conditions that affected average heights; a down turn in real wages in the early 1860s was followed by a decade and a half of stagnation (Weir, 1997).

Figure 3.12 shows that Japan opened the industrial era at the turn of the twentieth century with the smallest stature (about 157 cm) of any industrializing country. Hampered by a low protein diet, thereafter progress was slow and significantly correlated with per capita GDP but adversely affected by economic policy that diverted resources to the military (Honda, 1997). Its high level of urbanization and modest investments in public health were obstacles to human growth. Economic stagnation in the 1920s and the depression of the 1930s

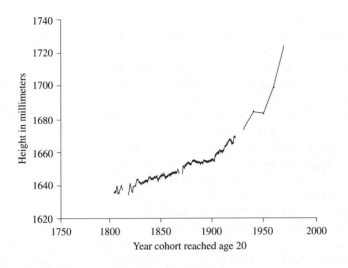

Fig. 3.11   Male height at age 20 in France, 1800–1980
Source: Weir, 1997

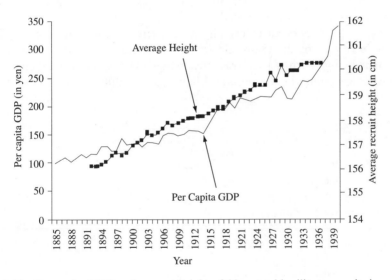

Fig. 3.12   Per capita GDP and average height of 20-year-old military recruits in
Japan, 1886–1940
Source: Honda, 1997

(which was rather mild in Japan) brought the modest gains in height to a halt in
the mid 1930s.

Germany and Australia realized gains in health during industrialization, but
progress was choppy, or otherwise interrupted by relatively brief cycles in height

(Twarog, 1997). Figure 3.13 shows the stature advantage of rural over urban residents that characterized all countries studied in this era. Adult males reached about 163.5 cm (average of rural and urban) in the province of Württemberg on the eve of industrialization, which began in the 1860s. A small spurt in average heights occurred during the 1870s, followed by decline and stagnation in the 1880s. This temporal pattern was related to the financial crash of 1873 and the subsequent depression that lasted into the early 1890s. Occupational differences in stature indicate that the professional classes were protected during the early phases of the economic depression and the loss in health was concentrated among the middle and lower classes. Thus, growing inequality played an important role in Germany's health trends during industrialization.

Figure 3.14 shows two features distinguish the Australian experience: the tall stature (about 172 cm) on the eve of modernization, followed by a large cycle in heights whereby the average height of the mid 1870s was not attained again until the second decade of the twentieth century (Whitwell *et al.*, 1997). The tall stature is undoubtedly related to an inexpensive and diverse diet that was also rich in protein, a phenomenon giving rise to the view that Australia was a working man's paradise. Even though the share living in urban areas was relatively high (about 50%), overall population density was low and the country and its major cities were relatively isolated.

But some troubles occurred even in these relatively idyllic circumstances. The height down turn of the 1880s and 1890s was the result of a double whammy. The share living in urban areas was already high (43% in 1881) and then jumped 8 percentage points in the decade following. A sanitary crisis followed and

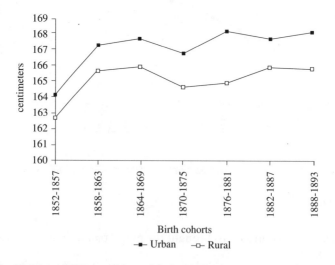

Fig. 3.13 Heights of Württemberg soldiers, 1852–57 to 1888–93 by urban-rural status. Source: Twarog, 1997

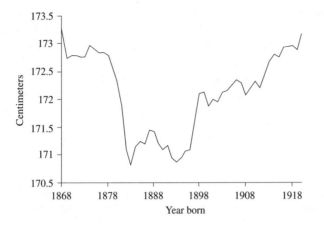

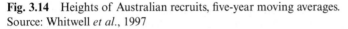

Fig. 3.14   Heights of Australian recruits, five-year moving averages.
Source: Whitwell *et al.*, 1997

typhoid fever, which disproportionately affected the young, was epidemic in the cities. Although the pace of urbanization fell considerably during the 1890s, GDP declined and remained relatively low for a decade, thereby dampening any hopes for quick recovery in heights and health.

Conclusion

Study of height and mortality patterns in countries diverse by time period of industrialization and by environmental factors indicates that a combination of general tendencies and idiosyncratic factors affected health during the industrial revolutions of the nineteenth and early twentieth centuries. In an era when public health policies were often lacking, or meagrely enlightened by theories of disease causation, urbanization was a widespread culprit in ill-health within countries studied in Europe and in the Pacific, and within the US. Height was inversely correlated with degree of urbanization across countries, and rising urbanization led to health deterioration, especially in England, Australia, and Japan.

Major business cycles also affected heights and health. France, the Netherlands, Germany, and Australia were victims of major down turns. Changing economic opportunities, in the form of growing inequality, adversely affected heights in Germany and the US.

Diets were important for health and human growth. Countries with the tallest men (Australia and the US) had excellent access to a variety of foods, some of which were rich in protein. Food was expensive and the diet was low in protein in the country with the smallest stature (Japan).

Lastly, public health policy (or lack thereof) was also important for health. Countries that industrialized early, such as the US and the UK, suffered the most, in part because the adverse effects of trade and population concentrations on health could not be offset by health policies informed by reliable theories of disease causation. Merely arriving late on the scene was no guarantee of protection against the by-products of industrialization, however, as shown by the Japanese case, where resources that could have been used for public health and human growth were diverted to the military.

Notes

1. To compare health status in situations where genetic differences are relevant, stature can be converted into percentiles of the appropriate (ethnic, regional, or country-specific) height standards.

2. An alternative view of stature is the 'small but healthy' paradigm emphasized by Sukhatme (1982), Seckler (1982), and others, in which it is claimed that many individuals adapt with low costs to nutritional deprivation. For critiques of this view see James (1987), Martorell (1989), and Dasgupta (1993).

3. Ingestion of toxic substances, such as alcohol or tobacco, *in utero* or in early childhood may create permanent stunting regardless of subsequent nutritional conditions.

4. Empirical models of the relationship between a country's per capita GNP and average height are discussed below. More elaborate models would consider a lagged relationship between income and stature, both at the household and the aggregate (national) level. For example, adult stature is a function of average income in each year from conception to maturity, and growth is more sensitive to income levels at ages when growth is ordinarily high, i.e. during early childhood and adolescence. For an application of this idea see Brinkman *et al.*, 1988.

5. Development economists have debated the effects of income on the diets of the poor. See Behrman and Deolalikar, 1987.

6. Of course, it is possible that higher incomes could purchase products such as alcohol, tobacco, or drugs that impair health.

7. The countries are Czechoslovakia, West Germany, the Netherlands, New Zealand, USA, Japan, South Korea, Egypt, India, Belgium, Denmark, Hungary, Italy, Argentina, and Australia. Three countries have two height studies conducted at different dates.

8. The log specification fits about as well as a quadratic or cubic polynomial, and given these results the log is preferred on grounds of simplicity.

REFERENCES

Behrman JR, Deolalikar AB. Will developing country nutrition improve with income? A case study for rural South India. *Journal of Political Economy*, 1987; **95**:492–507

Brinkman HJ, Drukker JW, Slot B. Height and income: a new method for the estimation of historical national income series. *Explorations in Economic History*, 1988; **25**:227–64

Costa D, Steckel RH. Long-term trends in health, welfare, and economic growth in the United States. In: Steckel RH, Floud R (eds) *Health and welfare during industrialization*. Chicago: University of Chicago Press, 1997, pp 47–89

Dasgupta P. *An inquiry into well-being and destitution*. New York: Oxford University Press, 1993

Drukker JW, Tassenaar V. Paradoxes of modernization and material well-being in the Netherlands during the nineteenth century. In: Steckel RH, Floud R (eds) *Health and welfare during industrialization*. Chicago: University of Chicago Press, 1997, pp 331–77

Eveleth PB, Tanner JM. *Worldwide variation in human growth*. Cambridge: Cambridge University Press, 1976

Eveleth PB, Tanner JM. *Worldwide variation in human growth*. 2nd edition. Cambridge: Cambridge University Press, 1990

Floud R. The heights of Europeans since 1750: a new source for European economic history. In: Komlos J (ed) *Stature, living standards, and economic development: essays in anthropometric history*. Chicago: University of Chicago Press, 1994, pp 9–24

Floud R, Harris B. Health, height, and welfare: Britain, 1700–1980. In: Steckel RH, Floud R (eds) *Health and welfare during industrialization*. Chicago: University of Chicago Press, 1997, pp 91–126

Fuchs VR. The contribution of health services to the American economy. In: Fuchs VR (ed) *Essays in the economics of health and medical care*. New York: National Bureau of Economic Research, 1972, pp 3–38

Honda G. Differential structure, differential health: industrialization in Japan, 1868–1940. In: Steckel RH, Floud R (eds) *Health and welfare during industrialization*. Chicago: University of Chicago Press, 1997, pp 251–84

James WPT. Research relating to energy adaptation in man. In: Schürch B, Scrimshaw NS (eds) *Chronic energy deficiency: consequences and related issues*. Lausanne: International Dietary Energy Consultancy Group, 1987, pp 7–36

Johnson P, Nicholas S. Health and welfare of women in the United Kingdom, 1785–1920. In: Steckel RH, Floud R (eds) *Health and welfare during industrialization*. Chicago: University of Chicago Press, 1997, pp 201–49

Komlos J. *Nutrition and economic development in the eighteenth-century Habsburg monarchy*. Princeton: Princeton University Press, 1989

Komlos J. Shrinking in a growing economy? The mystery of physical stature during the Industrial Revolution. *Journal of Economic History*, 1998; **58**:779–802

Malcolm LA. Ecological factors relating to child growth and nutritional status. In: Roche AF, Falkner F (eds) *Nutrition and malnutrition: identification and measurement*. New York: Plenum Press, 1974, pp 329–52 [Advances in Experimental Medicine and Biology, Vol. 49]

Margo RA, Steckel RH. Heights of native-born whites during the antebellum period. *Journal of Economic History*, 1983; **43**: 167–74

Martorell R. Body size, adaptation and function. *Human Organization*, 1989; **48**:15–20

Martorell R, Habicht J-P. Growth in early childhood in developing countries. In: Falkner F, Tanner JM (eds) *Human growth: a comprehensive treatise*, Vol. 3. New York: Plenum Press, 1986, pp 241–62

Mokyr J, Ó Gráda C. Poor and getting poorer? Living standards in Ireland before the Famine. *Economic History Review*, 1988; **41**:209–35

Nicholas S, Steckel RH. Tall but poor: nutrition, health, and living standards in pre-Famine Ireland. NBER Working Paper Series on Historical Factors in Long Run Growth, No. 39. Cambridge, Mass: National Bureau of Economic Research, 1992

Pope CL. Adult mortality in America before 1900: a view from family histories. In: Goldin C, Rockoff H (eds) *Strategic factories in nineteenth century American economic history*. Chicago: University of Chicago Press, 1992, pp 267–96

Sandberg LG, Steckel RH. Overpopulation and malnutrition rediscovered: hard times in nineteenth century Sweden. *Explorations in Economic History*, 1988; **25**:1–19

Sandberg LG, Steckel RH. Was industrialization hazardous to our health? Not in Sweden! In: Steckel RH, Floud R (eds) *Health and welfare during industrialization*. Chicago: University of Chicago Press, 1997, pp 127–59

Scrimshaw NS, Taylor CE, Gordon JE. *Interactions of nutrition and disease*. WHO Monograph Series, No. 52. New York: United Nations, 1968

Seckler D. Small but healthy: a basic hypothesis in the theory, measurement and policy of malnutrition. In Sukhatme PV (ed) *Newer concepts in nutrition and their implications for policy*. Pune: Maharashtra Association for the Cultivation of Science Research Institute, 1982, pp 127–37

Shay T. The level of living in Japan, 1885–1938: new evidence. In: Komlos J (ed) *Stature, living standards and economic development: essays in anthropometric history*. Chicago: University of Chicago Press, 1994, pp 173–201

Steckel RH. Height and per capita income. *Historical Methods*, 1983; **16**:1–7

Steckel RH. Stature and the standard of living. *Journal of Economic Literature*, 1995; **33**:1903–40

Steckel RH, Floud R. *Health and welfare during industrialization*. Chicago: University of Chicago Press, 1997

Sukhatme PV. *Newer concepts in nutrition and their implications for policy*. Pune: Maharashtra Association for the Cultivation of Science Research Institute, 1982

Summers R, Heston A. The Penn World Table (Mark 5): an expanded set of international comparisons, 1950–1988. *Quarterly Journal of Economics*, 1991; **106**:327–68

Tanner JM. Growth and physique in different populations of mankind. In: Baker PT, Weiner JS (eds) *The biology of human adaptability*. Oxford: Clarendon Press, 1966, pp 45–66

Tanner JM. *Fetus into man: physical growth from conception to maturity*. London: Open Books, 1978

Tanner JM. *A history of the study of human growth*. Cambridge: Cambridge University Press, 1981

Tanner JM, Hayashi,T, Preece MA, Cameron N. Increase in length of leg relative to trunk in Japanese children and adults from 1957 to 1977: comparisons with British and with Japanese Americans. *Annals of Human Biology*, 1982; **9**:411–23

Twarog S. Heights and living standards in Germany, 1850–1939: the case of Württemberg. In: Steckel RH, Floud R (eds) *Health and welfare during industrialization*. Chicago: University of Chicago Press, 1997, pp 285–330

US National Center for Health Statistics. *NCHS Growth Curves for Children, birth–18 years, United States*. Hyattesville, MD: DHEW Publication No. (PHS) 78–1650

Waterlow JC, Schürch B. Causes and mechanisms of linear growth retardation. *European Journal of Clinical Nutrition*, 1994; **48(Suppl)**: s1–s216

Weir DR. Economic welfare and physical well-being in France, 1750–1990. In: Steckel
    RH, Floud R (eds) *Health and welfare during industrialization.* Chicago: University
    of Chicago Press, 1997, pp 161–200
Whitwell G, de Souza C, Nicholas S. Height, health, and economic growth in Australia,
    1860–1940. In: Steckel RH, Floud R (eds) *Health and welfare during
    industrialization.* Chicago: University of Chicago Press, 1997, pp 379–422
World Bank. *World Development Report 1993: investing in health.* Washington, DC:
    World Bank, 1993

4 Common threads: underlying components of inequalities in mortality between and within countries

David A. Leon

Introduction

The study of inequalities in health has a long and distinguished history going back to the middle of the nineteenth century. Two strands may be clearly identified throughout. The first, and oldest, is concerned with differences in levels of health or disease between contrasting geographic areas. The second relates to differences between aggregates of individuals defined in terms of shared socio-economic characteristics including occupation, education, and income. In the much more recent past, there has been increasing attention paid to inequalities in health and disease according to gender (see Macintyre, this volume, chapter 14) and ethnicity. These different dimensions of inequalities in health do not exist in isolation, and there are examples in the literature of links being made between them. For example, there have been various attempts to look at how far ethnic differences in disease rates may be accounted for by underlying differences in education, income, and other socio-economic factors (Devesa and Diamond, 1980; McWhorter *et al.*, 1989; Davey Smith *et al.*, 1998a).

The study of health inequalities between socio-economic groups and between geographic areas have been particularly closely related. Some of the earliest studies within countries to investigate the link between health and wealth were based on contrasting mortality levels in different areas of the same city (Heron, 1907; Brown and Lal, 1914). These sorts of area-based investigations, or ecological studies, have become more sophisticated since they were first introduced. Modern studies typically use Census information to characterize small areas in terms of mean incomes, proportions of residents with certain levels of education, or other aggregate individual characteristics (Cohart, 1954; Kitagawa and Hauser, 1973; McLoone and Boddy, 1994). This information is then correlated with health outcomes such as mortality or cancer incidence. Most recently these techniques have been used to address the question of whether the socio-economic characteristics of an area have an impact upon the health of individuals over and above the individual characteristics of people living in each area (Eames *et al.*, 1993; Macintyre *et al.*, 1993; Sloggett and Joshi, 1994; Anderson *et al.*, 1997).

Geographic inequalities in health may be considered at widely varying levels of aggregation or scale. The analytic ecological studies already discussed, involving small areas, are at one extreme. At the other extreme are differences in health or mortality between global regions. The Global Burden of Disease project has generated estimates of the levels of major disease categories by region using a consistent methodology (Murray and Lopez, 1997*a*). An important rationale for the production of these global estimates is to provide a firm evidence base upon which to develop priorities for interventions and action. However, attention is now being turned to developing new tools that may be used to assess inequalities in the distribution of health within developing and developed countries, as the international policy agenda on health moves to incorporate issues of equity within countries. The current state of progress in this emerging area is discussed in chapter 10 by Murray and colleagues, and in chapter 11 by Gwatkin.

Explanations for the existence of differences in health and disease between global regions have tended to be framed in the most general terms. It is usually assumed that the underlying determinants of the enormous gap in life expectancy between North and South are to be found in the major differences in absolute poverty, deprivation, and education. Systematic attempts to analyse and explain the differences in health and mortality between specific countries across the globe have been far less frequent than studies that have simply described them. The work of Samuel Preston in the 1970s represented a watershed in this respect. He attempted to explain differences in mortality between a wide range of countries in terms of various macro-level economic and social indicators for each country. He found that GDP per capita was an important determinant of life expectancy, particularly among the poorer countries of the world (Preston, 1976). However, improvements in health status over time appeared to be partly related to advances in medicine and public health, independently of GDP.

The relationship between GDP per capita and life expectancy is not a linear one. As Preston observed, among high-income countries there is little relationship between GDP and mortality. This issue has been taken up more recently by Richard Wilkinson. He has been particularly intrigued by the absence of association between national wealth and life expectancy among high-income countries, given that within these same countries there were (and still are) well documented and strong positive associations between socio-economic level and health. This has led Wilkinson (1996) to hypothesize that variations in health between high-income countries are in fact related to inequities in income distribution rather than overall national wealth. The idea that income inequity, and the societal dysfunctions hypothesized to be associated with it, such as low levels of social capital and social cohesion (Kawachi and Kennedy, 1997), may be associated with health and mortality has attracted considerable attention. However, it remains a controversial area (Judge *et al.*, 1998), as discussed in chapter 8 by Kunitz in his account of the link between social capital and health.

A limitation of much of the work to explain variations in health and mortality between countries is the focus on analysing mortality as a whole. Far less attention has been given to analysing cause-specific patterns, thus ignoring the aetiological heterogeneity of specific causes of death that is clearly manifested in the variation between diseases in the strength and direction of socio-economic gradients within countries (see Davey Smith *et al.*, chapter 5).

It is from this perspective that the rest of this chapter explores the fine grain of cause-specific differences in mortality between countries, and examines how far these between-country differences parallel the cause-specific patterns of socio-economic variations within countries. This will throw light upon underlying mechanisms that may account for some of these patterns, and suggests that an in depth understanding of inequalities in health, whether within or between countries, requires greater sensitivity to and awareness of the temporal dimension of causal relationships.

Atemporal explanations

Many explanations of inequalities in health and disease within and between countries tend to neglect or ignore the temporal dimension of underlying mechanisms. At its most basic, this *atemporal* approach involves relating *current* levels of disease rates or mortality to *current* characteristics of the population or socio-economic group. For example, Preston (1976) in his pioneering work on the relationship between a country's national wealth (measured as GDP per capita) and mortality, focused on the cross-sectional relationships—correlating GDP per capita with mortality in the same calendar period. The more recent work by Wilkinson (1996) on the positive association between inequalities in income distribution and mortality does the same by correlating life expectancy with income inequity in the same period. The implicit assumption of these analyses is that current characteristics of a population provide a meaningful and adequate basis on which to explain concurrent differences in health.

For some diseases or causes of death, this assumption may not be problematic. For example, relating mortality levels from road traffic accidents to concurrent levels of per capita alcohol consumption implies a quite plausible immediacy between cause (alcohol intoxication) and effect (road traffic accident). Similarly, the finding that variations in mortality between US states from violence and alcohol-related disease is strongly related to income inequality, mediated in part through crime levels (Kawachi *et al.*, 1999), is also plausible from a temporal perspective. However, for many non-communicable diseases, such as cancer and cardiovascular disease, it is usually far less plausible that the rate of occurrence in a population or socio-economic group can be determined solely, or even primarily, by concurrent or even recent characteristics or exposures. This is a consequence of the fact that pathogenic processes preceding diagnosis may be spread over years or even decades.

The extended period over which many diseases develop is best illustrated in the case of cancer. It is very clear that there are long 'latent periods' between first exposure to a carcinogen and the diagnosis of the resultant malignancy. Thus, the distribution of lung cancer within a population today reflects smoking levels decades in the past, while in turn the distribution of smoking habits today will determine the pattern of lung cancer decades in the future (Peto *et al.*, 1996). This phenomenon has been particularly carefully studied in the case of occupational exposure to carcinogens, where, for example, latent periods of 30 or more years have been noted between exposure to chemicals in the dyestuffs industry and the onset of bladder cancer (Case, 1966). Similarly, a recent ecological study of alcohol-related malignancies found that changes in national drinking habits took two to three decades to manifest themselves in changes in mortality rates from cancers related to alcohol (Macfarlane *et al.*, 1996).

It is of course quite possible that current or recent circumstances may influence the length of survival from diagnosis to death, as is evident from socio-economic and regional differences in cancer survival (Kogevinas and Porta, 1997; Coleman *et al.*, 1999). Differences in survival, however, are generally going to have a considerably smaller influence on patterns of mortality, than are differences in disease incidence/occurrence.

Looking further back in time

A naïve approach to the temporal dimension of cardiovascular disease aetiology may well account for the celebrated 'French paradox' (Tunstall, 1988). Coronary heart disease (CHD) mortality in France is appreciably lower than in the UK today. In contrast, CHD risk factors, such as blood pressure and serum cholesterol, in the French population today are at the same level as, or are even less favourable than in the UK. A particularly popular explanation for this apparent paradox invokes a cardio-protective effect of the French habit of moderate alcohol consumption. However, this discrepancy may not constitute a paradox at all. It has been suggested that there could be a time 'lag-effect' between serum cholesterol levels and CHD mortality, such that mortality rates in a population today are going to reflect cholesterol levels in the past (Nestle, 1992). This is supported by the statistical observation that CHD mortality today is more closely related to risk factor levels several decades ago than to levels today (Law and Wald, 1999). This fits with the evidence for atherosclerotic lesions being initiated many years prior to the onset of clinically recognized disease (Enos *et al.*, 1953; McNamara *et al.*, 1971).

A more radical challenge to the notion that current inequalities in non-communicable diseases, particularly cardiovascular disease, may be adequately explained by reference to contemporary habits and exposures comes from the 'fetal origins' hypothesis (Barker, 1995). Starting from the observation that the persistent regional differences in mortality from stroke and CHD within the UK cannot be explained by contemporary variations in known risk factors, a series of studies have led to the proposition that circumstances *in utero* may 'programme' the susceptibility of individuals to diseases in adult life (Lucas, 1991; Barker, 1998). Hence, the current distribution of many diseases within and between populations may reflect *in utero* differences 60 or even 70 years ago. There is now good evidence from a wide range of experimental studies that in utero 'programming' is a biologically sound phenomenon (Waterland and Garza, 1999; Robinson *et al.*, 1999). Moreover, epidemiological studies in different countries conducted by a range of investigators show a relatively consistent picture linking impaired fetal growth with raised blood pressure (Leon and Koupilová, 2000), type II diabetes (McKeigue, 1997), and CHD (Leon and Ben-Shlomo, 1997). Although less conclusive, other work has suggested that *in utero* circumstances may also affect the risk of hormone-related cancers, including of the breast and prostate (Leon and Ben-Shlomo, 1997).

The rise of the 'fetal origins' hypothesis has been accompanied by development of a broader interest in the potential influence on later disease of factors operating across the entire life course from fetal to adult life (Kuh and Ben-Shlomo, 1997). The application of this life-course approach to understanding socio-economic differences in health is developed by Davey Smith and colleagues in chapter 5 (this volume).

Variation in life-expectancy between and within countries

Before proceeding further, it is worth looking at the extent of variation in mortality between and within countries. Differences in life expectancy between countries in the world today are considerable, as summarized by global region in Table 4.1. Data on variation in life expectancy within countries is generally only available from developed countries, as illustrated by data from England and Wales in Table 4.2. Not surprisingly, these social class variations within Britain are small, compared to the full range of variation between Global Regions in Table 4.1. However, they are of the same magnitude as seen between the Established Market and the Former Socialist Economies. Within-country variations, however, can be much larger, as has been vividly demonstrated by the fact that in the early 1980s mortality rates among men under 65 years in Harlem, New York, USA were higher than amongst men in Bangladesh (McCord and Freeman, 1990). Evidence of the substantial geographic variation in life expectancy within the US, pointing to profound inequalities in health, is presented by Murray and colleagues in chapter 10 (this volume). This parallels the large inequalities in mortality between small areas found in Britain today (Shear

Table 4.1 Life expectancy at birth in years by global region

Region	Females	Males
Sub-Saharan Africa	51.0	48.4
India	59.1	57.9
Middle-Eastern Crescent	63.4	60.3
Other Asia and Islands	64.9	60.8
Latin America + Caribbean	70.3	65.8
China	69.8	66.2
Former socialist economies of Europe	74.8	65.7
Established market economies	80.5	73.4

Source: Murray and Lopez, 1997b

Table 4.2 Life expectancy at birth in years by social class: England and Wales, 1987–91

Social class	Females	Males
IV + V	76.8	69.7
III manual	77.6	72.4
III non-manual	79.4	73.5
I+II	80.2	74.9

Source: Drever and Whitehead, 1997

et al., 1999). Socio-economic variations in life expectancy, therefore, within countries can be substantial even in the context of global variations in survival, a point also discussed by Sen in chapter 17 (this volume).

East–West differences in mortality

A current challenge to our understanding of determinants of inequalities in population health is the mortality gap between Eastern and Western European countries. For reasons that are far from clear, the former communist countries of Eastern Europe have higher mortality than the countries of Western Europe. This is illustrated in Fig. 4.1, which shows countries ordered according to their all-cause mortality rates divided along the East–West axis. For men aged 20–74, there is no overlap between East and West, while for women there is a very slight overlap of the East (Slovenia) with the West (Republic of Ireland). This East–West gap has a long history, being smallest in the mid-1960s and widening subsequently (Meslé and Hertrich, 1997). Since the fall of the Berlin Wall in 1990, Eastern countries have become particularly diverse in their trends (Chenet *et al.*, 1996), with mortality rates increasing sharply in many countries of the former Soviet Union (Leon *et al.*, 1997; Shkolnikov *et al.*, 1998). The link

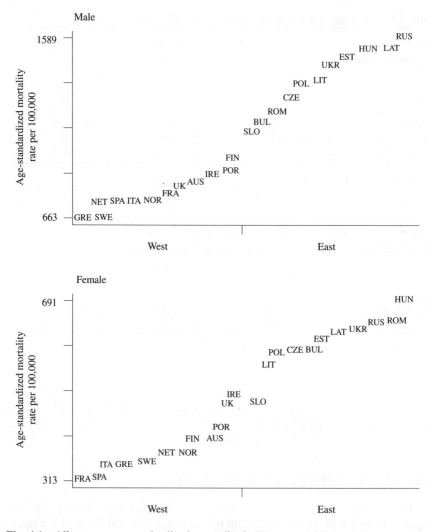

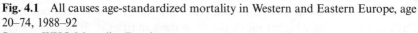

Fig. 4.1 All causes age-standardized mortality in Western and Eastern Europe, age 20–74, 1988–92
Source: WHO Mortality Database

between the collapse of the Soviet Union and the ensuing acute mortality crisis is dealt with in detail by McKee in chapter 2 (this volume).

Several studies have been undertaken to investigate the East–West mortality gap (Hertzman *et al.*, 1996). These tend to adopt an atemporal approach, focusing on identifying contemporary characteristics (including diet, smoking, alcohol consumption, and psycho-social stress) of East and West that may explain current differences in mortality (Bobák and Marmot, 1996). Little attention has been given to the possibility that differences in circumstances and conditions many decades or more in the past, rather than the present, may be crucial in explaining at least some of the current mortality differences across Europe.

Social class and East–West differences in mortality

Socio-economic differences in mortality within countries show a heterogeneous pattern by cause of death (see chapter 5, this volume). This has been particularly well documented for cancers (Davey Smith *et al.*, 1991; Kogevinas *et al.*, 1997). Although lower socio-economic groups have raised mortality from all causes combined, some causes of death show much stronger associations with socio-economic level than others. For example, mortality from causes such as tuberculosis shows very strong inverse associations with socio-economic level, while much weaker associations are generally found for mortality from cardiovascular disease. For a minority of causes, including cancer of the breast and prostate, mortality is greater in the upper compared to the lower socio-economic groups.

The heterogeneity by cause in the magnitude and direction of socio-economic differences in mortality within countries has a parallel in the heterogeneity by cause in the nature of differences in mortality between countries. A striking connection was found between the heterogeneous, cause-specific pattern of mortality by social class within Britain and mortality differences by cause between Eastern and Western Europe (Leon and Bobák, 1995). As shown in Figures 4.2 and 4.3, the cause-specific pattern of social class variation in mortality correlated closely with the cause-specific pattern of differences between East and

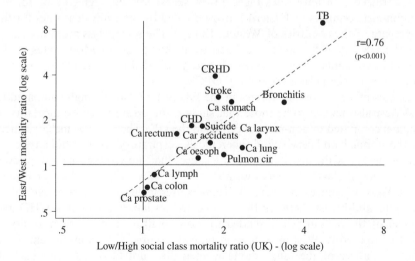

Fig. 4.2 East/West vs. social class age-standardized mortality rate ratios by cause, men aged 15–74
Source: OPCS, 1978

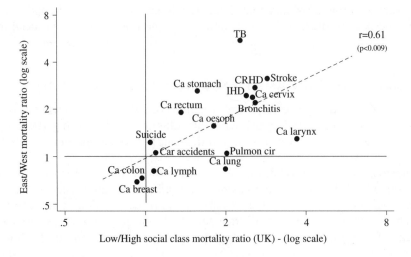

Fig. 4.3   East/West vs. social class age-standardized mortality rate ratios by cause, women aged 15–74

West. Similar correlations were found when the countries of the East were restricted to those, such as Hungary, Romania, and Czechoslovakia, that were outside the (then) Soviet Union.

In these figures, each point represents a specific cause of death. For each cause, the East–West mortality ratio (1987–9) was calculated from the age-standardized mortality rates (ages 15–74 years) for the aggregate of former communist countries of Eastern Europe divided by the equivalent rates for the aggregate of the countries of Western Europe. The social class mortality ratios for the UK (1979–83) were calculated from the age-standardized rates in the bottom two manual social classes (IV and V) divided by those for the top two non-manual social classes (I and II) (OPCS, 1978).

Causes of death for which rates in the East were relatively high compared to the West also tended to be those that showed the greatest relative mortality in manual compared to non-manual classes in the UK. These causes include cancer of the stomach and cervix, and tuberculosis, respiratory disease, and stroke. At the other end of the distribution, those causes that showed the smallest, or even reverse, social class differences were those that showed the smallest or reverse East–West differences in mortality. These causes included cancers of the colon, prostate, and breast. Between these two extremes lay causes such as CHD and cancer of the rectum, which tended to show small relative excess mortality in East compared to West as well as in manual compared to non-manual social classes. Cancer of the lung among women does not fit this general pattern. Although lung cancer rates are higher among manual compared to non-manual women, rates were lower among women in Eastern European than in Western Europe.

To throw further light on what might underlie the similar cause-specific patterning of mortality between East and West and by social class (in Britain) it will be helpful to consider a selection of specific causes one by one. While this approach may appear to risk missing the bigger picture, whereby socio-economic adversity generally leads to poorer health and higher mortality from a wide range of causes, the aetiological diversity that exists is potentially highly informative about the nature of underlying mechanisms.

Lung cancer

Lung cancer provides a good starting point. The vast majority of lung cancer cases and deaths in industrialized countries are accounted for by one factor—tobacco smoking. In addition, it is widely understood that differences in current rates between and within countries are not related to smoking habits today, but to the distribution of smoking habits decades in the past.

In most countries today for which data are available, lung cancer in men today shows a negative socio-economic gradient, with rates being highest in the lower socio-economic groups; Colombia and Brazil are the only exceptions to this pattern (Faggiano *et al.*, 1997). However, even in countries such as Britain, where there is a clearly established social class gradient, this has not always been the case. It is one of the very notable features of the development of the lung cancer epidemic in Britain, that social class differences among men (Fig. 4.4) and women only became fully developed in the 1950s.

By contrast, socio-economic differences in lung cancer among women today are particularly varied. Although, in many industrialized countries, lung cancer rates tend to be higher in the lower socio-economic groups, the opposite gradient is seen in quite a number of populations, including in Colombia, Greece,

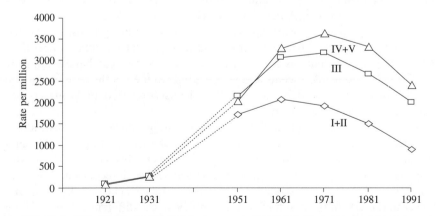

Fig. 4.4 Trends in social class differences in lung cancer mortality in England and Wales: men aged 55–64
Source: Logan, 1982; OPCS, 1986; Drever and Whitehead, 1997

Hungary, Italy and Brazil (Faggiano *et al.*, 1997). This shows that the social patterning of tobacco smoking among women in the past has been different in some countries to that seen for men.

The variable nature of the link between socio-economic factors and lung cancer is also demonstrated by gender differences in the East–West pattern of lung cancer mortality (Kubik *et al.*, 1995). Whereas lung cancer mortality in men in most Eastern European countries is higher than in Western European countries, for women this is not the case, with female rates in many Eastern countries being lower than in Western countries (Fig. 4.5). Indeed, lung cancer mortality among women in the UK and Republic of Ireland is higher than in any of the Eastern countries. Parallel gender contrasts are shown in the prevalence of adult smoking in countries of the WHO European region in the mid-1990s (Waller and Lipponen, 1997). For men, some of the highest smoking prevalences are in Eastern European countries, which also have some of the lowest smoking prevalences for women. Thus, in comparison with Western European countries, Eastern countries, particularly those of the former Soviet Union, have been and remain very gender divided with respect to smoking habit. It should be noted, however, that in Russia today there are indications that young women are smoking more than women born in earlier periods (McKee *et al.*, 1998).

A final illustration of the contingent link between socio-economic level and lung cancer and smoking is provided by intriguing data on racial differences in tobacco smoking in the US, presented in a 1998 report of the US Surgeon General (US DHHS, 1998). As is well known, African Americans in the US are socio-economically disadvantaged in comparison to Whites. They have higher rates of unemployment and lower levels of education and income. Nevertheless, in those aged less than 30 years, a higher proportion of Whites smoke than do African Americans. In 1994–5, among those aged 25–29 years, the prevalence of smoking among African Americans was 21%, while in Whites it was 32%. It should be noted that the reverse pattern is seen in older age groups, as reflected in the fact that overall African Americans have higher rates of lung cancer than Whites. However, it remains striking that, for cultural reasons that are not fully understood, among adolescents and young adults in the US the socio-economic disadvantage experienced by African Americans compared to Whites is not expressed in higher smoking rates.

In summary, today and in the recent past, lung cancer, in industrialized countries, in men, appears to be a disease of lower socio-economic groups and of Eastern rather than Western Europe. However, this consistency is not evidence of a necessary inverse association between socio-economic level and lung cancer. This is demonstrated by the absence of social class gradients in lung cancer in the UK in the first half of this century, in the different pattern of lung cancer among women within and between countries, and in the surprising racial differences in smoking among young people in the US today.

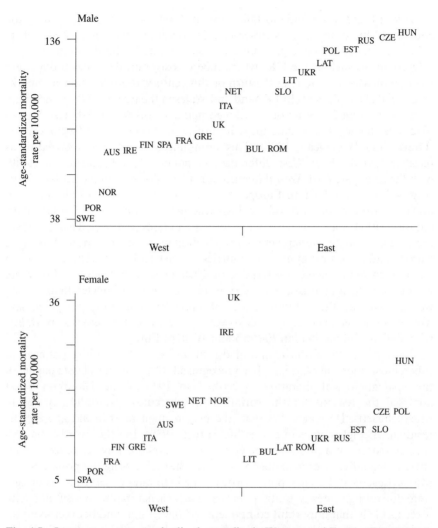

Fig. 4.5 Lung cancer age-standardized mortality in Western and Eastern Europe, age 20–74, 1988–92
Source: WHO Mortality Database

Tuberculosis

Tuberculosis contrasts sharply with lung cancer, in that there is abundant evidence that there is something intrinsic about poor socio-economic conditions that is associated with the disease. Tuberculosis shows one of the strongest and most persistent links with poor socio-economic and living conditions of any cause of death. Poor conditions of life, particularly standards of housing and overcrowding, as well as poor nutritional status and general health all increase the risk of tuberculosis and mortality from it (Cantwell *et al.*, 1998). During the course of this century, as socio-economic conditions have improved, tuberculosis mortality has undergone huge declines in industrialized countries.

In countries such as the UK, where tuberculosis mortality rates today are a fraction of what they were at the turn of this century, they still show a remarkable social class gradient. In England and Wales in the period 1991–3, mortality in the age group 20–64 among unskilled manual workers (social class V) was nine times higher than among those in professional occupations (social class I) (Drever and Whitehead, 1997). This pronounced social class association is paralleled in the East–West differences in pulmonary tuberculosis mortality with the aggregate East–West difference for tuberculosis being particularly large (Figs 4.2 and 4.3). Eastern European countries, however, do not all have high mortality from respiratory tuberculosis (the major component of total tuberculosis deaths), and show remarkable diversity in rates (Fig. 4.6). There is nevertheless only a slight overlap between the highest mortality countries of Western Europe and the lowest mortality countries of Eastern Europe. The well known sex differences in tuberculosis (Hudelson, 1996) are evident from Fig. 4.6, where in countries such as Russia mortality in men is ten times greater than among women. Despite these differences in absolute levels of mortality, men and women show relatively similar East–West patterns of tuberculosis mortality, with similar rankings within Eastern and Western Europe.

The importance of the temporal dimension in understanding patterns of tuberculosis mortality has long been recognized. In one of the classic papers of the epidemiological literature, published in 1939, Wade Hampton Frost analysed the reasons for the variation in tuberculosis mortality by age in Massachusetts. He concluded that 'the present high rates in old age are the residuals of higher rates in earlier life' (Frost, 1939). In other words, the age-specific pattern at a point in time could not be explained by reference to concurrent age differences in exposure or circumstances among the population of Massachusetts at the same point. Instead, the high rates observed at older ages were due to high rates of initial infection much earlier in life. In a similar vein, it seems likely that important components of the within- and between-country variations in tuberculosis mortality discussed above, may largely reflect substantial differences in the rates of tuberculosis infection in the past rather than current differences in the risk of being infected with tuberculosis today. The influence of historical conditions of life on current contrasts in tuberculosis mortality in different countries, and by analogy in different socio-economic groups within countries, is a theme that is taken up later in this chapter. It should be noted, however, that the balance between recent and historical influences on tuberculosis mortality may be decisively altered towards the recent past in countries with a high prevalence of HIV infection, which precipitates reactivation of an earlier acquired infection.

Thus, tuberculosis is classically an example of a disease that shows a particularly strong and direct link with absolute deprivation and poverty. In this respect

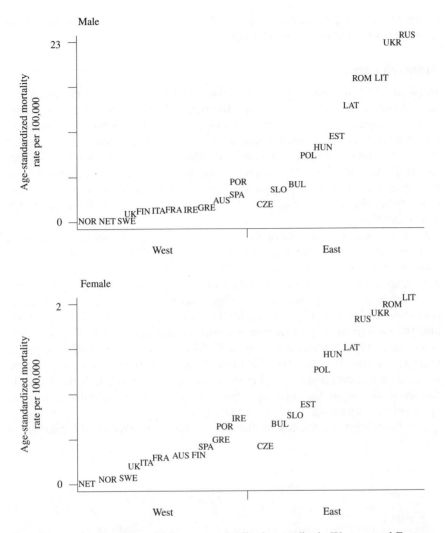

Fig. 4.6 Respiratory tuberculosis age-standardized mortality in Western and Eastern Europe, age 20–74, 1988–92
Source: WHO Mortality Database

it is in sharp contrast to lung cancer, which shows a more contingent link with poverty and deprivation. This is well illustrated by the relative position of Portugal in Figs 4.5 and 4.6. For lung cancer (Fig. 4.5), Portuguese mortality rates today are among some of the lowest in Europe, reflecting the way in which the relative poverty, poor standard of education, and isolation of the country earlier this century was associated with lower than average penetration of tobacco smoking. In contrast, Portugal's poor socio-economic level in the past is manifested today by the fact that it has one of the highest rates of tuberculosis mortality (Fig. 4.6) in Western Europe.

Stomach cancer

In all countries for which data is available, mortality from stomach cancer has been declining for decades, although the point at which the down turn began varies considerably from country to country. Despite these downward trends, on a global level, stomach cancer continues to be a major problem, accounting for the second largest number of cancer deaths in the world after lung cancer (Murray and Lopez, 1997a). Stomach cancer is still a relatively fatal malignancy, with over 85% of people dying within 5 years of diagnosis, and thus differences in mortality between countries are likely to reflect treatment differences to only a very small degree.

Stomach cancer shows one of the most consistent of all associations between socio-economic level and mortality of any cause (Kogevinas et al., 1997). Almost without exception, rates of incidence and mortality from stomach cancer are highest among those sections of any population who are the most socio-economically deprived. This has been well documented in a wide range of countries from Sweden to Colombia. The pronounced social class difference and the pattern of secular decline are both clearly apparent in Fig. 4.7. This shows mortality rates among men aged 55–64 by social class around each decennial Census from 1921 to 1991. What is striking is that the mortality rate in each social class has declined to roughly the same degree, leading to little change in the absolute size of the difference between social classes. Similar trends are apparent at younger ages and among women.

The East–West differences in stomach cancer are, predictably, marked as

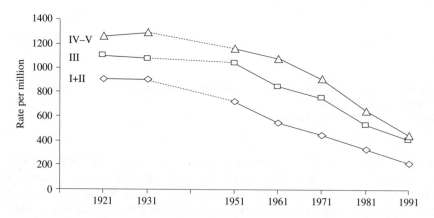

Fig. 4.7 Trends in social class differences in stomach cancer mortality in England and Wales: men aged 55–64
Source: Logan, 1982; OPCS, 1986; Drever and Whitehead, 1997

shown in Fig. 4.8. For both men and women, there is a very similar ranking of countries, with almost no overlap between East and West. As in the case of tuberculosis, Portugal is an outlier from the West, having rates that are greater than those for countries of Central and Southeastern Europe.

Our understanding of the causes of stomach cancer has developed considerably over the past 15 years since the isolation of *Helicobacter pylori*. This bacterium is now thought to play a central role in the aetiology of stomach cancer

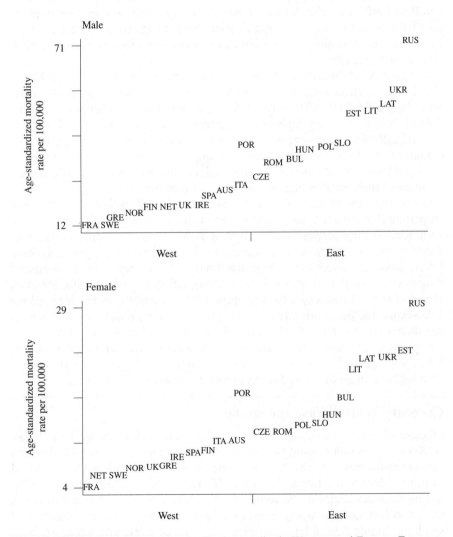

Fig. 4.8 Stomach cancer age-standardized mortality in Western and Eastern Europe, age 20–74, 1988–92
Source: WHO Mortality Database

(Parsonnett, 1999). *H. pylori* is generally acquired in childhood, and risk of infection is closely related to living conditions, hygiene, and housing standards. Geographic (EUROGAST Study Group, 1993), socio-economic (Malaty *et al.*, 1999), and secular variations in *H. pylori* prevalence fit well with the corresponding trends and differences in stomach cancer mortality rates between and within countries (Parsonnett, 1999). Factors related to poor sanitation in childhood in particular have been associated with stomach cancer (Barker *et al.*, 1990) and with *H. pylori* infection (Mendall *et al.*, 1992). The role of childhood infection, and the way in which this has changed over time in many countries as socio-economic circumstances have improved, is further exemplified by the relationship that stomach cancer mortality shows to period of birth (Hansson *et al.*, 1991).

The East–West differences in stomach cancer mortality shown in Fig. 4.8 are also likely to reflect long-term differences in the prevalence of *H. pylori* infection. In the EUROGAST study (1993), the only Central European country, Poland, had particularly high rates of infection compared to other European countries. Recent studies in parts of the former Soviet Union, including Estonia (Maaroos, 1995) and Russia (Malaty *et al.*, 1996), also show prevalences of *H. pylori* infection that are particularly high by international standards, corresponding to their notably high stomach cancer mortality rates.

Given the central role of a single causal agent, *H. pylori*, it is thus not surprising that stomach cancer has shown such a consistent inverse association with socio-economic position, or that it is higher in Eastern compared to Western Europe, where socio-economic levels in the past have generally been lower. Stomach cancer once more illustrates the importance of the temporal dimension, with the contrasts in rates today reflecting risk of infection with *H. pylori* many decades ago. In some important respects, the mechanism linking socio-economic deprivation to stomach cancer is very similar to that linking it to tuberculosis mortality. Both are directly mediated by poor environmental circumstances, particularly in childhood, that facilitate infection with the relevant infectious agent. This in turn results in strong social patterning of disease decades later, in adult life and into old age (Hansson *et al.*, 1991).

Coronary heart disease and stroke

Diseases of the circulatory system are a major cause of death in the world today. According to estimates from the Global Burden of Disease study, in 1990 CHD accounted for more deaths than any other single cause, with stroke in second position (Murray and Lopez, 1997a). CHD and stroke are clearly recognized as having distinct aetiologies. Nevertheless, they have a number of established risk factors in common, including raised blood pressure (hypertension), obesity, and smoking. In addition, it has been hypothesized that CHD and stroke are both linked to impaired fetal growth, hence references being made to the 'fetal origins of cardiovascular disease' (Barker *et al.*, 1993).

Data on time trends for cardiovascular disease rates as a whole conceal important differences between stroke and CHD (Uemura and Pisa, 1988). Mortality
from stroke has been declining in many Western countries over a long period of
time. In contrast, mortality rates from CHD in the West have not shown such a
consistent and steep pattern of decline. In the US, for example, stroke mortality
has been declining since 1900, whereas mortality from CHD rose dramatically
from the 1920s (Gale and Martyn, 1997), only starting to decline again in the
1960s. Trends in cardiovascular mortality in Eastern Europe, however, have been

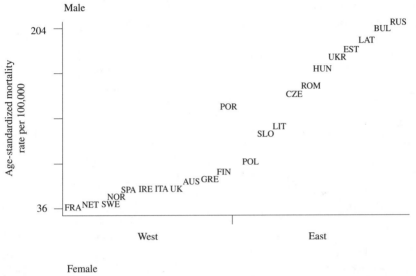

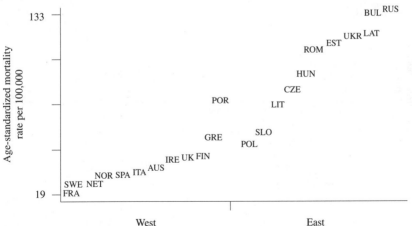

Fig. 4.9 Stroke age-standardized mortality in Western and Eastern Europe, age
20–74, 1988–92
Source: WHO Mortality Database

very different, with both stroke and CHD mortality tending to increase, particularly since the mid 1960s (Uemura and Pisa, 1988).

The higher mortality from stroke in Eastern compared to Western Europe is very evident in Fig. 4.9. As in the case of both stomach cancer and tuberculosis, there is very little overlap between East and West, with Portugal once more being the notable Western outlier. The variation in stroke mortality rates between Eastern countries is considerably larger than among Western countries.

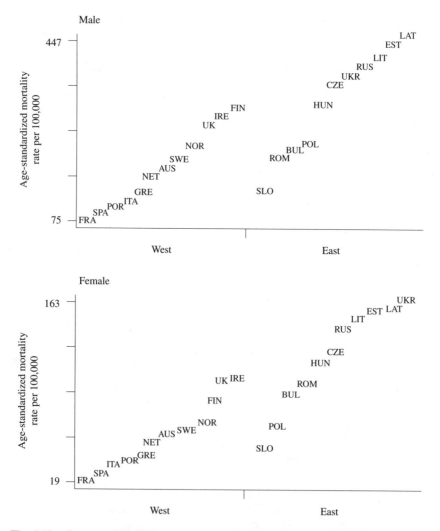

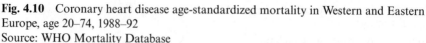

Fig. 4.10   Coronary heart disease age-standardized mortality in Western and Eastern Europe, age 20–74, 1988–92
Source: WHO Mortality Database

The East–West differences for CHD are shown in Fig. 4.10. Particularly for males, the contrast between the two halves of Europe is far less distinct than for stroke. Rates of CHD mortality in men are higher in Finland, the UK, and Ireland than they are in Poland, Bulgaria, Romania, and Slovakia. Moreover, compared to the picture for stroke mortality, there is much more heterogeneity between countries in the West. Of particular interest is Portugal, which has one of the lowest rates of CHD in Europe. This is in marked contrast to Portugal's position in Europe with respect to rates of mortality from tuberculosis, stomach cancer, and stroke. For these latter causes, mortality rates for both men and women in Portugal are intermediate between the East and West, with rates higher than other Western countries and a number of Eastern countries as well.

There is therefore a difference in the East–West patterns shown by stroke on the one hand and CHD on the other. This finds a parallel expression in the socio-economic variation shown by these two major components of cardiovascular disease. Based on work by Anton Kunst (1997), Fig. 4.11 shows the ratio of mortality in the manual social classes to that in the non-manual social classes for stroke and CHD in a range of countries. Despite variation in the size of the social class effect, in all countries mortality from stroke in manual men was appreciably higher than among non-manual men, parallel to the distinct separation between Eastern and Western countries for this cause. However, the social class pattern shown by CHD was less pronounced and consistent, parallel to the relatively indistinct pattern of East–West differences.

In summary, the within- and between-country patterns of mortality from stroke show interesting parallels, as do the patterns shown by CHD. However, the nature of mortality variation exhibited by stroke appears to have a number

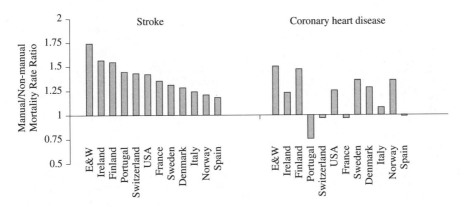

Fig. 4.11 Manual/non-manual differences in cardiovascular mortality for men aged 45–59 by country in the 1980s
Source: Kunst, 1997

of features that are similar to the pattern shown by tuberculosis and stomach cancer, which are not shared by CHD.

Prostate and breast cancers

In developed, industrialized countries, breast cancer is a major cause of death in women under the age of 50 years. Prostate cancer is one of the more important malignancies diagnosed in men, although unlike breast cancer it is rare under the age of 50 years. It is now well established that the aetiology of both cancers is intimately connected to hormonal factors. In the context of this chapter, they are both particularly unusual, in that, contrary to what is observed for many other major diseases, they tend to show positive socio-economic gradients. In other words, risk increases as one goes up the socio-economic scale, as illustrated for breast cancer in Fig. 4.12 for women aged 55–64 years.

Breast and prostate cancer provide further evidence that the pattern of socio-economic differences within countries parallels that between countries, particularly between Eastern and Western Europe. As seen in Fig. 4.13, they both show the atypical tendency for the highest rates to be in the West and the lowest in the East. While there is considerable overlap in the range of rates seen in the two halves of Europe, this pattern is in striking contrast to that seen for the other causes of death so far considered.

How can we explain these various contrasts? For breast cancer, one of the most well established risk factors is childbearing history. Risk goes up with increasing age at first birth and goes down the greater the number of children a woman gives birth to. Thus, some component of the within- and between-country differences described above are going to be related to underlying population differences in reproductive behaviour and childbearing patterns (Silva

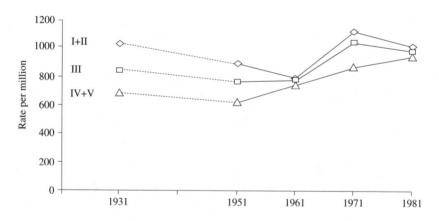

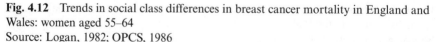
Fig. 4.12 Trends in social class differences in breast cancer mortality in England and Wales: women aged 55–64
Source: Logan, 1982; OPCS, 1986

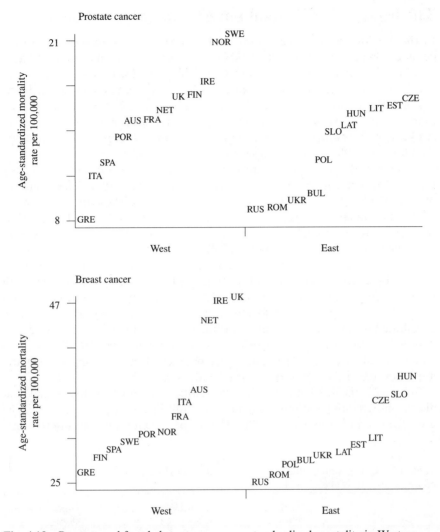

Fig. 4.13 Prostate and female breast cancer age-standardized mortality in Western and Eastern Europe, age 20–74, 1988–92
Source: WHO Mortality Database

and Beral, 1997). However, there is increasing evidence that growth *in utero* and childhood may also be positively related to breast cancer risk (see Davey Smith *et al.*, this volume, chapter 5). Circumstances *in utero*, childhood, and early adult life may thus once again play an important role in driving the contrasts in risk in adult life that we have outlined.

The legacy of childhood poverty and deprivation

In the previous section, the within- and between-country patterns for tuberculosis, stomach cancer, and stroke showed a number of similarities not shared by CHD. This impression is reinforced in Table 4.3, which shows the extent to which mortality rates from these causes in the 23 European countries (included in Fig. 4.1) are correlated with each other. It is evident from this table that CHD mortality is less strongly correlated with tuberculosis, stomach cancer, and stroke than these other diseases are correlated with each other. This is most evident for men, although it is also seen for women.

As already discussed, there are good reasons for believing that mortality patterns for tuberculosis and stomach cancer in adult life in part reflect patterns of risk of infection in childhood by specific pathogens. These risks in turn are related to standards of hygiene, sanitation, and living conditions. Is it possible that the contrasts in stroke may be related to poor childhood circumstances in the same way as tuberculosis and stomach cancer (Davey Smith et al., 1998b)?

One approach to this question is to identify an independent measure of the past socio-economic conditions of a country, particularly those associated with poor housing, hygiene, and sanitation. Infant mortality rates provide a proxy index of this sort, particularly for the early part of this century, where infection constituted the main cause of infant death. The link with poor hygiene and sanitation is particularly strong at this point in most countries, with deaths from diarrhoeal disease, dysentery, and other enteric infections being particularly important under the age of one year (Woods et al., 1988).

To examine the link between infant mortality (as a proxy for poor social conditions in early life) and mortality rates in adult life, a simple strategy may be used (Leon and Davey Smith, 2000). Cause-specific mortality rates in the early

Table 4.3 Correlation coefficients for mortality rates* between European countries by cause, aged 20–74, 1988–92

	Pulmonary tuberculosis	Stomach cancer	Stroke	Coronary heart disease
		Males		
Pulmonary tuberculosis	1.00			
Stomach cancer	0.87	1.00		
Stroke	0.83	0.88	1.00	
Coronary heart disease	0.39	0.53	0.57	1.00
		Females		
Pulmonary tuberculosis	1.00			
Stomach cancer	0.75	1.00		
Stroke	0.77	0.88	1.00	
Coronary heart disease	0.48	0.65	0.72	1.00

*Rates age-standardized to European population. Correlations estimated using log (rate)
Source: WHO Mortality Database

1990s (1991–3) among those aged 65–74 years define the mortality experience of people born around 1920 (1917–28, to be exact). We can therefore use infant mortality rates for 1921–3 (or 1920–4 when not available) as an indicator of social conditions (housing, hygiene, and sanitation) in infancy and early childhood for this particular birth cohort of people. The results of correlating infant mortality with adult mortality from a variety of causes are shown in Table 4.4.

The close relationship of infant mortality 1921–3 with stomach cancer rates 1991–3 for men aged 65–74 is shown in more detail in Fig. 4.14. The association seen for women is similar, as witnessed by the similar correlation coefficients for stomach cancer for men and women seen in Table 4.4. One of the striking features of Fig. 4.14 is that Japan and Russia are close to one another, both having historically very high rates of infant mortality and current high rates of stomach cancer. This proximity is particularly striking, given that today the countries are very different. In 1993, Japan was one of the most affluent nations and had the highest life expectancy of any country in the world, while Russia was in the throes of a major social and economic upheaval and had the lowest of any industrialized country. This reinforces the interpretation of the correlation between stomach cancer and infant mortality as being driven by specific factors in early life.

Table 4.4 Correlation coefficients (p-values) of adult mortality age 65–74 years in 1991–3 with infant mortality at time of birth and at time of death for 27 countries

	Infant mortality 1921–23		Infant mortality 1991–93	
	Males	Females	Males	Females
	Pearson correlation coefficients			
All causes	0.52 (0.005)	0.51 (0.007)	0.58 (0.002)	0.63 (<0.001)
Respiratory TB	0.77 (<0.001)	0.73 (<0.001)	0.40 (0.04)	0.33 (0.09)
Stomach cancer	0.83 (<0.001)	0.82 (<0.001)	0.39 (0.04)	0.44 (0.02)
Lung cancer	−0.10 (0.61)	−0.48 (0.01)	−0.02 (0.91)	−0.23 (0.24)
Coronary heart disease	−0.05 (0.81)	0.16 (0.42)	0.13 (0.53)	0.28 (0.16)
Stroke	0.66 (<0.001)	0.63 (<0.001)	0.61 (<0.001)	0.64 (<0.001)
	Partial correlation coefficients (see note at base of table)			
All causes	0.32 (0.11)	0.28 (0.17)	0.42 (0.03)	0.50 (0.009)
Respiratory TB	0.71 (<0.001)	0.69 (<0.001)	0.01 (0.96)	−0.07 (0.72)
Stomach cancer	0.80 (<0.001)	0.77 (<0.001)	−0.08 (0.71)	0.04 (0.87)
Lung cancer	−0.10 (0.60)	−0.43 (0.03)	0.04 (0.86)	0.02 (0.92)
Coronary heart disease	−0.13 (0.52)	0.03 (0.90)	0.18 (0.39)	0.23 (0.27)
Stroke	0.51 (0.008)	0.45 (0.02)	0.42 (0.03)	0.48 (0.01)

Notes: Sex and cause-specific correlations of adult mortality with infant mortality in one period adjusted for infant mortality in the other period. The 27 countries in the analyses were: Australia; Austria; Belgium; Bulgaria; Canada; Chile; Czechoslovakia; Denmark; Finland; France; Greece; Hungary; Ireland; Italy; Japan; Netherlands; New Zealand; Norway; Poland; Portugal; Romania; Russian Federation; Spain; Sweden; Switzerland; UK; US

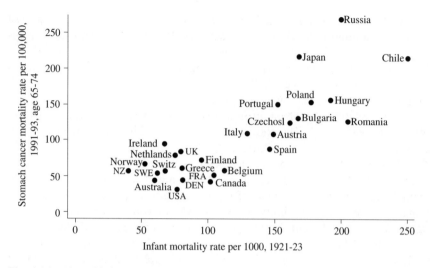

Fig. 4.14 Plot of infant mortality 1921–23 against stomach cancer mortality 1991–3 for men aged 65–74 in 27 countries
Source: Leon and Davey Smith (2000)

Could some of the correlation between infant mortality at time of birth with adult mortality be because countries that historically had poor socio-economic conditions still do so today—and it is current circumstances that are the main determinant of these correlations? To examine this possible confounding effect of current circumstances, Table 4.4 also shows correlations of adult mortality 1991–3 with infant mortality in the same period. For stomach cancer, these correlations are appreciable, but considerably smaller than with mortality at the time of birth. Partial correlation coefficients are also shown in the bottom half of the table, where the correlations of adult mortality with infant mortality in the two periods are mutually adjusted. These partial coefficients indicate that the association for stomach cancer is almost exclusively with infant mortality at the time of birth. Given what has already been discussed about tuberculosis mortality in the preceding sections, it is not surprising that it is also more strongly related to infant mortality at the time of birth than currently. In the countries covered in this analysis, most people dying of respiratory tuberculosis aged 65–74 years today will have been initially infected during their early years. Stroke mortality also shows the same sort of strong positive association with infant mortality at the time of birth as stomach cancer and tuberculosis, but also shows an association with current levels of infant mortality, unlike stomach cancer and tuberculosis. Most notable of all, however, in contrast to stomach cancer, tuberculosis, and stroke, CHD shows no systematic association with infant mortality, either at the time of birth, or concurrently.

Table 4.4 also shows correlation coefficients for two other causes of death. Lung cancer shows an appreciable inverse correlation with infant mortality at birth for women only, with historical levels of infant mortality being predictive of the position of women in society, which in turn is related to cohort differences in the uptake of tobacco smoking by women. This again fits in with what has already been said about the very contingent and variable nature of the link between socio-economic factors and lung cancer rates. Breast cancer shows a predictable inverse association with infant mortality around the time of birth, suggesting that risk factors may be influenced by early life and childhood circumstances through biological mechanisms (such as growth) as well as through cultural and social mechanisms that influence later patterns of childbearing.

These analyses suggest that poor infant and childhood environment, associated with high infant mortality, may explain some of the similarities in the patterns observed for stomach cancer, tuberculosis, and stroke. They also reinforce the fact that there are major differences in the aetiology of stroke and CHD (Gale and Martyn, 1997), with adverse early life circumstances being considerably more important for the former. The idea that within- and between-country variations in CHD mortality may reflect the influence of factors operating across the life course, some of which may be more or less strongly related to socio-economic circumstances, is developed by Davey Smith et al. in chapter 5 (this volume).

Conclusion

This chapter has considered a range of evidence that suggests that there are important common threads that underlie the pattern of inequalities in mortality within and between countries. Moreover, some of these common threads involve the action of factors that span the life course of individuals. The assumption that inequalities in health today, whether between or within countries, are caused by contemporaneous differences in circumstances of life is not sustainable for a range of important diseases that appear to be driven instead by poor socio-economic circumstances in early life and childhood. This insight has important implications for the assessment of the time-scale over which any public health interventions can be expected to reduce inequalities for specific causes. There is a need for a more nuanced approach to the way we think about the temporal dimension of cause and effect relationships. This is important, both for understanding the causes of inequalities and for developing effective and realistic strategies to ameliorate them.

Acknowledgements

The development of many of the ideas presented in this chapter has benefited from discussions with colleagues, in particular George Davey Smith and Martin McKee. I would also like to thank Susan Morton, Denny Vågerö, and Gill Walt for comments on an earlier draft.

REFERENCES

Anderson RT, Sorlie P, Backlund E, Johnson N, Kaplan GA. Mortality effects of community socioeconomic status. *Epidemiology*, 1997; **8**:42–7

Barker DJP. Fetal origins of coronary heart disease. *British Medical Journal*, 1995; **311**:171–4

Barker DJP. *Mothers, babies and health in later life*. Edinburgh: Churchill Livingstone, 1998

Barker DJ, Coggon D, Osmond C, Wickham C. Poor housing in childhood and high rates of stomach cancer in England and Wales. *British Journal of Cancer*, 1990; **61**:575–8

Barker DJP, Gluckman PD, Godfrey KM, Harding JE, Owens JA, Robinson JS. Fetal nutrition and cardiovascular disease in adult life. *Lancet*, 1993; **341**:938–41

Bobák M, .Marmot MG. East–West mortality divide and its potential explanations: proposed research agenda. *British Medical Journal*, 1996; **312**:421–5

Brown JW, Lal M. An inquiry into the relation between social status and cancer mortality. *Journal of Hygiene*, 1914; **14**:186–200

Cantwell MF, McKenna MT, McCray E, Onorato IM. Tuberculosis and race/ethnicity in the United States: impact of socioeconomic status. *American Journal of Respiratory and Critical Care Medicine*, 1998; **157**:1016–20

Case RAM. Tumours of the urinary tract as an occupational disease in several industries. *Annals of the Royal College of Surgeons of England*, 1966; **39**:213–35

Chenet L, McKee M, Fulop N *et al.* Changing life expectancy in central Europe: is there a single reason? *Journal of Public Health Medicine*, 1996; **s18**:329–36

Cohart EM. Socioeconomic distribution of stomach cancer in New Haven. *Cancer*, 1954; **7**:455–61

Coleman MP, Babb P, Damiecki P *et al. Cancer survival trends in England and Wales 1971–1995: deprivation and NHS region*. Series SMPS No. 61. London: The Stationery Office, 1999

Davey Smith G, Leon DA, Shipley MJ, Rose G. Socio-economic differentials in cancer among men. *International Journal of Epidemiology*, 1991; **20**:339–45

Davey Smith G, Neaton JD, Wentworth D, Stamler R, Stamler J. Mortality differences between black and white men in the USA: contribution of income and other risk factors among men screened for the MRFIT. MRFIT Research Group. Multiple Risk Factor Intervention Trial. *Lancet*, 1998a; **351**:934–9

Davey Smith G, Hart C, Blane D, Hole D. Adverse socioeconomic conditions in childhood and cause specific adult mortality: prospective observational study. *British Medical Journal*, 1998b; **316**:1631–5

Devesa SS, Diamond EL. Association of breast cancer and cervical cancer incidence with income and education among whites and blacks. *Journal of the National Cancer Institute*, 1980; **65**:515–28

Drever F, Whitehead M. *Health inequalities: decennial supplement*. Series DS No. 15. London: The Stationery Office, 1997

Eames M, Ben-Shlomo Y, Marmot MG. Social deprivation and premature mortality : regional comparison across England. *British Medical Journal*, 1993; **307**:1097–102

Enos WF, Holmes RH, Beyer J. Coronary disease among United States soldiers killed in action in Korea: preliminary report. *Journal of the American Medical Association*, 1953; **152**:1090–3

EUROGAST Study Group. An international association between Helicobacter pylori infection and gastric cancer. *Lancet*, 1993; **341**:1359–62

Faggiano F, Partanen T, Kogevinas M, Boffetta P. Socioeconomic differences in cancer. In: Kogevinas M, Pearce N, Susser M, Boffetta P (eds) *Social inequalities and cancer*. Lyon: International Agency for Research on Cancer, 1997, pp 65–176

Frost WH. The age selection of mortality from tuberculosis in successive decades. *American Journal of Hygiene*, 1939; **30**:91–6

Gale CR, Martyn CN. The conundrum of time trends in stroke. *Journal of the Royal Society of Medicine*, 1997; **90**:138–43

Hansson LE, Bergstrom R, Sparen P, Adami HO. The decline in the incidence of stomach cancer in Sweden 1960–1984: a birth cohort phenomenon. *International Journal of Cancer*, 1991; **47**:499–503

Heron D. Note on class incidence of cancer. *British Medical Journal*, 1907; **i**:621–2

Hertzman C, Kelly S, Bobák M. *East–West life expectancy gap in Europe: environmental and non-environmental determinants*. Dordrecht: Kluwer Academic Publishers, 1996

Hudelson P. Gender differentials in tuberculosis: the role of socio-economic and cultural factors. *Tubercle and Lung Disease*, 1996; **77**:391–400

Judge K, Mulligan JA, Benzeval M. Income inequality and population health. *Social Science and Medicine*, 1998; **46**:567–79

Kawachi I, Kennedy BP. Health and social cohesion: why care about income inequality? *British Medical Journal*, 1997; **314**:1037–40

Kawachi I, Kennedy BP, Wilkinson RG. Crime: social disorganization and relative deprivation. *Social Science and Medicine*, 1999; **48**:719–31

Kitagawa EM, Hauser PM. Differential mortality in the United States: a study in socioeconomic epidemiology. Cambridge, MA: Harvard University Press, 1973

Kogevinas M, Porta M. Socioeconomic differences in cancer survival: a review of the evidence. In: Kogevinas M, Pearce N, Susser M, Boffetta P (eds) *Social inequalities and cancer*. Lyon: International Agency for Research on Cancer, 1997, pp 177–206

Kogevinas M, Pearce N, Susser M, Boffetta P (eds). *Social inequalities and cancer*. Lyon: International Agency for Research on Cancer, 1997, pp 65–176

Kubik AK, Parkin DM, Plesko I *et al*. Patterns of cigarette sales and lung cancer mortality in some central and eastern European countries, 1960–1989. *Cancer*, 1995; **75**:2452–60

Kuh D, Ben-Shlomo Y. *A life course approach to chronic disease epidemiology*. Oxford: Oxford University Press, 1997

Kunst A. *Cross-national comparisons of socio-economic differences in mortality*. Rotterdam: Erasmus University, Department of Public Health, 1997

Law M, Wald N. Why heart disease mortality is low in France: the time lag explanation. *British Medical Journal*, 1999; **318**:1471–6

Leon DA, Ben-Shlomo Y. Pre-adult influences on cardiovascular disease and cancer. In Kuh D, Ben-Shlomo Y (eds) *A life course approach to chronic disease epidemiology*. Oxford: Oxford University Press, 1997, pp 45–77

Leon DA, Bobák M. *East–West differences in mortality: do they parallel socio-economic differences within the West?* Presentation at XVIIth ASPHER General Assembly, London School of Hygiene & Tropical Medicine, 6–8 September 1995 (unpublished)

Leon DA, Davey Smith G. Infant mortality, stomach cancer, stroke and coronary heart disease: ecological analysis *British Medical Journal*, 2000; **320**:1705–6

Leon DA, Koupilová I. Birth weight, blood pressure and hypertension: epidemiological studies. In: Barker DJP (ed) *Fetal origins of cardiovascular and lung disease.* Atlanta: National Institutes for Health, 2000

Leon DA, Chenet L, Shkolnikov VM *et al.* Huge variation in Russian mortality rates 1984–1994: artefact or alcohol or what? *Lancet*, 1997; **350**:383–8

Logan WPD. *Cancer mortality by occupation and social class 1851–1971.* London: HMSO, 1982

Lucas A. Programming by early nutrition in man. In: Bock GR, Whelan J (eds) *The childhood environment and adult disease. Ciba Foundation Symposium 156.* Chichester: Wiley, 1991, pp 38–50

Maaroos HI. Helicobacter pylori infection in Estonian population: is it a health problem? *Annals of Medicine*, 1995; **27**:613–6

McCord C, Freeman HP. Excess mortality in Harlem. *New England Journal of Medicine*, 1990; **322**:173–7

Macfarlane GJ, Macfarlane TV, Lowenfels AB. The influence of alcohol consumption on worldwide trends in mortality from upper aerodigestive tract cancers in men. *Journal of Epidemiology and Community Health,* 1996; **50**:636–9

Macintyre S, MacIver S, Sooman A. Area, class and health: should we be focussing on places or people? *Journal of Social Policy*, 1993; **22**:213–34

McKee M, Bobák M, Rose R, Shkolnikov V, Chenet L, Leon D. Patterns of smoking in Russia. *Tobacco Control*, 1998; **7**:22–6

McKeigue PM. Diabetes and insulin action. In: Kuh D, Ben-Shlomo Y (eds) *A life course approach to chronic disease epidemiology.* Oxford: Oxford University Press, 1997, pp 78–100

McLoone P, Boddy FA. Deprivation and mortality in Scotland, 1981 and 1991. *British Medical Journal*, 1994; **309**:1465–70

McNamara JJ, Molot MA, Stremple JF, Cutting RT. Coronary artery disease in combat casualties in Vietnam. *Journal of the American Medical Association*, 1971; **216**:1185–7

McWhorter WP, Schatzkin AG, Horm JW, Brown CC. Contribution of socioeconomic status to black/white differences in cancer incidence. *Cancer*, 1989; **63**:982–7

Malaty HM, Paykov V, Bykova O *et al.* Helicobacter pylori and socioeconomic factors in Russia. *Helicobacter*, 1996; **1**:82–7

Malaty HM, Graham DY, Wattigney WA, Srinivasan SR, Osato M, Berenson GS. Natural history of Helicobacter pylori infection in childhood: 12-year follow-up cohort study in a biracial community. *Clinical Infectious Diseases*, 1999; **28**:279–82

Mendall MA, Goggin PM, Molineaux N *et al.* Childhood living conditions and Helicobacter pylori seropositivity in adult life. *Lancet*, 1992; **339**:896–7

Meslé F, Hertrich V. Mortality trends in Europe; the widening gap between East and West. *International Population Conference Proceedings.* Beijing: IUSSP, 1997, pp 479–508

Murray CJL, Lopez AD. Mortality by cause for eight regions of the world: Global Burden of Disease Study. *Lancet*, 1997*a*; **349**:1269–76

Murray CJL, Lopez AD. Regional patterns of disability-free life expectancy and disability—adjusted life expectancy: global Burden of Disease Study. *Lancet*, 1997*b*; **349**:1347–52

Nestle M. Wine and coronary heart disease. *Lancet*, 1992; **40**:314–5

Office of Population Censuses and Surveys. *Occupational mortality. The Registrar General's decennial supplement for England and Wales, 1970–72*. Series DS No.1. London: HMSO, 1978

Office of Population Censuses and Surveys. *Occupational mortality. The Registrar General's decennial supplement for Great Britain, 1979–80, 1982–83*. Series DS No.6. London: HMSO, 1986

Parsonnett J. Helicobacter pylori and gastric adenocarcinoma. In: Parsonnet J (ed) *Microbes and malignancy. Infection as a cause of human cancers*. Oxford: Oxford University Press, 1999, pp 372–408

Peto R, Lopez AD, Boreham J, Thun M, Heath C, Jr., Doll R. Mortality from smoking worldwide. *British Medical Bulletin*, 1996; **52**:12–21

Preston SH. *Mortality patterns in national populations with special reference to recorded causes of death*. New York: Academic Press, 1976

Robinson JS, McMillen C, Edwards L *et al*. The effect of maternal nutrition on growth and development before and after birth. In: O'Brien PMS, Wheeler T, Barker DJP (eds) *Fetal programming: influences on development and disease in later life*. London: RCOG Press, 1999, pp 217–30

Shear CL, Dorling D, Gordon D, Davey Smith G. *The widening gap*. London: The Policy Press, 1999

Shkolnikov VM, Cornia AG, Leon DA, Meslé F. Causes of the Russian mortality crisis: evidence and interpretations. *World Development*, 1998; **26**:1995–2011

Silva IDS, Beral V. Socioeconomic differences in reproductive behaviour. In: Kogevinas M, Pearce N, Susser M, Boffetta P (eds) *Social inequalities and cancer*. Lyon: International Agency for Research on Cancer, 1997, pp 285–308

Sloggett A, Joshi H. Higher mortality in deprived areas: community or personal disadvantage? *British Medical Journal*, 1994; **309**:1470–4

Tunstall PH. Autres pays, autres moeurs [editorial]. *British Medical Journal,* 1988; **297**:1559–60

US Department of Health and Human Services. *Tobacco use among US racial/ethnic minority groups—African Americans, American Indians and Alaska Natives, Asian Americans and Pacific Islanders, and Hispanics: a report of the Surgeon General*. Atlanta, Georgia: US Department of Health and Human Services, Centres for Disease Control and Prevention, National Centre for Chronic Disease Prevention and Health Promotion, Office on Smoking and Health, 1998

Uemura K, Pisa Z. Trends in cardiovascular disease mortality in industrialized countries since 1950. *World Health Statistics Quarterly*, 1988; **41**:155–78

Waller M, Lipponen S (eds). *Smokefree Europe: a forum for networks*. Conference on Tobacco or Health, Helsinki, Finland, 2–4 October 1996. Helsinki: Finnish Centre for Health Promotion, 1997

Waterland RA, Garza C. Potential mechanisms of metabolic imprinting that lead to chronic disease. *American Journal of Clinical Nutrition*, 1999; **69**:179–97

Wilkinson RG. *Unhealthy societies: the afflictions of inequality*. London: Routledge, 1996

Woods RI, Watterson PA, Woodward JH. The causes of rapid infant mortality decline in England and Wales, 1861–1921. Part I. *Population Studies*, 1988; **42**:343–66

World Health Organization. Mortality database. http://www-nt.who.int/whosis/statistics 15 August 2000

5 Life-course approaches to socio-economic differentials in cause-specific adult mortality

George Davey Smith, David Gunnell, and Yoav Ben-Shlomo

There is now a considerable body of research on the origins of socio-economic differentials in health and mortality within high-income countries, much of it inspired by the publication of the report of the Black Committee in the UK (GB DHSS, 1980). This research has tended to focus on the four basic categories of explanation—artefact, health-related social selection, behavioural/cultural patterns (including use of health services), and material circumstances—and has led to varying conclusions regarding the relative importance of these in producing the observed health differentials (Whitehead, 1992; Davey Smith et al., 1994; Macintyre, 1997; Denton and Walters, 1999).

General susceptibility

When considering the origins of health inequalities, the specific factors contributing to the socio-economic distribution of particular causes of ill-health and death have been investigated in less detail than have the general categories of explanation listed above. This partly reflects the availability of data: most of the data sources used in documenting health inequalities do not contain detailed information regarding underlying social factors, potential mediators, and specific health outcomes in large enough samples to allow such analytical approaches (Hummer et al., 1998). However, the lack of attention to cause-specific analyses may also reflect the underlying models of disease causation which the investigators hold, particularly for those emphasizing the shared risk from many forms of ill-health seen among less favoured socio-demographic groups—a model sometimes referred to as 'general susceptibility' (Syme and Berkman, 1976; Najman and Congalton, 1979; Pearce et al., 1983; Marmot et al., 1984).

Several processes which could lead to increased susceptibility to disease in general amongst the less economically favoured have been proposed, including psycho-social stress, poor diet, inadequate coping resources, and genetic differences (Thurlow, 1967; Najman, 1980; Valkonen, 1987*a*). A wide range of physiological measures have been postulated to be potential mechanisms for the increased susceptibility, largely within the stress paradigm (Sterling and Eyer, 1981; Totman, 1987; Brunner, 1997). However, data from several sources suggest that the general susceptibility argument is inconsistent with the true complexity of socio-economic differentials in health. When particular causes of ill-health and death are examined, there is a considerable degree of heterogeneity in their association with socio-economic position. Figure 5.1 presents data relating to cancer from the Whitehall study of London civil servants, among whom there was a marked gradient in the association between employment grade and all-cause mortality (Marmot *et al.*, 1984). For overall cancer mortality, the lower grade civil servants (clerical and manual) had a 48% higher risk than the higher grades (administrators, professionals, and executives). However, for the thirteen specific cancer sites examined, grade-related risk varied by site. The low grade civil servants had a greater mortality risk for seven of the cancer sites, the higher grades had a greater risk for six (Davey Smith *et al.*, 1991). Similar findings with respect to the heterogeneity of site-specific cancer risk with socio-economic position have come from other studies (Faggiano *et al.*, 1997; Fernandez and Borrell, 1999).

In Table 5.1, data for a wider range of causes of death are presented from the mortality follow-up of a third of a million men in the US (Davey Smith *et al.*, 1996). Relative risks are given for mortality associated with $10,000 lower median income of the area of residence (Zip Code areas being used for this purpose). For some causes of death—including AIDS, homicide, respiratory disease, diabetes, and rheumatic heart disease—there are large differentials, with

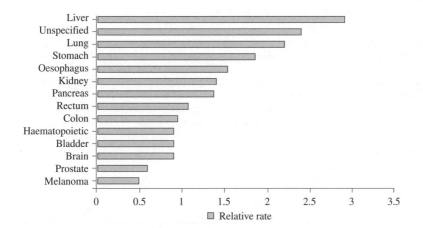

Fig. 5.1 Cancer by employment grade in the Whitehall Study
Source: Davey Smith *et al.*, 1991

relative risks greater than 1.5 per $10,000 lower Zip Code income. For other causes of death, including such major contributors to all-cause mortality as coronary heart disease, lung cancer, and stroke, the relative risks associated with $10,000 lower income were in the range 1.21–1.50. For a large number of causes of death—many of them relatively minor contributors to all-cause mortality—there were weak or reversed gradients between income and risk. The marked heterogeneity in the strength and even direction of the associations between socio-economic position and cause-specific mortality draws attention to the need for explanatory models which account for both the overall and the specific health effects of socio-economic position.

Fundamental and proximal causes of health inequalities

The Black Report committee made a distinction between fundamental and proximal causes of inequalities in health, concluding, for example, that 'smoking behaviour cannot be taken as a fundamental cause of ill-health, it is rather an epiphenomenon, a secondary symptom of deeper underlying features of economic society' (GB DHSS, 1980) and therefore policy makers needed to ask 'about the social and economic factors which explain … the prevalence of smoking in the first place, and whether these, independent of individual education and counselling, have to be given priority in reducing the differentials' (GB DHSS, 1980).

The notion of 'fundamental causes' stretches back to the beginnings of social

Table 5.1 Proportional increase in cause-specific mortality (relative risk) per $10,000 decrease in median income of area of residence (ZIP code) in US men screened in the MRFIT study

RR>1.50	RR 1.21–1.50	RR 1.00–1.20	RR<1.00
AIDS	Infection	Aortic aneurysm	Blood disease
Diabetes	Coronary heart disease	Suicide	Motor neurone disease
Rheumatic heart disease	Stroke	Nervous system disease	Flying accidents
Heart failure	Cirrhosis	Oesophageal cancer	Lymphoma
COPD	Genitourinary disease	Stomach cancer	Hodgkin's disease
Pneumonia/Influenza	Symptoms/signs	Pancreatic cancer	Melanoma
Homicide	Accidents	Prostate cancer	Bone/connective tissue cancer
	Lung cancer	Bladder cancer	
	Liver cancer	Kidney cancer	
	Colorectal cancer	Brain cancer	
		Myeloma	
		Leukaemia	

Source: Davey Smith *et al.*, 1996

epidemiology. For example, in *The condition of the working class in England*, Friedrich Engels considered that deficiencies in nutrition clearly contributed to the poor health of the labouring classes in the early 1840s (Engels, 1987). The financial straits of many families contributed to their poor nutrition, but beyond this there were many other ways in which the poor were disadvantaged with respect to diet. The payment of wages on Saturday evening meant that the workers could only buy their food after the middle class had had first choice during Saturday morning. When the workers reached the market:

> the best has vanished and, if it was still there they would probably not be able to buy it. The potatoes which the workers buy are usually poor, the vegetables wilted, the cheese old and of poor quality, the bacon rancid, the meat lean, tough, taken from old, often diseased, cattle, or such as have died a natural death, and not fresh even then, often half decayed.

The working classes were more likely to be sold adulterated food, Engels argued, because while the rich developed sensitive palates through habitual good eating and could detect adulteration, the poor had little opportunity to cultivate their taste. The poor also had to deal with small retailers who could not sell:

> even the same quality of goods so cheaply as the largest retailers, because of their small capital and the large proportional expenses of their business, must knowingly or unknowingly buy adulterated goods in order to sell at the lower prices required, and to meet the competition of the others.

Thus, according to Engels, the diet of the working class was clearly detrimental to their health, but this immediately begged the question as to why such a poor diet was consumed by the labouring classes. Data from several sources indicates that Engels' basic observation remains relevant today: those least able to purchase a healthy diet due to financial constraints are also those most likely to be disadvantaged with regard to access to healthy, micro-nutrient dense food. For example, a survey carried out in London in 1988 and repeated in 1995 found that at both times healthy food was more expensive in the deprived area while unhealthy food was slightly cheaper in the deprived area (Lobstein, 1995).

Recognition of the distinction between fundamental and proximal causes of health inequalities should broaden the explanatory framework and emphasize the need to account for the distribution of proximal causes, as well as demonstrate the role of these proximal causes in mediating between social factors and the distribution of disease. If, for example, it is shown that differences in dietary patterns between socio-economic groups account for at least some of the differentials in cardiovascular disease and cancer mortality, then the elements of social organization of dietary practices, discussed above, should be considered as the antecedent causes. These antecedents include inequitable income and wealth distribution, the profit-driven organization of food retailing, unequal educational opportunities and the failure of collective resistance to such inequities. The concentration of interventions upon proximal rather than fundamental causes of disease may underlie the disappointing outcomes of many health promotion programmes. Thus risk-factor modification approaches to reducing cardiovascular disease risk among the general population have had unimpressive effects (Ebrahim and Davey Smith, 1997; 1998), at the same time that secular changes in the social circumstances of population groups have been associated with dramatic decreases or increases in cardiovascular mortality. These secular mortality trends indicate that social change can result in sizeable changes in disease risk within populations, while interventions targeted at individuals have little impact on risk.

Socio-economic position across the life course and mortality

It is against this background that we enter into a discussion of the contribution of socially-patterned exposures across the life course to the production of health inequalities. While descriptive and analytical reviews are available of the socio-economic distribution of the major causes of death in adulthood (Kaplan and Keil, 1993; Kogevinas et al., 1997), existing studies have tended to focus on one phase of life—usually risk factors acting during adulthood, although recently there has also been an exclusive focus on the genesis of risk in very early life (Barker, 1991). We differ from these approaches by emphasizing the need to adopt a life-course approach to the development of chronic disease in adulthood (Kuh and Ben-Shlomo, 1997); an approach which we feel should also be applied to inequalities in health (Davey Smith, 1997a; 1997b). We therefore concentrate on studies which provide data about socio-economic circumstances and socially-patterned exposures at different stages of life.

A report on inequalities in health from the Department of Health for England and Wales concluded that 'it is likely that accumulative differential lifetime exposure to health-damaging or health-promoting physical and social environments is the main explanation for the observed variations in health and life expectancy' (GB Department of Health, 1995). However, while the socio-economic gradients in all-cause mortality among adults in high-income countries are very well described, few studies have empirical data regarding the effects on mortality of the cumulative experience of social disadvantage. In a prospective study in the West of Scotland (the Collaborative Study) it was possible to relate socio-economic position across the life course to mortality risk among men aged 35–64 who reported (a) details of their fathers' main occupation (as an index of social circumstances in childhood); (b) their own occupation at labour market entry; and (c) their current occupation (Davey Smith et al., 1997). A simple index of lifetime social circumstances was constructed, which ranged from those men with the least favourable socio-economic trajectories (with manual fathers and in a manual job themselves, both at labour market entry and in middle age), to those with the most favourable trajectories (non-manual fathers and non-manual jobs at labour market entry and middle age). Over a 21-year follow-up period, all-cause and cardiovascular disease mortality risk was strongly related to lifetime social circumstances (Table 5.2). Statistical adjustment for a wide range of risk factors measured in adulthood—including smoking, cholesterol, blood pressure, body mass index, and lung function—failed to account for much of this gradient.

Treated as single variables, the indicators of socio-economic position in childhood, early adulthood and middle age all predicted mortality in later adulthood (Table 5.3). The relative contribution of socio-economic circumstances at different stages of life was then investigated by entering social position at the three life course stages simultaneously into a multivariable model. Father's social class and current social class (at screening) both remained predictors of mortality, while social class at labour market entry became non-predictive. For all-cause mortality, the manual to non-manual relative risks were closely similar for father's social class and current social class. When different broad cause of death groups were examined, father's social class made a particular contribution to cardiovascular disease risk, while it was only weakly and non-significantly associated with cancer mortality once current social class was taken into account. For mortality from 'other' causes, current social class also appeared to be the more important socio-economic indicator.

These data indicate that socio-economic circumstances at different stages of the life course contribute to mortality risk in adulthood. They also show that these contributions differ between different broad cause-of-death groups. They suggest that deprivation in childhood increases the risk of cardiovascular disease in adulthood, but that adulthood circumstances also contribute to risk.

Table 5.2 Relative death rates (95% confidence intervals) by cumulative social class, adjusted for age and risk factors, for men in the West of Scotland Collaborative Study

	Cumulative Social Class				
	All three non-manual	Two non-manual, one manual	Two manual one non-manual	All three manual	p value for trend
All causes					
Age	1	1.29 (1.08, 1.56)	1.45 (1.21, 1.73)	1.71 (1.46, 2.01)	<0.0001
Age and risk factor*	1	1.30 (1.08, 1.57)	1.33 (1.11, 1.60)	1.57 (1.33, 1.85)	<0.0001
Cardiovascular causes					
Age	1	1.51 (1.16, 1.98)	1.90 (1.47, 2.45)	1.94 (1.53, 2.45)	<0.0001
Age and risk factor*	1	1.57 (1.20, 2.05)	1.78 (1.37, 2.31)	1.92 (1.51, 2.45)	<0.0001

* Adjusted for age, smoking, diastolic blood pressure, cholesterol concentration, body mass index, adjusted FEV_1, angina, bronchitis and ECG ischaemia
Source: Davey Smith *et al.*, 1997

Table 5.3 Mortality by social class at three different stages of the life course in the West of Scotland Collaborative Study

Age-adjusted relative rates for manual compared with non-manual social class locations, with individual and simultaneous adjustments for each social class indicator

	Father's social class	First social class	Current social class
All cause			
Individual	1.44 (1.27 – 1.64)	1.29 (1.16 – 1.43)	1.40 (1.27 – 1.55)
Simultaneous	1.28 (1.11 – 1.47)	1.01 (0.89 – 1.16)	1.29 (1.14 – 1.47)
Cardiovascular disease			
Individual	1.58 (1.32 – 1.89)	1.35 (1.16 – 1.56)	1.38 (1.20 – 1.59)
Simultaneous	1.41 (1.15 – 1.72)	1.08 (0.90 – 1.30)	1.20 (1.01 – 1.43)
Cancer			
Individual	1.26 (1.02 – 1.56)	1.25 (1.04 – 1.50)	1.35 (1.13 – 1.61)
Simultaneous	1.11 (0.87 – 1.41)	1.04 (0.82 – 1.31)	1.28 (1.03 – 1.60)
Non cardiovascular, non cancer			
Individual	1.45 (1.07 – 1.98)	1.18 (0.92 – 1.53)	1.59 (1.24 – 2.03)
Simultaneous	1.28 (0.91 – 1.80)	0.80 (0.58 – 1.10)	1.67 (1.22 – 2.28)

Source: Davey Smith *et al.*, 1997

They also suggest that, for the aggregate category of other causes of death, socially-determined exposures in adulthood are of key importance, although, as we will see, for some specific causes within this grouping this is not the case.

In the same study, data were also available on age at leaving full-time education. Education was related to mortality risk (all causes) and broad cause-of-death groups (Davey Smith *et al.*, 1998a) and, as with the cumulative socio-economic position measure, these associations could not be explained by risk factors measured in adulthood (Davey Smith and Hart, 1998) (Table 5.4). Education was related to both early-life and later-life socio-economic position, and further analyses demonstrated that it acts similarly to father's social class, in being more strongly associated with cardiovascular disease mortality than with the other cause-of-death categories (Davey Smith *et al.*, 1998a). It therefore seems that educational level serves, in part at least, as an indicator of socio-economic experience in childhood. This conclusion is the same as one drawn 30 years ago by Hinkle and colleagues in their classic study of coronary heart disease among employees of the Bell telephone company (Hinkle *et al.*, 1968). They observed the particular dependence of risk on education and considered this to indicate that 'some aspects of the origin of coronary heart disease must be sought for in childhood or adolescence, if not earlier'.

The above data suggest that the relative importance of socially patterned exposures at different stages of life will differ between particular causes of death. We therefore now review the evidence on this issue for several specific adulthood diseases.

Table 5.4 Age-adjusted all-cause and cardiovascular disease (CVD) relative mortality rates according to social class and education, adjusted for age and risk factors,* in the West of Scotland Collaborative Study

Mortality			Social Class				
	I	II	IIIN	IIIM	IV	V	
All cause mortality							
Age-adjusted RR (95% CI)	1	1.07 (0.88–1.31)	1.45 (1.20–1.76)	1.65 (1.38–1.97)	1.63 (1.35–1.97)	1.74 (1.34–2.26)	
Multivariate RR (95% CI)*	1	1.05 (0.86–1.29)	1.42 (1.17–1.73)	1.52 (1.26–1.83)	1.50 (1.23–1.83)	1.65 (1.26–2.17)	
CVD mortality							
Age-adjusted RR (95% CI)	1	1.47 (1.09–1.97)	1.84 (1.38–2.46)	2.03 (1.55–2.66)	2.00 (1.50–2.66)	1.86 (1.25–2.70)	
Multivariate RR (95% CI)*	1	1.45 (1.08–1.95)	1.84 (1.38–2.47)	1.99 (1.51–2.63)	2.02 (1.50–2.71)	1.96 (1.30–2.95)	

Mortality	Age Leaving Full-time Education, y				
	19+	17–18	15–16	12–14	
All cause mortality					
Age-adjusted RR (95% CI)	1	1.20 (0.93–1.55)	1.40 (1.12–1.75)	1.67 (1.35–2.00)	
Multivariate RR (95% CI)*	1	1.23 (0.95–1.59)	1.37 (1.09–1.72)	1.56 (1.26–1.30)	
CVD mortality					
Age-adjusted RR (95% CI)	1	1.55 (1.06–2.26)	1.79 (1.28–2.51)	2.03 (1.47–2.80)	
Multivariate RR (95% CI)*	1	1.67 (1.14–2.44)	1.68 (1.34–2.64)	2.07 (1.49–2.30)	

*Adjusted for age, smoking, diastolic blood pressure, cholesterol concentration, body mass index, adjusted FEV$_1$, angina, bronchitis, and ECG ischaemia
Source: Davey Smith and Hart, 1998

Coronary heart disease (CHD)

Coronary heart disease is the major single cause of death among men in most of the industrialized world, and an increasingly important cause of death in urban areas of industrializing countries. In some ways, it can be seen as the cause of death which illustrates the life-course perspective *par excellence*, since risk is associated with parental health, with intrauterine development, with growth and health in childhood, and with several socio-economic and behavioural factors in adulthood. While the social patterning of CHD according to adulthood social position has been investigated extensively—and, in most industrialized countries, marked gradients of increasing risk with worsening social circumstances are seen—there has been relatively little investigation of life-course socio-economic influences on CHD risk.

Life-course influences on CHD risk

The importance of childhood and adulthood social circumstances can be illustrated with data from the West of Scotland Collaborative Study. In this study, father's social class as a measure of childhood social circumstances was predictive of CHD mortality, with a relative risk of 1.52 (95% confidence intervals 1.24–1.87) for men whose fathers were in manual occupations, compared to those with non-manual fathers (Davey Smith *et al.*, 1998*b*). There were three measures of adulthood social position available—own occupation in middle age, deprivation level of the area of residence, and car driving (as an indicator of car access, a useful marker for available income in UK studies). Adjustment for these markers of adulthood social circumstances reduced the strength of the association between father's social class and CHD mortality to 1.28 (95% C.I. 1.03–1.61). This adjusted effect, however, may be an under-estimation of the importance of early-life social circumstances. Early- and later-life social circumstances are linked, and the measures of adulthood circumstances are clearly superior, both in being multidimensional and in being likely to contain less measurement error than father's occupation reported by middle-aged men. The data therefore provide evidence that both early-life and later-life social circumstances contribute to CHD risk.

Studies in several other countries have examined the association between childhood social circumstances and CHD risk. Most have found a link that is apparently not purely due to adverse socio-economic destinations of those born into poor circumstances (Gillum and Paffenbarger, 1978; Burr and Sweetnam, 1980; Notkola *et al.*, 1985; Kaplan and Salonen, 1990; Vågerö and Leon, 1994; Gliksman *et al.*, 1995; Wannamethee *et al.*, 1996), although several have not (Hasle, 1990; Lynch *et al.*, 1994). In a Swedish census follow-up, men with fathers in manual occupations had considerably higher CHD mortality risk than those whose fathers were in non-manual occupations (Vågerö and Leon, 1994). For all-cause mortality, the association with father's social class was less clear, with mortality being dependent on adult social class to a considerably greater degree than childhood social class. The particular dependence of CHD risk in comparison to some other causes of death on childhood socio-economic circumstances has also been observed in area-based studies from Finland (Valkonen, 1987b; Koskinen, 1994).

Interest in the possible specific effects of socio-economic deprivation in early life on later health was stimulated by the work of Forsdahl (1977; 1978), and subsequently developed by Barker and Osmond (Barker and Osmond, 1986), who demonstrated that areas with high infant mortality rates earlier this century had high CHD rates currently. Forsdahl interpreted this as demonstrating that deprivation in early life, followed by later affluence, worked together to increase coronary risk. As Table 5.5 indicates, there is no evidence that later affluence is required to translate poor social circumstances in childhood into increased CHD risk in adulthood. Other studies which have looked for an interaction between childhood and adulthood social circumstances have also failed to find evidence to support this component of the Forsdahl hypothesis (Burr and Sweetnam, 1980; Notkola et al., 1985; Wannamethee et al., 1996).

Lifetime social circumstances and CHD risk factors

In the West of Scotland Collaborative Study, other potential pathways between social position in childhood and CHD risk in adulthood were examined, by analysing conventional risk factors in relation to father's (childhood) and own (adulthood) social class (Blane et al., 1996). Men with manual social class fathers had lower, rather than higher, serum cholesterol concentrations, compared with men with non-manual social class fathers. Behavioural risk factors, such as smoking and exercise, were more dependent on adulthood social position than parental social class. This supports the notion that such activities are powerfully influenced by the social environment experienced during adult life, and that modifying such behaviours is dependent upon the presence of the social circumstances required for maintaining favourable health-related behaviours. Blood pressure and lung

Table 5.5 Relative rates of mortality from CHD according to social class at screening and fathers' social class in the West of Scotland Collaborative Study

	Subject non-manual at screening		Subject manual at screening	
	Non-manual father	Manual father	Non-Manual father	Manual father
Age	1	1.51 (1.16–1.96)	1.68 (1.09–2.58)	1.82 (1.43–2.32)
Risk factors*	1	1.43 (1.10–1.86)	1.59 (1.02–2.48)	1.67 (1.27–2.13)

*Age, smoking, diastolic blood pressure, cholesterol, body mass index, adjusted FEV$_1$, deprivation category, and car
Source: Davey Smith et al., 1998

function are associated with both current and parental social class, but more strongly with the former. This suggests that exposures—such as smoking and occupational exposures for lung function, or alcohol and other dietary factors for blood pressure—are more dependent upon adult than childhood social circumstances.

Body mass index (BMI) and triglyceride levels, on the other hand, were dependent on childhood social class rather than current social class: men with manual fathers had higher body mass indices and higher triglyceride levels than men with non-manual fathers and, once father's social class was taken into account, there was no association of current social class with BMI and a reverse association for triglycerides—i.e. higher triglyceride levels amongst the men in non-manual rather than manual occupations in adulthood (Davey Smith and Hart, 1997). High BMI and elevated triglycerides are components of the insulin resistance syndrome. This is compatible with some studies that have indicated that the concomitants of adverse childhood socio-economic circumstances are associated with an elevated risk of diabetes and impaired glucose tolerance in adulthood (Alvarsson et al., 1994; Lehingue, 1996). The components of insulin resistance syndrome cluster in childhood (Bao et al., 1994; Raitakari et al., 1994) and this clustering tracks into adulthood. This suggests that a common factor, already active in young childhood, underlies the risk of syndrome X from early life onwards.

There is, therefore, evidence that some, but not all, conventional risk factors measured in adulthood are influenced by childhood socio-economic circumstances. In the Collaborative Study, the CHD differentials according to father's social class were attenuated, but not abolished, by adjustment for adult risk factors (Davey Smith et al., 1998b), suggesting that outcomes of social environment in childhood could have a long-term influence on CHD risk in adulthood. In the Boyd Orr cohort, leg length in childhood—an indicator of early-life growth and nutritional status—was inversely associated with risk of CHD mortality occurring over the subsequent 60 years (Gunnell et al., 1998a). Infections acquired in childhood could also increase the risk of CHD many years later. Socio-economic position in childhood is related to birthweight, with lower birthweights on average among those born into a less favourable social environment, and several studies have found low birthweight to be related to increased CHD risk (Barker, 1998). Thus, these various outcomes of childhood and pre-childhood social circumstances could contribute to socio-economic differentials in CHD.

Explanations for CHD inequalities according to adulthood social position

In the first Whitehall study, much of the large gradient in CHD mortality risk according to employment grade could not be accounted for by differences in smoking behaviour, blood pressure, plasma cholesterol, BMI, or CHD existing at the time of study entry (Marmot et al., 1984). Similarly, a prospective study of a third of a million men screened for the Multiple Risk Factor Intervention Trial between 1970 and 1973, with 16 years of mortality follow-up, found a strong inverse association between the income level of the area of residence of the men and their risk of mortality from CHD and stroke (Davey Smith *et al.*, 1996). While adjustment for smoking, cholesterol levels, blood pressure, and diabetes somewhat attenuated these associations, it did not remove them. Prospective studies from Sweden, Finland, Denmark, and the US, using a variety of indices of social position, have reached essentially the same conclusions for both men and women.

It has been suggested that the residual associations seen between social class and CHD incidence are due to the inaccuracy inherent in using single measurements of risk factors as proxy measures of lifetime exposure (Pocock *et al.*, 1987). Whilst measurement imprecision in these factors renders the exploration of causes of differentials problematic (Phillips and Davey Smith, 1991), it is also the case that the use of social class alone leads to a marked underestimation of the strength of the relationship between socio-economic position and mortality (Davey Smith *et al.*, 1990). Studies with more precise classification of socio-economic circumstances demonstrate much greater differentials than those using cruder measures, such as occupational class in adulthood alone. Studies with precise measurement of life-course socio-economic position and risk factors are required to take this issue forward. In the Collaborative Study, for example, the substantial differentials in cardiovascular mortality according to lifetime social circumstances were little altered by adjustment for a wide range of behavioural and physiological risk factors measured in adulthood (Table 5.2; Davey Smith *et al.*, 1997).

A study of Finnish men constitutes the most detailed prospective investigation of factors contributing to the socio-economic gradient in cardiovascular mortality undertaken to date (Lynch *et al.*, 1996). The risk of all-cause and cardiovascular disease mortality across quintiles of adulthood income showed 2.5–3-fold differences. It was possible to adjust for 22 possible risk factors— plasma fibrinogen, serum HDL cholesterol, serum apolipoprotein B, blood leukocytes, serum copper, mercury in hair, serum ferritin, blood haemoglobin, serum triglycerides, systolic blood pressure, BMI, height, cardiorespiratory fitness, cigarette smoking, alcohol consumption, leisure time physical activity, depression, hopelessness, cynical hostility, participation in organizations, quality of social support, and marital status (Lynch *et al.*, 1996). On adjustment for all these factors, the association between social position and cardiovascular disease mortality was greatly attenuated, while the associations between social position and all (fatal and non-fatal) CHD incidence remained substantial. As the authors acknowledge, it is difficult to interpret such analyses, for several reasons. First, some of the factors adjusted for may be markers of disease presence (e.g. blood leukocytes, fibrinogen), and statistical adjustment for these could, in essence, be adjusting for the presence of cardiovascular disease, which is itself produced by social factors. The reduction in relative risks in the lower income groups which occurs on adjustment for these factors cannot be taken as demonstrating the 'explanation' of why the social distribution of cardiovascular mortality exists, although it may help identify potential mediating mechanisms. Second, some factors—e.g. height, BMI, and serum triglycerides—may be the outcome of socio-economic processes which act in early life. Adjusting for them similarly fails to account for the reasons for the social distribution in cardio-vascular mortality, since it automatically leads to questions as to how childhood social conditions may influence insulin resistance syndrome and thus coronary disease risk. Finally, as we have discussed earlier, the reasons for the social dis-tribution of certain behaviours—e.g. smoking and exercise—should themselves become a target for explanation.

The development of CHD risk over the life course

The long incubation period for CHD has been recognized for many years (Rose, 1982), and a life-course approach to its aetiology is a natural extension of this view. In this discussion, we have focused on studies for which the main focus is the social patterning of CHD risk. However, most of the important risk factors identified for CHD are socially patterned. The combined effects of exposures acting at different stages of the life course on CHD risk have been investigated for illustrative purposes in the Collaborative Study. Table 5.6 presents the com-bined effects of father's social class (as a marker of early-life circumstances) and behavioural and socio-economic factors acting in adulthood on CHD mortality. In each case, the influence of both early-life socio-economic factors and later-life behaviours or social environment can be seen. Table 5.7 summarizes factors which are established CHD risk factors and/or are of particular interest from a life-course perspective, according to their period of influence. It is clear that

Table 5.6 Age-adjusted relative rates of CHD mortality by father's social class and later-life risk indicators in the West of Scotland Collaborative Study

Father's social class	Smoking	
	Other	Current cigarette
Non manual	1	2.01 (1.46–2.77)
Manual	1.56 (1.18–2.07)	2.78 (2.12–3.63)
	Alcohol	
	<15 units/week	≥15 units/week
Non manual	1	1.17 (0.80–1.70)
Manual	1.44 (1.18–1.75)	1.86 (1.50–2.31)
	Screening social class	
	Non manual	Manual
Non manual	1	1.53 (1.06–2.21)
Manual	1.46 (1.18–1.82)	1.78 (1.45–2.17)

Table 5.7   Life-course risk factors for CHD

Maternal health, development, and diet before and during pregnancy
Parental history of CHD
Low birthweight
Socio-economic deprivation from childhood onward
Poor growth in childhood
Short leg length in childhood
Obesity in childhood
Certain infections acquired in childhood
Diet from childhood onwards
Blood pressure in late adolescence
Serum cholesterol in late adolescence
Smoking from late adolescence onwards
Little physical activity from late adolescence onwards
Job insecurity
Blood pressure in adulthood
Serum cholesterol in adulthood
Obesity in adulthood
Short stature in adulthood
Binge alcohol drinking in adulthood
Diabetes and components of syndrome X in adulthood
Certain infections acquired in adulthood

CHD can be considered the archetype of diseases whose determinants should be sought across the entire life course—from conditions existing at the time of conception and during intrauterine development, through nutrition, growth, and health in childhood, to social conditions, occupation, diet, physical activity, and smoking throughout adult life. Socio-economic inequalities in CHD can only be understood through consideration of how these factors are influenced by social circumstances, how this social dependence leads to them clustering across time such that some individuals are adversely influenced by a wide array of risk factors, and thus how the accumulation of—and interaction between—influences acting at different stages of life determines the pattern of CHD within and between populations.

Stroke

Stroke is a heterogenous clinical entity, and aetiologial studies need to distinguish ischaemic, haemorrhagic, and other sub-types of stroke. Ischaemic stroke is commonest in older populations, and therefore most epidemiological studies that have examined all combined strokes are essentially determining associations with this type, despite some misclassification. (Ebrahim and Harwood, 1999). Most work on risk factors for stroke have identified physiological and behavioural factors predominantly acting during adult life, such as hypertension, obesity, smoking, physical inactivity, serum lipids, and diabetes. Most of these are related in the same direction with CHD risk (Ebrahim and Harwood,

1999). Stroke also shows the same association with socio-economic position as CHD, lower socio-economic position being associated with increased risk. The Collaborative Study, mentioned above, found an increased risk of cardio-vascular disease (including CHD and stroke) with cumulative periods of socio-economic deprivation (Davey Smith et al., 1997). This observation is unsurprising, and a simplistic explanation would argue that, as both diseases are different phenotypic manifestations of the same underlying pathophysiological process, atherosclerosis, they should manifest the same associations. The social patterning of these exposures would therefore predict similar associations with stroke, and these have been discussed above. However, there are also interesting differences between the two diseases, which complicate this argument (Charlton et al., 1997). First, the international ecological correlation for CHD and stroke mortality is relatively weak (0.22). Certain countries, such as Japan and France, have relatively high stroke rates but paradoxically low CHD rates, whilst this pattern is reversed for other countries such as Israel, Romania, and Cuba (Charlton et al., 1997). Second, temporal trend data in Britain from the turn of the century show a rise and fall in CHD, in contrast to the relatively steady decline in stroke mortality seen throughout the twentieth century. Third, gender differences are far more marked for CHD than for stroke. Further evidence suggesting that stroke and CHD have distinct aetiologies is discussed by Leon in chapter 4 (this volume).

Factors contributing to socio-economic differentials in stroke risk according to adult social circumstances have been investigated considerably less thoroughly than in the case of CHD, but similar conclusions apply, since most studies find differentials remain, although they are attenuated, after conventional risk factors—such as smoking and blood pressure—have been taken into account (van Rossum et al., 1999; Hart et al., in press a). Many studies examining mortality associations with both childhood and adult socio-economic position have not presented data specifically on stroke, but rather the broader category of cardiovascular disease (e.g. Lynch et al., 1994), which may be misleading. Data from the Collaborative Study supports a differential relationship between life-course socio-economic position for CHD and for stroke (Davey Smith et al., 1998b). Whilst adjustment for adult social circumstances considerably attenuated the relationship between childhood conditions and CHD (see above), it had little influence with respect to stroke. Indeed, the stroke rate differences between men with manual and non-manual fathers were essentially identical in those who themselves had manual or non-manual occupations (Table 5.8). These findings highlight the particular importance of adverse circumstances in early life for stroke risk. Similarly, a small case control study indicated that stroke cases were more likely to come from poorer homes, and to have had an infant or perinatal death in a sibling, although none of these associations were statistically significant (Coggon et al., 1990a). Previous ecological studies have observed an association between maternal mortality rates in the past and current stroke mortality (Barker and Osmond, 1987), and maternal constraint on intrauterine develop-

Table 5.8 Relative rates of mortality from stroke according to social class at screening and father's social class in the West of Scotland Collaborative Study

Adjustment	Subject non-manual at screening		Subject manual at screening	
	Non-manual father	Manual father	Non-manual father	Manual father
Age	1	1.84 (1.04–3.28)	1.74 (0.97–3.12)	1.88 (1.09–3.24)
Risk factors*	1	1.74 (0.97–3.12)	0.94 (0.30–2.91)	1.65 (0.90–3.03)

*Age, smoking, diastolic blood pressure, cholesterol, body mass index, adjusted FEV_1, deprivation category, and car
Source: Davey Smith *et al.*, 1998*b*

ment has been identified as a risk factor for stroke (Martyn *et al.*, 1996). However, a detailed temporal analysis of stroke mortality in South East England and Greater London concluded that although there was a cohort effect, this did not appear to be consistent with past maternal or neonatal mortality rates (indexing intrauterine experiences) (Maheswaran *et al.*, 1997). Childhood, rather than intrauterine, circumstances may therefore be of particular importance. This is consistent with studies that have shown an inverse association between height and stroke (Leon *et al.*, 1995; Njolstad *et al.*, 1996; Parker *et al.*, 1998; Davey Smith *et al.*, 2000), although this has not always been seen (Wannamethee *et al.*, 1998). Early-life influences on stroke risk do not seem to be produced entirely through conventional risk factors, since adjustment for these had relatively little influence on the elevated risk of stroke among men with manual as compared to non-manual fathers (Davey Smith *et al.*, 1998*b*). However, factors related to development of blood pressure level prior to adulthood seem importantly to influence stroke risk, since blood pressure in early adulthood (around 18 to 20 years of age) predicts subsequent risk of stroke (Paffenbarger and Wing, 1967).

A greater dependence on early-life exposures for stroke than for CHD may explain the differences seen in the epidemiology of these two conditions (Davey Smith and Ben-Shlomo, 1997); in particular, the largely continuous decline in stroke mortality seen over this century in the UK may reflect a condition which is responsive to improvements in circumstances influencing early life development, health and nutrition, while in the case of CHD the rise and fall seen over this century indicates that improvements in these factors do not have, on their own, an unequivocally beneficial influence on disease risk.

Non-smoking related cancers

Socio-economic differences in cancer incidence and mortality are well documented, although, as already described, patterns of risk vary with cancer site (see Fig. 5.1). The most robust socio-economic differentials in cancer are the gradients of increasing risk with worsening social circumstances seen for stomach cancer, and a reverse gradient to this seen for breast cancer. For smoking-related cancers, the gradient largely depends upon the socio-economic gradient in smoking which exists in a particular locale (Faggiano et al., 1997). Because of both the profound effect of smoking and the marked social patterning of smoking behaviour, our focus here will mainly be on those cancers whose aetiology is not thought to be related to smoking. As seen with the other disorders discussed in this review, pathways underlying the socio-economic gradients in cancer may involve a number of mechanisms ranging from socio-economic inequalities in access to early detection and treatment facilities (Kogevinas and Porta, 1997) to socially-patterned exposure to risk factors—such as diet and smoking—over the life course (Leon and Ben-Shlomo, 1997). Socio-economic differences in access to diagnostic and treatment services are of importance in terms of the organization and management of health services, whereas socio-economic variations in cancer incidence (which is the focus of this chapter) are of aetiological importance.

Cancer is thought to arise as a result of DNA damage at a number of specific loci important in the regulation of the cell cycle (Weinberg, 1996). Unrepaired DNA damage accumulates throughout life, and thus cancer epidemiology lends itself to life-course analyses, as damage from exposures before birth may be as important in the pathway of risk development as damage occurring in old age. Much research to date has focused on single-site cancers. However, some of the mechanisms underlying the development of malignancies may be common to many cancers. Specific genes appear to be important in regulating the cell cycle, and thus their mutation may lead to an increased risk of cancers at a number of sites. This view is supported by the observation that some family patterns of increased cancer risk are seen for cancers arising in several sites (Rodriguez et al., 1998). Likewise, raised levels of insulin-like growth factor-1 (IGF-1) and low levels of binding protein IGFBP-3 diminish cell apoptosis, thus impairing one of the body's natural defences against malignancy. Recent research has demonstrated that raised levels of IGF-I are associated with increased risk of prostate (Chan et al., 1998), breast (Hankinson et al., 1998), and colorectal (Ma et al., 1999) cancers.

Few studies have specifically investigated the importance of early-life social circumstances in relation to cancer risk. Their importance is suggested by migrant studies and analyses of associations between anthropometry and cancer. Migrant studies indicate that women migrating out of their area of birth take their risk of breast cancer with them, suggesting the importance of exposures operating before adulthood (Buell et al., 1973; Barbone et al., 1996), although this effect is not seen in all studies (Adelstein et al., 1979). More direct evidence of the importance of early-life exposures comes from studies examining associations between anthropometry at various stages of development and later cancer incidence. Birthweight reflects the adequacy of fetal growth; height, as well as reflecting genetic endowment, also gives an indication of the cumulative effect of nutrition and health over the growing years (Tanner, 1978). A number of studies have found associations between birthweight and later risk of prostate, ovarian, and breast cancer and, although there is some inconsistency in this evidence, most research indicates that raised birthweight is associated with increased risk of these cancers (Le Marchand *et al.*, 1988; Ekbom *et al.*, 1992; Ekbom *et al.*, 1995; Tibblin *et al.*, 1995; Sanderson *et al.*, 1996; Lawson, 1998). More consistent evidence of the role of early-life factors in the development of cancer risk comes from studies showing associations between measures of stature either in childhood (Gunnell *et al.*, 1998*b*) or adulthood (Albanes *et al.*, 1988; Leon *et al.*, 1995; Hebert *et al.*, 1997; Davey Smith *et al.*, 2000) and later cancer risk. After adjustments for age and adult socio-economic position, analyses of the Whitehall, Renfrew/Paisley, and Boyd Orr cohorts indicate that mortality from cancers thought not to be associated with smoking increases with height (Gunnell *et al.*, 1998*b*; Davey Smith *et al.*, 1998*c*; Davey Smith *et al.*, 2000). Site-specific relative risks associated with a 6-inch difference in height in members of the Whitehall cohort are shown in Table 5.9. A possible explanation for the observed height–cancer associations is that childhood exposures which influence height may permanently influence adult growth factor levels, which are in turn related to cancer risk (see above) (Holly *et al.*, 1999). Socio-economic differences in childhood diet may underlie these associations, and recent analyses of the Boyd Orr cohort, where data on childhood diet are available for subjects who are now in their late sixties/early seventies, suggest that childhood calorie consumption is associated with increased risk of cancers whose aetiology is not thought to be related to smoking (Frankel *et al.*, 1998).

Later-life risk factors for cancer development are thought to include diet, alcohol consumption, exposures to some infections, and occupation. In women, age at menarche, use of contraceptives, and number of children are also important with respect to breast cancer. Many of these exposures are socially patterned and are likely to contribute to socio-economic differences in cancer incidence and mortality (Faggiano *et al.*, 1997). Few analyses have sought specifically to

Table 5.9 Relative rates of cancer associated with a 6-inch increase in height in the Whitehall Study

	Relative rate
Oesophagus	0.47
Colon	0.93
Pancreas	0.93
Stomach	0.93
Bladder	1
Rectum	1.03
All sites	1.1
Leukaemia	1.1
Lung	1.12
Prostate	1.43
Brain	1.79
Lymphoma	1.89

Source: Leon *et al.*, 1995

partition the relative effects of early-life and later-life influences on cancer risk. This is an area where more detailed research is certainly required. Since most is known about the association of lifetime social circumstances with breast and stomach cancer, these are briefly reviewed here.

Breast cancer

Cancer of the breast is a major source of morbidity and mortality in the developed world (Forbes, 1997). Unlike many other diseases, breast cancer is generally regarded as showing a positive association with socio-economic position, so that it is more common amongst affluent women. A recent review of 37 populations in 21 countries found this association to be remarkably consistent (Faggiano *et al.,* 1997). The best established risk factors for cancer of the breast are parity, age at first birth, age at menarche, and family history. Risk increases with a longer period of fertility and fewer episodes of pregnancy (Rosner *et al.,* 1994). Apart from family history, these factors are socially patterned so that one would expect that higher socio-economic position, or educational level, would be associated with greater risk. In a study focused on explaining socio-economic differentials in breast cancer, risk adjustment for these factors in multivariable models progressively attenuates the association, and the residual association could at least in part be explained by measurement imprecision in the risk factors (Heck and Pamuk, 1997). Less well-established risk factors include:

(1) physical activity in childhood (Marcus *et al.*, 1999);

(2) dietary fat (Wynder *et al.*, 1994);

(3) obesity and weight gain (Huang *et al.*, 1997);

(4) alcohol consumption (Talamini *et al.*, 1984);

(5) birth weight, (Michels *et al.*, 1996; Sanderson *et al.,* 1996);

(6) neonatal jaundice, (Ekbom *et al.*, 1997) and

(7) pre-eclampsia. (Ekbom *et al.*, 1992).

Pregnancy increases the risk of breast cancer transiently after the pregnancy but the longer-term effect is to decrease risk (Adami *et al.*, 1998). Most (Wang *et al.*, 1997; Ziegler, 1997; Cold *et al.*, 1998; Galanis *et al.*, 1998) but not all studies (Kaaks *et al.*, 1998; Tavani *et al.*, 1998; Davey Smith *et al.*, 2000) show positive associations with adult height.

Some of these factors may show differential associations with pre- and post-menopausal cancers. For example, the significant trend between birthweight and risk of breast cancer was only seen for women under the age of 50 years (Michels *et al.*, 1996). Similarly, an association with obesity has been noted for post-menopausal cancers in women who have never used hormone replacement therapy, but not for pre-menopausal cancers, which, if anything, show an inverse association with degree of obesity (Huang *et al.*, 1997). There is clearly an association between age at puberty, peak height velocity, and attained adult height. However, one study has suggested that, rather than actual height, it is the age of maximum height attainment which is a more important determinant of breast cancer risk, even after adjustment for age at menarche (Li *et al.*, 1997).

Studies that have reported associations between adult socio-economic position and breast cancer do not provide data on childhood social circumstances, so the long-term influence of childhood conditions has not been investigated directly. Recently, several reports have suggested that the social distribution of breast cancer may be changing, such that the social differences are becoming attenuated or perhaps even reversing. Studies from the Netherlands (van Loon *et al.*, 1994), the US (Wagener and Schatzkin, 1994), and the UK (Brown *et al.*, 1997) suggest either an absent social gradient or a reduction in the gradient. These observations are both interesting and challenging. Given detection bias—affluent women are more likely to get screened for breast cancer—we may be underestimating the extent to which the socio-economic distribution of breast cancer is changing. The UK Longitudinal Study provides data for trends in cancer incidence for women aged less than 65 years (Brown *et al.*, 1997) (see Fig. 5.2). Between 1976 to 1989, the manual to non-manual rate ratios for younger cases of breast cancer have reversed from 0.92 to 1.09. In contrast, the ratios for older cases, aged 65 years or over, have remained relatively constant at 0.85. One possible explanation is that these divergent patterns seen for pre- and post-menopausal cancers reflect the different role of endocrine factors such as IGF-1. This has been shown to have no association with post-menopausal cancers but a strong four-fold association for the top versus bottom tertile for cancers diagnosed at less than 50 years. (Hankinson *et al.*, 1998). The long-term determinants of adult IGF-1 levels remain unclear, but patterns of adolescent growth (Juul *et al.*, 1994) and intrauterine influences (Fall *et al.*, 1995) may be important. In particular, restrained intrauterine growth (indexed by low birthweight) followed by catch-up growth is associated with higher IGF-1 levels. (Fall

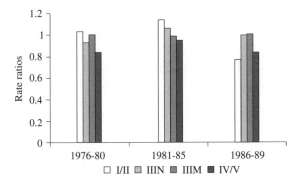

Fig. 5.2 Trends in incidence rates for breast cancer under the age of 65 years by social class
Source: Brown *et al.*, 1997

et al., 1995) More speculatively, increasing overall affluence this century with a continuing social class gradient in birthweight may have resulted in a changing socio-economic gradient in IGF-1 levels and, consequently, a changing gradient in pre-menopausal breast cancer incidence.

Current understanding of breast cancer aetiology indicates that it is a condition which is influenced by socially-patterned exposures acting across the life course (Krieger, 1989; Colditz and Frazier, 1995; Adami *et al.*, 1998). These models base their mechanistic understanding on the suggestion that with maturation of mammary ductal tissue from a less differentiated to a more differentiated form, susceptibility to carcinogens is reduced. Susceptibility is, on the other hand, increased by exposure to hormonal signals for cell division (especially oestrogens), since dividing cells are liable to malignant transformation, and by growth factors (such as IGF-1), which prevent apoptosis (cell death) of transformed cells and thus increase the risk of established malignancy. These mechanisms would account for why certain factors increase risk of breast cancer by increasing the window of exposure to high levels of oestrogens (early menarche, late menopause, exogenous oestrogens, and alcohol consumption) or possibly by programming levels of ovarian hormones and/or IGF-1 in later life (physical activity and calorie intake in childhood), through direct effects or through influencing age at menarche. Pregnancy has a dual influence, transiently increasing breast cancer risk through oestrogen and IGF-1 elevation during pregnancy, but decreasing risk in the longer term by stimulating terminal differentiation of ductal tissue into a less susceptible form. Clearly, age at menarche, age at menopause, age at first pregnancy, total number of pregnancies, and dietary and exercise patterns from childhood onwards are both socially patterned and exert their influences from early life through to late adulthood. The interrelationships of such exposures demonstrate the complexity which may exist with respect to disease development over the life course (Krieger, 1989; 1994).

Stomach cancer

Stomach cancer is a cause of death which shows striking socio-economic gradients in most places where its socio-economic distribution has been studied (Faggiano *et al.*, 1997). The incidence of and mortality from stomach cancer has also declined dramatically in the UK and many other high-income countries over several decades (Howson *et al.*, 1986). Migrant studies suggest that stomach cancer risk is in part determined during early life (Coggon *et al.*, 1990b) and current mortality correlates with markers of adverse socio-economic circumstances earlier in the twentieth century (Barker *et al.*, 1990; Ben-Shlomo and Davey Smith, 1991; Swerdlow and dos Santos Silva, 1991; Leon and Davey Smith, 2000). Analyses of cohort effects seen in mortality trends support the hypothesis that exposure to causative factors early in life is important in the development of stomach cancer (Hansson *et al.*, 1991).

In the Collaborative Study, stomach cancer mortality risk demonstrated a striking gradient with father's social class, with the risk in those men whose fathers were in social class IV and V occupations being nearly three times that of the men whose fathers were in social class I and II (Davey Smith *et al.*, 1998*b*). Adjustment for social class in adulthood of these men had no effect on this association. Conversely, social class in adulthood was essentially unrelated to stomach cancer mortality, once childhood social class was taken into account.

Helicobacter pylori infection has been implicated in the causation of stomach cancer (Forman *et al.*, 1991; Parsonnet, 1999). *H. pylori* infection in adulthood is related to various indicators of poor socio-economic circumstances in childhood (Mendall *et al.*, 1992; Whitaker *et al.*, 1993), and little new infection seems to occur in adulthood. Number of siblings—which may be related to risk of acquisition of infection—is also positively related to stomach cancer risk (Hansson *et al.*, 1994). In the UK, there has been a striking decline in the prevalence of *H. pylori* infection among adults, and this demonstrates similar cohort patterns to those that have been seen with relation to the decline in stomach cancer mortality (Banatlava *et al.*, 1993).

Thus stomach cancer in adulthood could be the late sequelae of an infection acquired in childhood, with the risk of infection being increased by overcrowding, large family size, and the inability to maintain adequate hygiene standards. If this is the case, it follows that the socio-economic distribution in stomach cancer among adults is created by differentials in material circumstances in early life.

Suicide and depression

Suicide accounts for only 1% of all deaths in England and Wales but, because it is one of the commonest causes of death in young people, is an important contribution to premature mortality and lost potential life years (Gunnell, 2000). The aetiology of suicide is complex; suicidal behaviour arises from an interaction between personality factors predisposing to suicide and a number of quite distinct disease and social processes which may trigger suicide attempts.

Few cohorts are of sufficient size, or contain adequate exposure data, to study life-course influences on suicide risk. However, persuasive evidence of the importance of socio-economic influences at various stages of the life course on risk comes from a number of sources. Childhood adversity—including economic hardship and loss of a parent through death or divorce—has been shown to increase susceptibility to mental illness in later life (Rodgers, 1990; Lundberg, 1993; Maughan and McCarthy, 1997; Sadowski *et al.*, 1999). Cohort studies indicate that, in the longer term, these factors are also associated with an increased risk of suicide (Allebeck *et al.*, 1988; Neeleman *et al.*, 1998). Further back in the life course, prenatal under-nutrition and birth complications, both of which are socially patterned, have been shown to increase the risk of later schizophrenia (Jones, 1997), a disorder which accounts for 10% of all suicides.

In adulthood, a number of social stressors such as unemployment and relationship breakdown are associated with increased suicide risk (Gunnell, 2000). In Britain, cohort studies (Lewis and Sloggett, 1998) and time series analyses (Gunnell et al., 1999) have demonstrated the effect of unemployment on an individual's suicide risk, and of economic recession on national suicide rates. Unemployed individuals are at two-fold increased risk of suicide (Lewis and Sloggett, 1998) and, during the two great recessions of the twentieth century, suicide rates increased by around 50% in young people. Likewise analyses of national mortality data show gradients of increasing suicide risk in relation to lower socio-economic position (Drever and Whitehead, 1997). The situation is complex and, in analyses of the Longitudinal Study, those in social class I and V were shown to be at increased risk compared to other groups (Charlton et al., 1993). Furthermore, in a long-term follow-up of 41,000 university students in the US, risks were significantly increased in those whose parents had college education and whose fathers were in professional occupations (Paffenbarger and Asnes, 1966). It is possible that, amongst those privileged to receive higher education, stresses were greater amongst those whose parents were successful.

To date, the life-course aspects of suicide risk have not been studied in sufficient detail. Further research, based on large cohorts and followed up over long periods, is required to understand the complex issues underlying suicidal behaviour. Evidence to date suggests that socio-economic adversity in early life may increase vulnerability to risk factors associated with suicide risk in later life.

Respiratory function and obstructive airways disease

There are marked socio-economic gradients for respiratory function (FEV_1) (Davey Smith et al., 1990), respiratory morbidity, respiratory disease consultations (McCormick et al., 1995), and mortality (Ebi-Kryston, 1989). Much of this pattern can be explained by smoking behaviour, which is known to explain the faster rate of decline of FEV_1 seen amongst smokers compared to non-smokers. Former smokers have rates of FEV_1 decline that are similar to the rates for lifelong non-smokers, although they do not make up most of the FEV_1 lost as a result of their previous cigarette consumption (Fletcher et al., 1976). However, studies have shown associations of socio-economic position with measures of ventilatory function, independent of current smoking habit (Blane et al., 1996). Furthermore, as Strachan has observed (Strachan, 1997), bronchitis mortality in the 1920s showed a strong social class gradient long before there was any substantial variation in smoking behaviour by social class (see Fig. 5.3.)

Several studies have shown the importance of childhood social conditions and highlighted potential early exposures (Shaheen, 1997). In the Collaborative

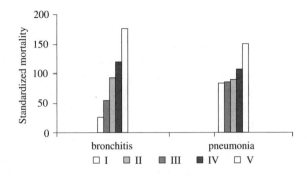

Fig. 5.3 Standardized mortality rates for bronchitis and pneumonia of men aged 20 to 65 years by social class from the 1921 Decennial supplement

Study, childhood social class was related to FEV_1 independently of adult social class (Blane *et al.*, 1996), and respiratory mortality risk was related to childhood social class after adulthood social class and adulthood risk factors had been taken into account (Davey Smith *et al.*, 1998*b*). In a similar fashion, analyses of the 1946 birth cohort showed associations between measures of childhood social circumstances and adult lung function (peak expiratory flow rate) (Mann *et al.*, 1992).

Measures of childhood social circumstances clearly can act as a proxy for a wide variety of potentially important exposures; poor intrauterine development, childhood infections, impaired growth in childhood, outdoor and indoor air pollution, housing with damp and mould, passive smoke exposure, and poor nutrition (in particular low anti-oxidant intake). Much interest has focused on the potential role of childhood infections during a critical period in early life. The 1946 Birth Cohort (Mann *et al.*, 1992), and studies from Derbyshire (Shaheen *et al.*, 1994), Hertfordshire (Barker *et al.*, 1991), and St Andrews (Shaheen *et al.*, 1998), have found associations between recorded respiratory infections, especially within the first two years of life, and deficits in adult lung function. Intrauterine development has also been a focus of interest: the Hertfordshire study (Barker *et al.*, 1991) and a study from India (Stein *et al.*, 1997) have also demonstrated a graded deficit in FEV with a decrease in weight at birth, but this was not seen for the St Andrews study (Shaheen *et al.*, 1998). In the Renfrew and Paisley Offspring Study, maternal (but not paternal) smoking was related to lung function in adulthood, suggesting an intrauterine influence of maternal smoking on later lung health (Upton *et al.*, 1998). Interpreting these associations is problematic, as several possible explanations exist (Strachan, 1997). Chest infections may produce long-term lung damage and subsequent disease. Impaired lung development *in utero*, as crudely measured by birthweight, may result in an increased risk of childhood infections, which then results in adult disease. Conversely, however, chest infections in childhood may simply be a marker of poor lung growth (which is related to adult disease), and infections may not themselves have an aetiological role.

The clustering of adverse exposures for individuals brought up in poor social circumstances and their continuity across the life course due to social and biological pathways may result in cumulative lung damage and disease (see Fig. 5.4). For example, repeated childhood infections may not only lead to lung damage and further infections, but also to school absence and therefore poor educational attainment, which in turn may influence smoking behaviour, diet, and occupational exposures. Disentangling the relative—independent, interactive, and cumulative—effects of such correlated exposures presents a serious analytical challenge to attempts to carry out life course analyses. However, lung function measurements may serve as useful ramp-sum indices of exposure to many noxious elements over the life course and, in turn, be an important contributor to mortality risk.

Conclusions

Our review of selected specific health problems indicates that socio-economic position at different stages of the life course can influence particular conditions

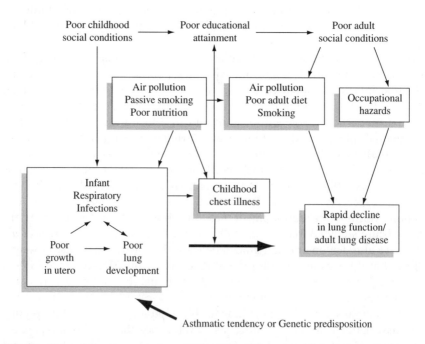

Fig. 5.4   Schematic representation of life course influences on respiratory disease (taken from presentation by Ben-Shlomo Y. and Kuh D., Life course approach to chronic disease, at *Synthetic Biographies: State of the art and developments* international workshop, Pisa, 1999)

in particular ways. Two of the conditions—stroke and stomach cancer—appear to be particularly responsive to early-life influences while others—CHD, chronic obstructive respiratory disease, breast cancer, and suicide—appear to be influenced by socially-patterned exposures acting right across life. Some conditions which we have not reviewed—for example, lung cancer—appear to be mostly determined by socially patterned factors acting in adulthood. Thus, there is no single answer to the question which we posed rhetorically ten years ago on whether deprivation in childhood or adulthood is a more important determinant of adult mortality risk (Ben-Shlomo and Davey Smith, 1991). Not only is there a difference between particular health conditions at one point in time with respect to early- or later-life determination of risk, but the relative importance of factors can change over time. For example, tuberculosis (TB) morbidity and mortality in adulthood has long been considered to reflect infection acquired in childhood (Frost, 1939; Springett, 1952), with social conditions in early life therefore being of key importance in determining adulthood TB risk. However, with the advent of HIV infection, in many places the major driving force for resurgent adulthood TB rates will be an adulthood phenomenon—acquisition of HIV.

The changing importance of early- and later-life determinants of adulthood mortality risk can be seen in the long-term trends in mortality in Britain over the last 160 years. In 1934, Kermack and colleagues (Kermack *et al.*, 1934) demonstrated that all-cause mortality began to decline after about 1850 in a cohort-specific manner, with falls being seen first in young children, then in young adults, and then in older adults. The mortality rates behaved as if people who were children after around 1850 took with them, as they aged, better health potential, which had been established in early life. Interestingly, Kermack and colleagues pointed out that, as infant mortality did not decline until the turn of the century, it was unlikely that this improvement in mortality reflected improved intrauterine development; they therefore interpreted their data as suggesting that nutrition and health in childhood determined later health. Thus, over the period 1850–1930, mortality risk in adulthood appeared to be importantly influenced by childhood environment. After 1930, however, serious disruption to the cohort-specific mortality trends occurred (Kuh and Davey Smith, 1993), with middle-aged or over mortality rates falling less and younger age mortality rates falling much faster than anticipated. This suggests that environmental factors acting in adulthood were of importance. The rise of smoking in the British population is one obvious candidate here, leading to adverse trends in older-age mortality. Another is the introduction of medical therapies which favourably influenced mortality risk. A change in the balance of causes of death, such that diseases with predominantly early-life determination (including TB, stomach cancer, rheumatic heart disease, and stroke) decreased in importance, while those with adulthood determination (including lung cancer and accidental/violent death) or determination over the life course (including CHD and breast cancer) became of relatively greater importance, also occurred. After

1930, therefore, the dominance of the early-life determination of mortality risk seems to have been replaced by a greater contribution of adulthood influences.

Our review suggests that specific patterns of life-course exposure are related to specific diseases. We find little support for a simple model of general susceptibility entrained by psycho-social stress. Inequalities in overall health status result from the tendency for the important causes of ill-health—for example, CHD, stroke, lung cancer, and respiratory disease—to show large socio-economic differentials. The social processes which concentrate the exposures which increase the risk of these diseases on particular disadvantaged groups therefore underlie inequalities in overall health status.

The social structure leads to clustering—over time and cross-sectionally— of multiple factors within the lives of the same individuals. Furthermore, the coexistence of a series of exposures within one person's life may generate greater health problems than would be anticipated from the known effect of single exposures. For example, the combination of an occupational exposure (arsenic or asbestos) and smoking generates a greater risk of lung cancer than would be expected from the single addition of the known effects of the exposures experienced on their own (Hertz-Picciotto et al., 1992; Erren et al., 1999). This synergistic effect of combined exposures would contribute to the poor health outcomes of people who experience disadvantage in several components of their lives.

A striking phenomenon, mentioned above, is the tendency for the most important causes of death to demonstrate the most marked socio-economic gradients. Indeed, as particular causes of death have become more important health problems over the course of this century, the tendency for them to be concentrated among the most deprived tends to become greater. Table 5.10 presents data on male lung cancer from 1931–91. In 1931, when lung cancer caused 1% of deaths, it showed no social class gradient; by 1991, there was a marked gradient—with the mortality rate in social class V men being 4.6 times that of social class I men. A similar picture could be seen with respect to social class differences in CHD during the period of rapid increase in this condition as a cause of death. This reflects the way that more favourable social circumstances provide

Table 5.10 Lung cancer mortality 1931–91: social class differences and contribution to total mortality among men of working age

	Social class							% all deaths
	I	II	IIIn		IIIm	IV	V	
1931	1.07	0.96		1.01		0.91	1.12	1.0%
1951	0.81	0.82		1.07		0.91	1.18	2.5%
1971	0.53	0.68	0.84		1.18	1.23	1.43	11.7%
1991	0.45	0.61	0.87		1.38	1.32	2.06	9.9%

Note: Before 1971, social class III was not divided into IIIn (IIInon-manual) and IIIm (IIImanual)
Source: Logan 1982; Drever and Whitehead, 1997

people with the ability to avoid identified noxious exposures. The influence of these exposures occurs against the background of less avoidable exposures (for example poor growth, health, and development in childhood) to determine the overall pattern of disease. It should be remembered in this regard that even lung cancer—a disease for which a particularly important adult risk factor can be identified—shows socio-demographic differentials over and above those created by smoking (Davey Smith *et al.*, 1995; Hart *et al.*, 2000).

While 'general susceptibility' as a unitary biological phenomenon does not appear to underlie health inequalities, it is certainly possible to identify social processes which lead to unfavourable exposures being concentrated on those in less privileged social circumstances, from birth to death. Human bodies in different social locations become crystallized reflections of the social experiences within which they have developed. The socially-patterned nutritional, health, and environmental experiences of the parents, and of the individuals concerned, influence birthweight, height, weight, and lung function, for example, which are in turn important indicators of future health prospects. These biological aspects of bodies (and the histories of bodies) should be viewed as frozen social relations, rather than as asocial explanations of health inequalities which, once accepted, exclude the social from consideration (Najman and Davey Smith, 2000). The life-course approach to health inequalities views the physical and the social as being mutually constitutive, since aspects of bodily form can influence social trajectory in the same way that social experiences become embodied. Comprehending the ways in which the social becomes biological—and the biological in turn becomes part of the social world—must be a central aspect of an agenda aimed at improved understanding of how health inequalities arise and how they can potentially be reduced.

Acknowledgements

We would like to thank David Leon for editorial help and Liz Humphries for assistance in preparation of the manuscript and Carole Hart for analyses reproduced in Table 5.6.

REFERENCES

Adami HO, Signorello LB, Trichopoulos D. Towards an understanding of breast cancer etiology. *Cancer Biology*, 1998; **8**:255–62

Adelstein AM, Staszewski J, Muir CS. Cancer mortality in 1970–1972 among Polish born migrants to England and Wales. *British Journal of Cancer*, 1979; **40**:464–75

Albanes D, Jones DY, Schatzkin A *et al.* Adult stature and risk of cancer. *Cancer Research*, 1988; **48**:1658–62

Allebeck P, Allgulander C, Fisher LD. Predictors of completed suicide in a cohort of 50465 young men: role of personality and deviant behaviour. *British Medical Journal*, 1988; **297**:176–8

Alvarsson M, Efendic S, Grill VE. Insulin responses to glucose in healthy males are associated with adult height but not with birth weight. *Journal of Internal Medicine*, 1994; **236**:275–9

Banatvala N, Mayo K, Megraud F, Jennings R, Deeks JJ, Feldman RA.The cohort effect and Helicobacter pylori. *Journal of Infectious Diseases*, 1993; **168**:219–21

Bao W, Srinivasan SR, Wattigney WA, Berenson GS. Persistence of multiple cardio-vascular risk clustering related to syndrome X from childhood to young adulthood. *Archives of Internal Medicine*, 1994; **154**:1842–7

Barbone F, Filiberti R, Franceschi S *et al.* Socioeconomic status, migration and the risk of breast cancer in Italy. *International Journal of Epidemiology*, 1996; **25**:479–87

Barker DJP. Foetal and infant origins of inequalities in health. *Journal of Public Health Medicine*, 1991; **13**:64–8

Barker DJP. *Mothers, babies and health in later life*. Edinburgh: Churchill Livingstone, 1998

Barker DJP, Osmond C. Infant mortality, childhood nutrition, and ischaemic heart disease in England and Wales. *Lancet*, 1986; **i**:1077–81

Barker DJP, Osmond C. Death rates from stroke in England and Wales predicted from past maternal mortality. *British Medical Journal*, 1987; **295**:83–6

Barker DJP, Coggon D, Osmond C, Wickham C. Poor housing in childhood and high rates of stomach cancer in England and Wales. *British Journal of Cancer*, 1990; **61**:575–8

Barker DJP, Godfrey KM, Fall C *et al.* The relation of birthweight and childhood respiratory infection to adult lung function and death from chronic obstructive air-ways disease. *British Medical Journal*, 1991; **303**:671–5

Ben-Shlomo Y, Davey Smith G. Deprivation in infancy or in adult life: which is more important for mortality risk? *Lancet*, 1991; **337**:530–4

Blane D, Hart CL, Davey Smith G, Gillis CR, Hole DJ, Hawthorne VM. The associa-tion of cardiovascular disease risk factors with socioeconomic position during child-hood and during adulthood. *British Medical Journal*, 1996; **313**:1434–8

Brown J, Harding S, Bethune A, Rosato M. Incidence of Health of the Nation cancers by social class. *Population Trends*, 1997; **90**:40–7

Brunner E. Stress and the biology of inequality. *British Medical Journal*, 1997; **314**:1472–6

Buell P. Changing incidence of breast cancer in Japanese-American women. *Journal of the National Cancer Institute*, 1973; **51**:1479–83

Burr ML, Sweetnam PM. Family size and paternal unemployment in relation to myocardial infarction. *Journal of Epidemiology and Community Health*, 1980; **34**:93–5

Chan JM, Stampfer MJ, Giovannucci E, *et al.* Plasma insulin-like growth factor-I and prostate cancer risk: a prospective study. *Science*, 1998; **279**:563–6

Charlton J, Kelly S, Dunnell K, Evans B, Jenkins R. Suicide deaths in England and Wales: trends in factors associated with suicide deaths. *Population Trends*, 1993; **71**:34–42

Charlton J, Murphy M, Khaw K-T, Ebrahim S, Davey Smith G. Cardiovascular diseases. In: Charlton J, Murphy M (eds) *The health of adult Britain 1841–1994*. London: The Stationery Office, 1997

Coggon D, Margetts B, Barker DJ *et al.* Childhood risk factors for ischaemic heart disease and stroke. *Paediatric and Perinatal Epidemiology*, 1990a; **4**:464–9

Coggon D, Osmond C, Barker DJP. Stomach cancer and migration within England and Wales. *British Journal of Cancer*, 1990*b*; **61**:573–4

Cold S, Hansen S, Overvad K, Rose C. A woman's build and the risk of breast cancer. *European Journal of Cancer*, 1998; **34**:1163–74

Colditz GA, Frazier AL. Models of breast cancer show that risk is set by events of early life: prevention efforts must shift focus. *Cancer Epidemiology, Biomarkers and Prevention*, 1995; **4**:567–71

Davey Smith G. Socioeconomic differentials. In: Kuh D, Ben-Shlomo Y (eds) *A life course approach to chronic disease epidemiology*. Oxford: Oxford University Press, 1997*a*, pp 242–73

Davey Smith G. Down at heart—the meaning and implications of social inequalities in cardiovascular disease. *Journal of the Royal College of Physicians*, 1997*b*; **31**:414–24

Davey Smith G, Ben-Shlomo Y. Geographical and social class differentials in stroke mortality—the influence of early-life factors: comment on papers by Maheswaran and colleagues. *Journal of Epidemiology and Community Health*, 1997; **51**:134–7

Davey Smith G, Harding S. Is control at work the key to socio-economic gradients in mortality? *Lancet*, 1997; **350**:1369–70

Davey Smith G, Hart C. Insulin resistance syndrome and childhood social conditions. *Lancet*, 1997; **349**:284

Davey Smith G, Hart C. Socioeconomic factors and determinants of mortality. *Journal of the American Medical Association*, 1998; **280**:1744–5

Davey Smith G, Shipley MJ, Rose G. Magnitude and causes of socioeconomic differentials in mortality: further evidence from the Whitehall study. *Journal of Epidemiology and Community Health*, 1990; **44**:265–70

Davey Smith G, Leon D, Shipley MJ, Rose G. Socioeconomic differentials in cancer among men. *International Journal of Epidemiology*, 1991; **20**:339–45

Davey Smith G, Blane D, Bartley M. Explanations for socio-economic differentials in mortality: evidence from Britain and elsewhere. *European Journal of Public Health*, 1994; **4**:131–44

Davey Smith G, Shipley M, Hole D *et al.* Explaining male mortality differentials between the west of Scotland and the south of England. *Journal of Epidemiology and Community Health*, 1995; **49**:541

Davey Smith G, Neaton JD, Wentworth D, Stamler R, Stamler J. Socioeconomic differentials in mortality risk among men screened for the Multiple Risk Factor Intervention Trial: I. White Men. *American Journal of Public Health*, 1996; **86**:486–96

Davey Smith G, Hart C, Blane D, Gillis C, Hawthorne V. Lifetime socioeconomic position and mortality: prospective observational study. *British Medical Journal*, 1997; **314**:547–52

Davey Smith G, Hart C, Hole D *et al.* Education and occupational social class: which is the more important indicator of mortality risk? *Journal of Epidemiology and Community Health*, 1998*a*; **52**:153–60

Davey Smith G, Hart C, Blane D, Hole D. Adverse social circumstances and cause-specific mortality: prospective observational study. *British Medical Journal*, 1998*b*; **316**:1631–5

Davey Smith G, Shipley M, Leon DA. Height and mortality from cancer among men: prospective observational study. *British Medical Journal*, 1998*c*; **317**:1351–2

Davey Smith G, Hart C, Upton M, *et al.* Height and risk of death among men and women: aetiological implications of associations with cardiorespiratory disease and cancer mortality. *Journal of Epidemiology and Community Health*, 2000; **54**:97–103

Denton M, Walters V. Gender differentials in structural and behavioural determinants of health: an analysis of the social production of health. *Social Science and Medicine*, 1999; **48**:1221–35

Drever F, Whitehead M (eds). *Health inequalities: decennial supplement*. London: The Stationery Office, 1997

Ebi-Kryston K. Predicting 15 year chronic bronchitis mortality in the Whitehall Study. *Journal of Epidemiology and Community Health*, 1989; **43**:168–72

Ebrahim S, Davey Smith G. Systematic review of randomised controlled trials of multiple risk factor interventions for preventing coronary heart disease. *British Medical Journal*, 1997; **314**:1666–74

Ebrahim S, Davey Smith G. Health promotion for coronary heart disease: past, present and future. *European Heart Journal*, 1998; **19**:1751–7

Ebrahim S, Harwood R. *Stroke: epidemiology, evidence and clinical practice*, (2nd edn). Oxford: Oxford University Press, 1999.

Ekbom A, Trichopoulos D, Adami HO, Hsieh CC, Lan SJ. Evidence of prenatal influences on breast cancer risk. *Lancet,* 1992; **340**:1015–8

Ekbom A, Thurjell E, Hsieh CC, Trichopoulos D, Adami HO. Perinatal characteristics and adult mammographic patterns. *International Journal of Cancer*, 1995; **61**:177–80

Ekbom A, Hsieh C, Lipworth L, Adami HO, Trichopoulos D. Intrauterine environment and breast cancer risk in women: a population-based study. *Journal of the National Cancer Institute*, 1997; **89**:71–6

Engels F. *The Condition of the Working Class in England*. Harmondsworth: Penguin, 1987 (1st edn 1845)

Erren TC, Jacobsen M, Piekarski C. Synergy between asbestos and smoking on lung cancer risks. *Epidemiology*, 1999; **10**:405–11

Faggiano F, Partanen T, Kogevinas M, Boffetta P. Socioeconomic differences in cancer incidence and mortality. In: Kogevinas M, Pearce N, Susser M, Boffeta P (eds) *Social Inequalities in Cancer*. IARC Scientific Publications No. 138. Lyon: IARC, 1997, pp 65–176

Fall CHD, Pandit AN, Law CM *et al.* Size at birth and plasma insulin-like growth factor-1 concentrations. *Archives of Disease in Childhood*, 1995; **73**:287–93

Fernandez E, Borrell C. Cancer mortality by educational level in the city of Barcelona. *British Journal of Cancer*, 1999; **79**:684–9

Fletcher C, Peto R, Tinker C *et al. The natural history of chronic bronchitis and emphysema*. Oxford: Oxford University Press, 1976

Forbes JF. The incidence of breast cancer: the global burden, public health considerations. *Seminars in Oncology*, 1997; **24(S1)**:20–35

Forman D, Newell DG, Fullerton F *et al.* Association between infection with Helicobacter pylori and risk of gastric cancer: evidence from a prospective investigation. *British Medical Journal*, 1991; **302**:1302–5

Forsdahl A. Are poor living conditions in childhood and adolescents an important risk factor for arteriosclerotic heart disease? *British Journal of Preventive and Social Medicine*, 1977; **31**:91–5

Forsdahl A. Living conditions in childhood and subsequent development of risk factors for arteriosclerotic heart disease. *Journal of Epidemiology and Community Health*, 1978; **32**:34–7

Frankel S, Gunnell DJ, Peters T, Maynard M, Davey Smith G. Childhood energy intake and adult mortality from cancer: the Boyd Orr cohort. *British Medical Journal,* 1998; **316**:499–504

Frost WH. The age selection of mortality from tuberculosis in successive decades. *American Journal of Hygiene,* 1939; **30**:91–6

Galanis DJ, Kolonel LN, Lee J, Le Marchand L. Anthropometric predictors of breast cancer incidence and survival in a multi-ethnic cohort of female residents of Hawaii, United States. *Cancer Causes and Control,* 1998; **9**:217–24

Gillum RF, Paffenbarger RS. Chronic disease in former college students. XVII Socio-cultural mobility as a precursor of coronary heart disease and hypertension. *American Journal of Epidemiology,* 1978; **108**:289–98

Gliksman MD, Kawachi I, Hunter D *et al.* Childhood socioeconomic status and risk of cardiovascular disease in middle aged US women: a prospective study. *Journal of Epidemiology and Community Health,* 1995; **49**:10–15

Great Britain Department of Health. *Variations in health.* London: Department of Health, 1995

Great Britain Department of Health and Social Security. *Inequalities in health: report of a research working group.* London: DHSS, 1980

Gunnell D. The epidemiology of suicide. *International Review of Psychiatry,* 2000; **12**:21–6

Gunnell D, Davey Smith G, Frankel S *et al.* Childhood leg length and adult mortality: follow up of the Carnegie (Boyd Orr) Survey of Diet and Health in Pre-War Britain. *Journal of Epidemiology and Community Health,* 1998a; **52**:142–52

Gunnell DJ, Davey Smith G, Holly JMP, Frankel SJ. Leg length and risk of cancer in the Boyd Orr cohort. *British Medical Journal,* 1998b; **317**:1350–1

Gunnell DJ, Lopatatzidis A, Dorling D, Wehner H, Southall H, Frankel S. Suicide, unemployment and gender—an analysis of trends in England and Wales: 1921–1995. *British Journal of Psychiatry,* 1999; **175**:263–70

Hankinson SE, Willett WC, Colditz GA. Circulating concentrations of insulin-like growth factor-I and risk of breast cancer. *Lancet,* 1998; **351**:1393–6

Hansson LE, Bergström R, Sparén P, Adami HO. The decline in the incidence of stomach cancer in Sweden 1960–1984: a birth cohort phenomenon. *International Journal of Cancer,* 1991; **47**:499–503

Hansson LE, Baron J, Nyren O *et al.* Early-life risk indicators of gastric cancer. A population-based case-control study in Sweden. *International Journal of Cancer,* 1994; **57**:32–7

Hart CL, Hole DJ, Davey Smith G. The contribution of risk factors to stroke differentials by adulthood socioeconomic position among men and women in the Renfrew/Paisley Study. *American Journal of Public Health* (in press *a*)

Hart CL, Hole DJ, Gillis CR, Davey Smith G, Watt GCM, Hawthorne VM. Social class differences in lung cancer: risk factor explanations using two Scottish cohort studies. *International Journal of Epidemiology* (in press *b*)

Hasle H. Association between living conditions in childhood and myocardial infarction. *British Medical Journal,* 1990; **300**:512–3

Heck KE, Pamuk ER. Explaining the relation between education and postmenopausal breast cancer. *American Journal of Epidemiology,* 1997; **145**:366–72

Herbert PRP, Ajani U, Cook NR, Lee I-M, Chan KS, Henneckens CH. Adult height and incidence of cancer in male physicians. *Cancer Causes and Control,* 1997; **8**:591–697

Hertz-Picciotto I, Smith AH, Holtzman D, Lipsett M, Alexeeff G. Synergism between occupational arsenic exposure and smoking in the induction of lung cancer. *Epidemiology*, 1992; **3**:23–31

Hinkle LE, Whitney H, Lehman EW, Dunn J *et al.* Occupation, education and coronary heart disease. *Science*, 1968; **161**:238–46

Holly JP, Gunnell DJ, Davey Smith G. Growth hormone, IGF-I and cancer. Less intervention to avoid cancer? More intervention to prevent cancer? *Journal of Endocrinology*, 1999; **162**:321–30

Howson CP, Hiyama T, Wynder EL. The decline in gastric cancer: epidemiology of an unplanned triumph. *Epidemiologic Reviews*, 1986; **8**:1027

Huang Z, Hankinson SE, Colditz GA *et al.* Dual effects of weight and weight gain on breast cancer risk. *Journal of the American Medical Association*, 1997; **278**:1407–11

Hummer RA, Rogers RG, Eberstein IW. Sociodemographic differentials in adult mortality: a review of analytical approaches. *Population and Development Review*, 1998; **24**:553–78

Jones P. The early origins of schizophrenia. *British Medical Bulletin*, 1997; **53**:135–55

Juul A, Bang P, Hertel NT *et al.* Serum insulin-like growth factor-I in 1030 healthy children, adolescents, and adults: relation to age, sex, stage of puberty, testicular size, and body mass index. *Journal of Clinical Endocrinology and Metabolism,* 1994; **78**:744–52

Kaaks R, Van Noord PA, Den Tonkelaar I, Peeters PJH, Riboli E, Grobbee DE. Breast-cancer incidence in relation to height, weight and body-fat distribution in the Dutch 'DOM' cohort. *International Journal of Cancer*, 1998; **76**:647–51

Kaplan GA, Keil JE. Socioeconomic factors and cardiovascular disease: a review of the literature. *Circulation*, 1993; **88**:1973–98

Kaplan GA, Salonen JT. Socioeconomic conditions in childhood and ischaemic heart disease during middle age. *British Medical Journal*, 1990; **301**:1121–3

Kermack WO, McKendrick AG, McKinlay PL. Death rates in Great Britain and Sweden: Some general regularities and their significance. *Lancet*, 1934; **226**:698–703

Kogevinas M, Porta M. Socioeconomic differences in cancer survival: a review of the evidence. In: Kogevinas M, Pearce N, Susser M, Boffeta P (eds) *Social inequalities in cancer*. IARC Scientific Publications No. 138. Lyon: IARC, 1997

Kogevinas M, Pearce N, Susser M, Boffeta P (eds). *Social inequalities in cancer*. IARC Scientific Publications No. 138. Lyon: IARC, 1997

Koskinen S. Origins of regional differences in mortality from ischaemic heart disease in Finland. National Research and Development Centre for Welfare and Health Search Report 41. Helsinki: NAWH, 1994

Krieger N. Exposure, susceptibility and breast cancer risk: a hypothesis regarding exogenous carcinogens, breast tissue development, and social gradients, including black/white differences, in breast cancer incidence. *Breast Cancer Research and Treatment*, 1989; **13**:205–23

Krieger N. Epidemiology and the web of causation: has anyone seen the spider? *Social Science and Medincine*, 1994; **39**:887–903

Kuh D, Ben-Shlomo Y (eds). *A life course approach to chronic disease epidemiology*. Oxford: Oxford University Press, 1997

Kuh D, Davey Smith G. When is mortality risk determined? Historical insights into a current debate. *Social History of Medicine*, 1993; **6**:101–23

Lawson JS. Prostate cancer, birthweight, and diet. *Epidemiology*, 1998; **9**:217

Lehingue Y. Fetal environment and coronary ischemia risk: review of the literature with particular reference to syndrome X. *Revue d'Epidemiologie et de Santé Publique*, 1996; **44**:262–77

Le Marchand L, Kolonel LN, Myers BC, Mi M-P. Birth characteristics of pre-menopausal women with breast cancer. *British Journal of Cancer*, 1988; **57**:437–9

Leon D, Ben-Shlomo Y. Preadult influences on cardiovascular disease and cancer. In: Kuh D, Ben-Shlomo Y (eds) *A life course approach to chronic disease epidemiology*. Oxford: Oxford University Press, 1997, chapter 3

Leon DA, Davey Smith G. Infant mortality, stomach cancer, stroke and coronary heart disease: ecological analysis. *British Medical Journal*, 2000; **320**:1705–6

Leon DA, Davey Smith G, Shipley M, Strachan D. Adult height and mortality in London: early life, socioeconomic confounding, or shrinkage? *Journal of Epidemiology and Community Health*, 1995; **45**:5–9

Lewis G, Sloggett A. Suicide, deprivation and unemployment. *British Medical Journal,* 1998; **317**:1283–6

Li CI, Malone KE, White E, Daling JR. Age when maximum height is reached as a risk factor for breast cancer among young US women. *Epidemiology*, 1997; **8**:559–65

Lobstein T. The increasing cost of a healthy diet. *Food Magazine*, 1995; **31**:17

Logan WPD. *Cancer mortality by occupation and social class 1851–1971*. London: HMSO, 1982

Lundberg O. The impact of childhood living conditions on illness and mortality in adulthood. *Social Science and Medicine*, 1993; **36**:1047–52

Lynch JW, Kaplan GA, Cohen RD. Childhood and adult socioeconomic status as predictors of mortality in Finland. *Lancet*, 1994; **343**:524–7

Lynch JW, Kaplan GA, Cohen RD, Tuomilehto J, Salonen JT. Do known risk factors explain the relation between socioeconomic status, risk of all-cause mortality, cardiovascular mortality and acute myocardial infarction? *American Journal of Epidemiology*, 1996; **144**:934–42

Ma J, Pollak MN, Giovannucci E *et al.* Prospective study of colorectal cancer risk in men and plasma levels of insulin-like growth-factor (IGF-I) and IGF-Binding-Protein 3. *Journal of the National Cancer Institute*, 1999; **91**:620–5

McCormick A, Fleming D, Charlton J. *Morbidity statistics from general practice. Fourth National Study 1991–1992*. London: HMSO, 1995

Macintyre S. The Black Report and beyond: what are the issues? *Social Science and Medicine*, 1997; **44**:723–45

Maheswaran R, Strachan DP, Elliott P, Shipley MJ. Trends in stroke mortality in Greater London and south east England—evidence for a cohort effect? *Journal of Epidemiology and Community Health*, 1997; **51**:121–6

Mann SL, Wadsworth MEJ, Colley JRT. Accumulation of factors influencing respiratory illness in members of a national birth cohort and their offspring. *Journal of Epidemiology and Community Health*, 1992; **46**:286–92

Marcus PM, Newman B, Moorman PG, Millikan RC, Baird DD. Physical activity at age 12 and adult breast cancer risk (United States). *Cancer Causes and Control*, 1999; **10**:293–302

Marmot MG, Shipley MJ, Rose G. Inequalities in death—specific explanations of a general pattern? *Lancet*, 1984; **i**:1003–6

Martyn CN, Barker DJP, Osmond C. Mothers' pelvic size, fetal growth, and death from stroke and coronary heart disease in men in the UK. *Lancet*, 1996; **348**:1264–8

Maughan B, McCarthy G. Childhood adversities and psychosocial disorders. *British Medical Bulletin*, 1997; **53**:156–69

Mendall MA, Goggin PM, Molineaux N, Levy J, Toosy T, Strachan D, Northfield TC. Childhood living conditions and *Helicobacter pylori* seropositivity in adult life. *Lancet*, 1992; **339**:896–7

Michels KB, Trichopoulos D, Robins JM, *et al.* Birthweight as a risk factor for breast cancer. *Lancet*, 1996; **348**:1542–6

Najman JM. Theories of disease causation and the concept of general susceptibility: a review. *Social Science and Medicine*, 1980; **14A**:231–7

Najman JM, Congalton AA. Australian occupational mortality, 1965–1967: cause specific or general susceptibility? *Sociology of Health and Illness*, 1979; **1**:158–76

Najman JM, Davey Smith G. The embodiment of class-related and health inequalities: Australian policies. *Australia and New Zealand Journal of Public Health*, 2000; **24**:3–4

Neeleman J, Wessely S, Wadsworth M. Predictors of suicide, accidental death, and premature natural death in a general-population cohort. *Lancet*, 1998; **351**:93–7

Njolstad I, Arnesen E, Lund-Larsen PG. Body height, cardiovascular risk factors, and risk of stroke in middle-aged men and women. A 14-year follow-up of the Finnmark Study. *Circulation*, 1996; **94**:2877–82

Notkola V, Punsar S, Karvonen MJ, Haapakaski J. Socio-economic conditions in childhood and mortality and morbidity caused by coronary heart disease in adulthood in rural Finland. *Social Science and Medicine*, 1985; **21**:517–23

Paffenbarger RS, Asnes DP. Chronic disease in former college students III. Precursors of suicide in early and middle life. *American Journal of Public Health*, 1966; **56**:1026–36

Paffenbarger RSJ, Wing AL. Characteristics in youth predisposing to fatal stroke in later years. *Lancet*, 1967; **i**:753–4

Parker DR, Lapane KL, Lasater TM, Carleton RA. Short stature and cardiovascular disease among men and women from two southeastern New England communities. *International Journal of Epidemiology*, 1998; **7**:970–5

Parsonnet J. *Microbes and malignancy. Infection as a cause of human cancers.* Oxford: Oxford University Press, 1999

Pearce NE, Davis PB, Smith AH, Foster FH. Mortality and social class in New Zealand II: male mortality by major disease groupings. *New Zealand Medical Journal*, 1983; **96**:711–6

Phillips A, Davey Smith G. How independent are independent effects? Relative risk estimation when correlated exposures are measured imprecisely. *Journal of Clinical Epidemiology*, 1991; **44**:1223–31

Pocock SJ, Shaper AG, Cook DG, Phillips AN, Walker M. Social class differences in ischaemic heart disease in British men. *Lancet*, 1987; **ii**:197–201

Raitakari OT, Porkka KVK, Rasanen L, Ronnemaa T, Viikari JSA. Clustering and six year cluster-tracking of serum total cholesterol, HDL-cholesterol and diastolic blood pressure in children and young adults. *Journal of Clinical Epidemiology,* 1994; **47**:1085–93

Rodgers B. Adult affective disorder and early environment. *British Journal of Psychiatry*, 1990; **157**:539–50

Rodríguez C, Calle EE, Tatham LM, *et al.* Family history of breast cancer as a predictor for fatal prostate cancer. *Epidemiology*, 1998; **9**:525–9

Rose G. Incubation period of coronary heart disease. *British Medical Journal*, 1982; **284**:1600–1

Rosner B, Colditz GA, Willett WC. Reproductive risk factors in a prospective study of breast cancer: the Nurses' Health Study. *American Journal of Epidemiology*, 1994; **139**:819–35

Sadowski H, Ugarte B, Kolvin I, Kaplan C, Barnes J. Early life and family disadvantages and major depression in adulthood. *British Journal of Psychiatry*, 1999; **174**:112–20

Sanderson M, Williams MA, Malone KE *et al.* Perinatal factors and risk of breast cancer. *Epidemiology*, 1996; **7**:34–7

Shaheen S. The beginnings of chronic airflow obstruction. *British Medical Bulletin*, 1997; **53**:58–70

Shaheen SO, Barker DJP, Shiell AW *et al.* The relationship between pneumonia in early childhood and impaired lung function in late adult life. *American Journal of Respiratory and Critical Care Medicine*, 1994; **149**:616–9

Shaheen SO, Sterne JA, Florey CD. Birth weight, childhood lower respiratory tract infection, and adult lung function. *Thorax*, 1998; **53**:549–53

Springet VH.An interpretation of statistical trends in tuberculosis. *Lancet*, 1952; **i**:521–5; 575–80

Stein CE, Kumaran K, Fall CH, Shaheen SO, Osmond C, Barker DJ. Relation of fetal growth to adult lung function in south India. *Thorax*, 1997; **52**:895–9

Sterling P, Eyer J. Biological basis of stress-related mortality. *Social Science and Medicine*, 1981; **15E**:3–42

Strachan DP. Respiratory and allergic diseases. In: Kuh D, Ben-Shlomo Y (eds) *A life course approach to chronic disease epidemiology*. Oxford: Oxford University Press, 1997, pp 15–41

Swerdlow AJ, dos Santos Silva I. Geographical distribution of lung and stomach cancers in England and Wales over 50 years: changing and unchanging patterns. *British Journal of Cancer*, 1991; **63**:773–81

Syme SL, Berkman LF. Social class, susceptibility and sickness. *American Journal of Epidemiology*, 1976; **104**:1–8

Talamini R, La Vecchia C, Decarli A *et al.* Social factors, diet and breast cancer in a northern Italian population. *British Journal of Cancer*, 1984; **49**:723–9

Tanner JM. *Foetus into man*. Cambridge, MA: Harvard University Press, 1978

Tavani A, Braga C, La Vecchia C, Parazzini F, Talamini R, Franceschi S. Height and breast cancer risk. *European Journal of Cancer*, 1998; **34**:543–7

Thurlow HJ. General susceptibility to illness: a selective review. *Canadian Medical Association Journal*, 1967; **97**:1397–404

Tibblin G, Eriksson M, Cnattingius S, Ekbom A. High birthweight as a predictor of prostate cancer risk. *Epidemiology*, 1995; **6**:423–4

Totman R. *Social causes of illness*. London: Souvenir Press, 1987

Upton MN, Watt GC, Davey Smith G, McConnachie A, Hart CL. Permanent effects of maternal smoking on offspring's lung function. *Lancet*, 1998; **352**:453

Vågerö D, Leon D. Effect of social class in childhood and adulthood on adult mortality. *Lancet*, 1994; **343**:1224–5

Valkonen T. Social inequality in the face of death. In: *European Population Conference*. Helsinki: Central Statistical Office of Finland, 1987*a*, pp 201–61

Valkonen T. Male mortality from ischaemic heart disease in Finland, relation to region of birth and region of residence. *European Journal of Population*, 1987*b*; **3**:61–83

van Loon AJ, Goldbohm RA, Van den Brandt PA. Socioeconomic status and breast cancer incidence: a prospective cohort study. *International Journal of Epidemiology*, 1994; **23**:899–905

van Rossum CTM, van de Mheen H, Breteler MB, Grobbee DE, Mackenbach JP. Socioeconomic differences in stroke among Dutch elderly women. The Rotterdam Study. *Stroke*, 1999; **30**:357–62

Wagener DK, Schatzkin A. Temporal trends in the socioeconomic gradient for breast cancer mortality among US women. *American Journal of Public Health*, 1994; **84**:1003–6

Wang DY, DeStavola BL, Allen DS *et al.* Breast cancer risk is positively associated with height. *Breast Cancer Research and Treatment*, 1997; **43**:123–8

Wannamethee SG, Whincup PH, Shaper G, Walker M. Influence of fathers' social class on cardiovascular disease in middle-aged men. *Lancet*, 1996; **348**:1259–63

Wannamethee SG, Shaper AG, Whincup PH, Walker M. Adult height, stroke, and coronary heart disease. *American Journal of Epidemiology*, 1998; **148**:1069–76

Weinberg RA. How cancer arises. *Scientific American*, 1996; **September**:32–40

Whitaker CJ, Dubiel AJ, Galpin OP. Social and geographical risk factors in Helicobacter pylori infection. *Epidemiology and Infection*, 1993; **111**:63–70

Whitehead M. The health divide. In: Townsend P, Davidson N, Whitehead M (eds) *Inequalities in health: the Black Report and the Health Divide*. Harmondsworth: Penguin, 1992

Wynder EL, Coham LA, Rose DP, Stellman SD. Dietary fat and breast cancer: where do we stand on the evidence? *Journal of Clinical Epidemiology*, 1994; **47**:217–22

Ziegler RG. Anthropometry and breast cancer. *Journal of Nutrition*, 1997; **127**:924S–928S.

6 The impact of health interventions on inequalities: infant and child health in Brazil

Cesar G. Victora, Fernando C. Barros, and
J. Patrick Vaughan

Da Humana Condição
Custa o rico a entrar no céu
(Afirma o povo e não erra)
Porém muito mais difícil
É um pobre ficar na terra.

On the Human Condition
It is hard for a rich man to go to Heaven
(With no blunder the people assert)
However, much harder it seems to be
For a poor man to remain on Earth.
Mario Quintana, Brazilian poet, 1986.

Although there is much debate in developed countries about levels and trends of health inequities (Lancet editorial, 1997; Mackenbach *et al.*, 1997; Williams, 1998), data from developing countries are limited and—even when available—are not fully explored (Braveman, 1998). In particular, data on time trends in inequities are very scarce. This chapter reports on the findings of two population-based birth cohort studies carried out eleven years apart in the same Brazilian city, providing unique data for examining health inequities in the country with the second worst income distribution in the world (World Bank, 1999).

In this chapter, we will refer to inequities rather than inequalities, because the former represent inequalities that are judged to be unfair and unjust, leaving out inequalities that are biologically inevitable (Whitehead, 1992; Braveman, 1998).We also restrict the discussion to real-life interventions that are made available to the general population and that are not specifically targeted at high-risk groups. The analyses are focused on proximate health sector interventions (such as drugs, vaccines, or technologies), as opposed to broad changes in public policy that may also have health implications.

Almost 30 years ago, Julian Tudor-Hart proposed the now well-known 'inverse care law', stating that 'the availability of good medical care tends to vary inversely with the need for it in the population served' (Hart, 1971). In Brazil, this law has been repeatedly demonstrated to hold (Barros *et al.*, 1986; Victora *et al.*, 1992), and this is probably true for other market economies.

A possible corollary to this law is that 'new health interventions will tend to increase inequities', since they will be applied preferentially to those with better baseline health status and therefore will tend to increase existing gaps, at least initially. Based on this corollary, several hypothetical scenarios may be devised. Figure 6.1 shows a set of curves, where the following sequence of events can be observed:

(1) there is an initial gap (inequity) in the outcome measure between the wealthy and the poor;

(2) the new intervention is firstly picked up by the wealthy (the inverse care law);

(3) as a consequence, the outcome improves rapidly among the wealthy, since a high coverage is reached within a short time;

(4) the outcome measure stabilizes, at a very low level, among the wealthy, since no further reductions are possible—the minimum achievable plateau has been reached;

(5) the intervention trickles down through the social scale;

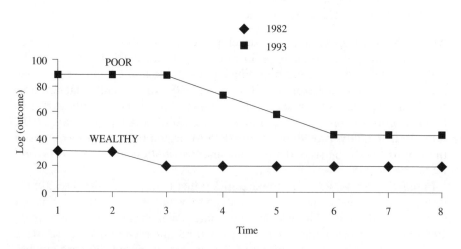

Fig. 6.1 Hypothetical set of curves showing incidence trends in poor and wealthy sub populations

(6) the outcome improves among the poor, but more slowly than it did among the wealthy, since uptake of the intervention is slower; and

(7) since there was greater scope for improvement among the poor, due to their higher baseline level, the final gap narrows.

Figure 6.2 shows that, depending on when the assessment takes place, one may conclude that the intervention led to increased inequity (for example at time points 3 or 4), to no change in the inequity ratio (at time point 5), or to a narrowing of the gap (at time points 6 and 7).

These figures show a simplified scenario in which a single intervention is being implemented in a setting where outcome levels were previously stable both for the poor and the wealthy. In real life, several interventions are usually being promoted concomitantly, at different stages of implementation.

Before examining how well this scenario explains a real life situation in Brazil, a note is required regarding the scale to be used for measuring inequities. Inequity gaps may be measured on absolute (difference) or relative (ratio) scales. For example, if the infant mortality rates (IMRs) are equal to 80 deaths per thousand live births among the poor and to 20 among the rich, the absolute gap is equal to 60 deaths per thousand, and the ratio is equal to 4. If, as a consequence of an intervention, the IMRs become respectively 50 and 10, the difference decreases to 40 deaths per thousand but the ratio increases to 5. Therefore, according to the scale being used, one may have an apparent increase or decrease in the inequity gap.

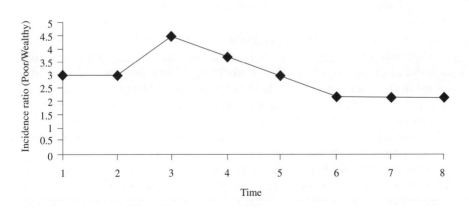

Fig. 6.2 Incidence ratios between poor and wealthy subpopulations corresponding to incidence ratios in Figure 6.1

Using absolute or difference scales will very often lead to apparent reductions in inequity gaps, because baseline rates that are already low—such as those for wealthy—are unlikely to decrease in absolute terms as fast as those among the poor, who start out at a much higher baseline level. Ratio scales, on the other hand, take into account the different baseline levels, and are thus more appropriate for examining time trends.

Population and methods

Pelotas is a 350,000-inhabitant city located in the extreme south of Brazil near the Uruguayan border. The average annual per capita income is US$2700, and Rio Grande do Sul state, where Pelotas is situated, has the highest quality of life index in the country, according to the 1999 Human Development Report by the United Nations' Development Programme.

Over 99% of all births take place in hospitals, so that hospital-based birth cohorts may be regarded as representative of the whole population. Two such studies were carried out 11 years apart, in 1982 and 1993. In the 1982 cohort, children were examined soon after birth, and their mothers were interviewed. When the children were approximately 12 months old, a 33% sub-sample were sought at home using the addresses obtained at the hospital, and 82.3% of them were located. In an attempt to increase this follow-up rate, both in 1984 and 1986 all 70,000 households in the city were visited in search of all children born in 1982. Respectively 87.3% and 83.5% of the original cohort were located. In all three follow-up visits, at least 80% of children in all family income groups were located, and the proportions traced were very similar for the lowest and highest income groups. During the home visits, mothers were interviewed and children were weighed using portable scales. Deaths were monitored through monthly visits to all hospitals, cemeteries, and registries. Further details of the methodology are available elsewhere (Barros et al., 1990).

In 1993, again all maternity hospitals were visited daily during the whole year. A systematic sub-sample of approximately 20% of all children born were visited at home at the age of 12 months, of whom 93.4% were located—92.3% in the lowest income group and 95.5% in the highest group. Mortality data are available for the whole cohort using the same methodology as in 1982. Further methodological details are available elsewhere (Victora et al., 1996; 1998). Table 6.1 shows the numbers of children included in each cohort, according to family income groups in minimum wages per month as reported by the mother in the hospital interview (one minimum wage was then approximately equivalent to US$50). The percentage of children in the poorest and wealthiest categories were similar for both studies, so that it is possible to compare time trends in these groups.

In the eleven years between the two studies, there were several important

Table 6.1   Distribution of children in 1982 and 1983 according to income

Year	Number of children (%) according to family income groups in monthly minimum wages[a]					Total number
	<= 1	1.1–3	3.1–6	6.1–10	>10	
1982	1288	2789	1091	382	335	5914
	(21.8%)	(47.4%)	(18.5%)	(6.5%)	(5.7%)	
1993	967	2148	1203	433	385	5249
	(18.8%)	(41.8%)	(23.4%)	(8.4%)	(7.5%)	

[a] Family income information was missing for 29 children in 1982 and for 113 children in 1993.

changes in health care delivery in the city. The number of first-level governmental health facilities—providing free primary health care, and located mostly in low-income boroughs—increased from less than ten to over 50. In 1982, there were no neonatal intensive care units, but by 1993 the three major maternity hospitals in the city had such units. In addition, the decade witnessed an important expansion of governmental expenditure in preventive and curative health programmes. Pelotas seems to be fairly typical of a middle-sized Brazilian city, where several health interventions were made available to the general population, but were not specifically targeted at the poorest.

Results

The changes in health care provision described above strongly affected inequities in programme coverage. Antenatal care attendance is almost universal in Pelotas, but adequate care requires that medical care should start early in pregnancy. Figure 6.3 shows that, in 1982, 74% of women in the lowest income group had their first attendance before the fifth month of pregnancy, and that this proportion increased to 84% in 1993. Among women from the wealthiest families, this proportion was already 98% in 1982, and remained at this level in 1993. Paraphrasing the notion of a 'minimum achievable level' for disease occurrence presented above, it appears that the wealthy had already reached in 1982 the 'maximum achievable level' for intervention coverage, so that the gap had to narrow given any improvement among the poor.

A similar picture is observed for vaccine coverage (Fig. 6.4). Coverage with three doses of DPT vaccine (diphtheria, pertussis, and tetanus) was already at a very high level among the wealthy in 1982, and this hardly changed in 1993. Substantial improvement, from 72% to 84%, however, was observed among the poor, resulting in a closing gap. Similar findings were observed for other vaccines.

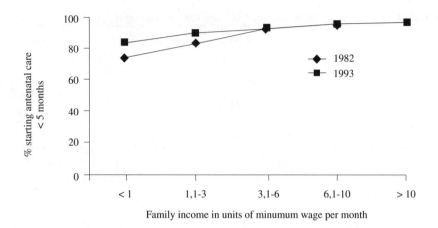

Fig. 6.3 Percentages of women giving birth who had started antenatal care before fifth month of pregnancy by family income, Pelotas, Brazil, 1982 and 1993

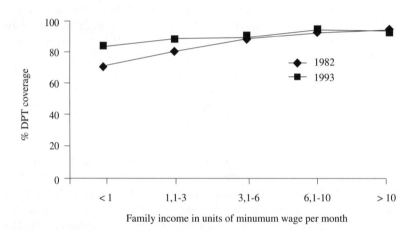

Fig. 6.4 Percentages of children aged 12 months who had received three doses of DPT vaccine by family income, Pelotas, Brazil, 1982 and 1983

For both coverage indicators, therefore, the gap closed during the decade. Given the theoretical scenario described in the first section, the closing gaps in coverage indicators might suggest that inequities in health impact outcomes— like nutrition, morbidity, or mortality—would also start to close in time.

A major impact indicator studied in both cohorts was the prevalence of low weight-for-age at 12 months, defined as being below -2 z-scores relative to the NCHS reference (WHO Expert Committee on Nutrition, 1995). The overall prevalence of underweight decreased from 5.4% in 1982 to 3.7% in 1993, reflecting the general secular decrease in malnutrition that is taking place in Brazil (Monteiro *et al.*, 1993).

Figure 6.5 shows that, already in 1982, prevalences in the three highest income categories were around 1%. In a well-nourished population, 2.3% of the children are expected to be underweight according to the normal distribution (WHO Expert Committee on Nutrition, 1995), and thus there was little room for improvement among the three highest income categories. According to the hypothetical scenario, in this situation the inequity ratio is likely to be reduced, since the wealthy have already reached the minimum achievable level. Figure 6.5 confirms that this was indeed the case, since prevalences in the wealthiest group remained unchanged but those in the poorest group decreased from 14% to 9%.

A different picture appeared for the infant mortality ratio (IMR), which dropped from 36 to 21 per thousand between 1982 and 1993, mostly due to reductions in post-neonatal mortality and in infectious diseases. Figure 6.6 shows that, in spite of such overall improvement, the IMR ratio between the poor and wealthy, which was equal to 7 in 1982, was of exactly the same magnitude in 1993.

To investigate why this gap remained, these data were stratified by birthweight, the major proximate determinant of infant mortality. Percent reductions in mortality between 1982 and 1993 were calculated for four combinations of birthweight (below 2500 g versus 2500 g or more) and family income (3 minimum wages or less versus over 3 minimum wages). To ensure sufficient sample sizes, only two family income groups were used. The results were striking.

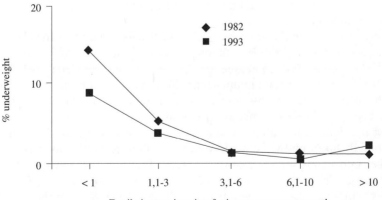

Fig. 6.5   Percentages of children aged 12 months below −2 z-score weight for age by family income, Pelotas, Brazil, 1982 and 1993

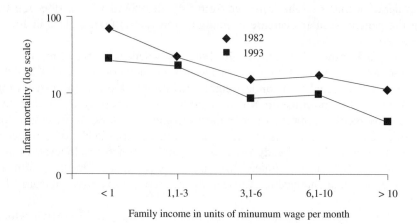

Fig. 6.6   Infant mortality rates per thousand live births (log scale) by family income, Pelotas, Brazil, 1982 and 1993

Among children with an appropriate birthweight (2500 g or more), there was no mortality reduction in the wealthy group, since their IMR was already 5 per thousand in 1982, close to the minimum achievable level, and remained at this level in 1993. Mortality among poor infants with appropriate birthweight, however, fell from 25 to 12, a 52% reduction. The mortality gap was thus reduced from a 5-fold to a 2.4-fold difference between 1982 and 1993, as predicted by the hypothetical curves for interventions that had already been in place for sufficient time. In this case, the interventions that are efficacious against mortality of appropriate-birthweight infants relate mainly to the post-neonatal period, particularly the prevention and management of infectious diseases delivered by primary health services.

A very different picture emerged for low-birthweight infants. Mortality rates, which were already lower in 1982 among the wealthy, fell by a further 68% (from 148 to 48 per thousand), compared to a 36% reduction (from 220 to 141) among the poor. Obviously, the minimum achievable level had not been reached by the wealthy in 1982. The gap thus increased, from 1.5 times in 1982 to 2.9 times in 1993. The most likely interpretation is that the new technologies introduced during the decade, including neonatal intensive care and surfactant therapy, were rapidly taken up by the wealthy and are still to reach the poor. Interviews with key informants suggest that this is indeed the case, since few intensive care beds were available and private patients had priority access to these. According to the hypothetical set of curves, the gap will start to close when the poor have greater access to these technologies that resulted in decreased mortality among wealthy low-birthweight infants.

It should be noted, however, that not every type of health inequality is harmful to the poorest. Figure 6.7 shows the rates of Caesarean sections for Pelotas in both years, by family income groups. Assuming that no more than 15% of all births should be Caesarean sections, all income groups in Pelotas are at an increased risk of unnecessary surgery, particularly the wealthiest group, in which women are now more likely to undergo a Caesarean section than a vaginal delivery! (Barros *et al.*, 1991; 1996).

Discussion

In summary, the data from Pelotas show that the coverage of preventive programmes improved, particularly for the poorest mothers and children. The gap in malnutrition prevalence also diminished, since the poor improved and the wealthy just could not get any better. For mortality, where reductions for the wealthy were still possible, the gap persisted with the same magnitude, but this was due to a combination of a closing gap in mortality of children with an appropriate birthweight and to an increasing gap in the mortality of low-birthweight babies. In future years, one might expect the mortality gap to also close, since the current IMR among the wealthiest category—about 5 per thousand—is similar to that found in the lowest mortality countries in the world.

The present analyses showed that the inverse care law is still operating at full force in southern Brazil. Good quality care is most available to those who need it least. The proposed corollary to this law—that new interventions will tend to increase inequity since they will initially reach those who are already better

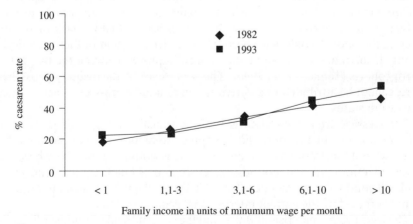

Fig 6.7   Caesarean section rates (% of deliveries) by family income, Pelotas, Brazil, 1982 and 1993

off—also appears to hold, at least until the wealthy reach a level beyond which little progress can be made. As a result, inequity gaps will increase with new technologies, but may eventually decrease as these trickle down the social scale.

The hypothetical curves shown in Figs 6.1 and 6.2 seem to fit the data described above well. A fundamental issue in the evaluation of the impact of interventions on equity, therefore, is the timing factor, since apparently contradictory results may be found at different stages of implementation.

It may be argued that, if interventions are strictly aimed to reach the poorest, inequity gaps may be reduced immediately. While there is no doubt that this might work under experimental trial conditions, it is less clear that it will be so in real life. The authors' study of the Brazilian health scene over more than 20 years suggests that most interventions reach the private sector (and therefore the wealthy) years before they are made available to the general population through government health services. This has been the case for vaccines, antibiotics, surfactant therapy, neonatal intensive care, antenatal screening, and many other technologies. Secondly, even in the rare event when new interventions are delivered through the governmental system but are not available commercially, the wealthy are also entitled to use them, and—being better informed—will acquire access to these technologies before the poor.

Analyses and interpretations of time trend data are made more complex by the fact that there are several interventions taking place at the same time. As was shown for the IMR, interventions that are now being picked up by the poor have already have had their maximum impact on the wealthy, but—at the same time—mortality among the latter is now being further reduced by new interventions that have not yet reached the poor.

Mortality and morbidity obviously depend not only on health sector interventions but also on concomitant changes in socio-economic, demographic, and environmental factors—factors which also interact with the interventions themselves. In this case study, there is no reason to believe that the lack of progress among the poorest could have been due to a deterioration in their standard of living. If anything, the stake of the poorest improved between the two Pelotas birth cohorts (Tomasi et al., 1996). The persistence of the inequity gaps, therefore, cannot be attributed to a deterioration in non-health-sector factors affecting health status.

The message from these data is both pessimistic and optimistic. It is pessimistic because interventions did not appear to reduce inequity ratios until the wealthy could just not improve any more. It is optimistic, however, because it shows that mortality and morbidity rates seem to be falling for all social groups, and will continue to do so in the future if the availability of social programmes is not curtailed by the current international economic crisis.

The recent economic crisis in Brazil and the current trend toward neo-liberalism —resulting in major cuts in health programmes—cast some doubts on whether the achievements among the poorest stratum of mothers and children can be sustained in the future.

REFERENCES

Barros FC, Vaughan JP, Victora CG. Why so many Caesarean sections? The need for a further policy change in Brazil. *Health Policy and Planning*, 1986; **1**:19–29

Barros FC, Victora CG, Vaughan JP. The Pelotas birth cohort study, 1982–1987. Strategies for following up 6,000 children in a developing country. *Paediatric and Perinatal Epidemiology*, 1990; **4**:205–20

Barros FC, Vaughan JP, Victora CG, Huttly SRA. An epidemic of caesarian sections in Brazil? The influence of tubal ligations and socioeconomic status. *Lancet*, 1991; **338**:167–9

Barros FC, Victora CG, Morris SS. Caesarian sections in Brazil (letter). *Lancet*, 1996; **347**:839

Braveman P. Monitoring equity in health: a policy-oriented approach in low- and middle-income countries. Geneva: World Health Organization (Division of Analysis, Research and Assessment), 1998

Hart JT. The inverse care law. *Lancet*, 1971; **i**:405–12

Lancet Editorial. Health inequality: the UK's biggest issue. *Lancet*, 1997; **349**:1185

Mackenbach JP, Kunst AE, Cavelaars AE, Groenhof F, Geurts JJ. Socioeconomic inequalities in morbidity and mortality in Western Europe. The EU Working Group on Socioeconomic Inequalities in Health. *Lancet*, 1997; **349**:1655–9

Monteiro CA, Benicio MHD, Iunes R, Gouveia NC, Taddei JAAC, Cardoso MAA. ENDEF e PNSN: para onde caminha o crescimento físico da criança brasileira? *Cadernos de Saude Publica*, 1993; **9(suppl 1)**:85–95

Tomasi E, Barros FC, Victora CG. Situação socioeconômica e condições de vida: comparação de duas coortes de base populacional no sul do Brazil. *Cadernos de Saude Publica*, 1996; **12 (suppl 1)**:15–9

UNDP. *1999 World Development Report.* http://www.undp.org.br/HDR/HDR99.htm, 24 January 2000

Victora CG, Barros FC, Vaughan JP. *Epidemiologia de la Desigualdad.* Washington: Pan-American Health Organization, 1992

Victora CG, Barros FC, Tomasi E *et al.* Tendencias e diferenciais na saude materno-infantil: delineamento e metodologia das coortes de 1982 e 1993 de mães e crianças de Pelotas, RS. *Cadernos de Saude Publica*, 1996; **12(suppl 1)**:7–14

Victora CG, Morris SS, Barros FC, Horta BL, Weiderpass E, Tomasi E. Breastfeeding and growth in Brazilian infants. *American Journal of Clinical Nutrition*, 1998; **67**:452–8

Whitehead M. The concepts and principles of equity and health. *International Journal of Health Services*, 1992; **22**:429–45

Williams RB. Lower socioeconomic status and increased mortality: early childhood roots and the potential for successful interventions. *Journal of the American Medical Association*, 1998; **279**:1745–6

World Bank. *World Development Report 1998/99: knowledge for development.* Washington DC: World Bank, 1999

World Health Organization Expert Committee on Nutrition. *Physical status, uses and interpretation of anthropometry.* WHO Technical Report Series No. 854. Geneva: World Health Organization, 1995

7 Children's health in developing countries: issues of coping, child neglect and marginalization

Claudio F. Lanata

Public health interventions aimed at reducing the burden of infectious diseases in children in developing countries are frequently developed and implemented on the basis of a number of often unstated assumptions. In particular, it is assumed that the provision of health services with trained professionals and the implementation of specific effective interventions (such as oral rehydration, immunization, and fortified foods) will lead to a uniform improvement of health status throughout the population. However, these assumptions are not necessarily true, and have been called into question by work we have conducted since 1982 in Canto Grande, a densely populated area of low socio-economic status in peri-urban Lima, Peru (Lopez de Romaña, 1987; Yeager, 1991).

It has long been recognized that if a large group of children living in the same community are followed to identify the frequency by which they develop diarrhoeal diseases, the distribution of the diarrhoeal episodes detected is not uniform. Some children have many repeat episodes while others (around 20% in peri-urban Lima) will not develop any diarrhoeal episode detected by the home surveillance system in place. Preliminary observations in Lima have indicated that the group of children with the highest incidence and prevalence of diarrhoea also have the highest prevalence of respiratory illnesses. These children are not necessarily the poorest or those living at worst conditions within the population. While poor immune status (due, for example, to micro-nutrient deficiency) may be a factor, other mechanisms may also be involved.

Some insight into the nature of these other mechanisms has been provided by field workers who have been conducting frequent home visits to detect diarrhoeal diseases in children participating in community-based studies of diarrhoeal diseases in peri-urban Lima. They reported that children who developed malnutrition, or died from diarrhoeal or respiratory illnesses, often appeared to be the ones not wanted by their parents. Indeed, some field workers were confident that they were able to predict the health and survival of a woman's offspring before they were born, simply on the basis of their assess-ment of the nature of the home environment and the attitudes and capabilities of the parents. In several cases, having been alerted by field workers, study doctors and field co-ordinators attempted to intervene at an early stage, offering help in an attempt to avoid poor outcomes. However, this help was frequently rejected by parents.

One such case involves a malnourished child who was admitted to the Nutri-tion Research Institute with the agreement of the family. However, after the child had successfully recovered, the mother cried when the child was discharged to go home, expressing her distress at the difficulties of raising the child. She perceived the health care and the successful recovery of her child as a hostile action towards her. It could be said that she had wished her child would die at the Nutrition Institute. Another similarly dramatic case reported by a field worker involved twins, both of whom developed an acute diarrhoeal episode and died with acute dehydration within 24 hours of each other. The deaths occurred despite the fact that the field worker had previously explained in detail to the mother and family about the preparation and use of oral rehydration solutions, and had left several envelopes of dehydration formula at the home, had given advice about early signs of dehydration, and had urged the mother to take the twins to the nearest health facility if symptoms developed. It became clear when interviewing the mother during the following home visits that the twins had not been adequately cared for, that they were left untended for long periods of time, that no oral rehydration was given, and that they were not taken to the nearby hospital when they became dehydrated.

Since these early anecdotal reports, we have come to recognize through several community-based studies (Black et al., 1989; Lanata et al., 1989; 1991; 1992; 1996a; 1996b; Huttly et al., 1998; WHO/CHD Immunization-linked Vitamin A Supplementation Study Group, 1998; Penny, 1999) that the majority of deaths due to respiratory illnesses, diarrhoea, or malnutrition in this community are occurring in unwanted or neglected children. Child neglect per se is a risk factor that is not detected by the health system and is not registered in the vital statis-tics of the country. Moreover, the dramatic cases outlined above suggest that effective and available interventions are not sufficient to prevent the develop-ment of life-threatening conditions in these unwanted children, because their parents, whether intentionally or not, end up secluding them from the help available.

Despite these dramatic cases, it is nevertheless clear that, in general, the health of children does improve as a consequence of frequent home visits by field workers. Thus, the overall infant mortality rates observed in the study popula-tion has always been lower when compared to the nearby communities not visited by field workers. In addition the severity of diarrhoeal episodes tends to be lower than expected, in children under surveillance. Even though field workers are trained only to obtain specific information required by the study during these home visits, and to provide primary health care, they often establish a strong and positive personal relationship with the mother of the study children. This relationship in many cases has stimulated mothers to provide more attention to, and better care of, their children. This effect may partly explain the frequently recognized observation that effective interventions have a greater efficacy in populations participating in controlled studies, as compared with those not part of the study, or those who refuse to participate in it (Clemens *et al.*, 1993).

The importance of the quality of care provided to children living in poor communities was also indicated by preliminary observations reported in a meeting by another group of investigators (Gambirazo C, personal communication) although, unfortunately, this study was never published. As part of a longitudinal, community-based study of children in peri-urban areas of Puno, a Peruvian city located on the edge of Lake Titicaca at 4100 metres above sea level, several variables were measured at baseline in a group of children who were followed to identify risk factors for poor nutritional growth. The best predictor of better growth in this poor community, after controlling for socio-economic and other variables measured in the study, was the presence in the home of the mother or a mother-substitute who was classified as a good care-provider at baseline, based on the love and affection given to the child as observed by a study psychologist. Children who did not have a person who cared for them had worse nutritional status and worse health in the period under follow-up.

Anecdotal information reported by feminist groups in Peru has indicated the potential for some effective ways of intervening in the case of unwanted or neglected children (Galdos S, personal communication). While concentrating their efforts and interventions on women usually affected by home violence, alcohol, and other social problems, they noticed that once they succeeded in improving the self-esteem of these women, the frequency of visits to the study clinic by their children was reduced, even though no intervention was given to them, other than providing free health care. This effect occurred even when mothers spent less time with their children in order to participate in community activities introduced by them. Improving maternal self-esteem may be an important intervention in these high-risk groups.

A conceptual model

Based on the preliminary, anecdotal information outlined above, and on reports from the literature (mostly from developed countries), a conceptual model has been developed to help understand the variables that may be playing a role in this complex scenario of child neglect in poor communities in developing countries, their social marginalization and their seclusion from the health care available to them.

We suggest that the capacity to care for and nurture children in the adverse social conditions prevailing in many poor communities in developing countries is a neglected issue that has several components. The individual characteristics of the child and the mother and, more importantly, the nature and quality of the mother–child interaction, seems essential for the healthy development of the child. The mother–child relationship is affected by the presence of the father or any other family member who may function in that role, especially for the support to the mother. These essential players function within the constraints and influences of the socio-cultural environment in which they live (Fig. 7.1). When these conditions are not favourable, the mother–child–father relationship is placed under strain.

Some parents or carers under these circumstances are able to make best use of all the individual, familial, and communal resources available to them in order to protect their own welfare and that of their children. Although the limitations of the environment in the area where they live (food availability, job opportunities, access to health services, and so on) may not be optimal, it is these children who are most likely to survive. We suggest that the parents of these children are people who are most likely to be members of social groups available in the community, like mother clubs or community kitchens, who work towards community development, education, health or nutrition, and who get involved in adult education.

Under the same stresses and strains, however, other parents and carers are not able to cope or make use of the available resources. This may be associated with family disruption (linked to increased violence and alcohol or drug abuse), low maternal self-esteem, and depression. These factors then affect the development and health of the child. Children who die as a consequence of this sort of neglect will rarely have child abuse or neglect stated as the cause of death. Instead,

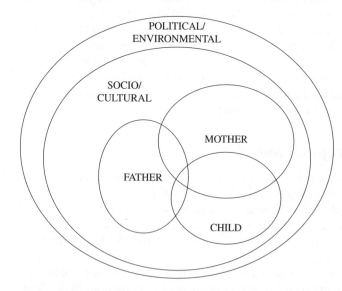

Fig. 7.1 Conceptual model on the relationships existing between the principal elements involved with child neglect and social marginalization in developing countries

the cause of death may well be given as one of the diseases that are prevalent in the area, like respiratory or diarrhoeal diseases and malnutrition. We suggest that the parents and carers involved in such tragedies may be unlikely to be part of any social organization available in their community. This is not only because they may lack the energy and resources to participate, but also because they may be rejected by other members of the community for failing to show an adequate level of participation and commitment. For the same reasons they also are very unlikely to respond to the call from organized social groups or existing organizations (health, education, etc.), remaining 'silent', marginalized, and secluded in their community until a serious event develops. Those children who manage to survive in those conditions will have a price to pay in terms of their personal development, characteristics, and well-being, having permanent disabilities, and the tendency to perpetuate their condition once they became parents, replicating the circle.

In reality, the capabilities of parents and carers in any community span a wide range, with the types described above constituting only a minority at either end of the distribution. However, public health programmes do not generally take into account this important dimension of variation within the communities they are trying to help. Public health does not generally recognize the importance of the essential players within a family, and the factors that influence their functioning. Instead, efforts are usually concentrated towards the child or the mother, taken out of context of the nature of their interactions. However, in order to optimize the success of public health interventions, these programmes need to incorporate the mother–child–father (or substitute) participants in their activities, and be sensitive to the presence of hostile conditions from their environment and the subgroup of families and individuals who will exclude themselves from their action. Further research is needed better to understand the nature of the relationship between maternal self-esteem and depression with child development and health in developing countries, in order to develop specific interventions.

In the rest of this chapter we will explore the extent to which our conceptual model involving the role of child neglect as an important determinant of child health is supported by the available information.

Child factors

It is known that children born with lower birthweight, or prematurely, have a higher incidence of infectious diseases and are at greater risk of death (Barros *et al.*, 1992). This may be due, in part, to biological factors, as indicated by the lower mortality observed in children born with lower birthweight that received a daily zinc supplement during the first nine months of life (Sazawal *et al.*, 1999). Non-biological factors may also play a role. The sex of the child could be a risk factor for greater mortality, as observed in some societies with strong cultural preferences for males (Thein and Goh, 1991). In some cases, active female infanticide may occur, as reported in north India (Miller, 1987), Bangladesh (Fauveau, 1991), and China. However, unwanted children may die without any of these risk factors. Pioneer work done in shanty towns in Brazil described the occurrence of child deaths in families exposed to harsh social conditions (Sheper-Hughes, 1991*a*). *Death without weeping* (Sheper-Hughes, 1991*b*), a detailed recollection of cases observed, illustrates how deaths were attributed to several cultural reasons (infants born weak, or influenced by bad spirits, etc.) that justified not trying to save them, making the families and their social group more amenable to dealing with these early losses. These deaths do not occur randomly throughout the community. They cluster among some high-risk families, who frequently have more than one death in the same family (Das Gupta, 1990; Madise and Diamond, 1995). It is possible that children born in these high-risk families are neglected and exposed to psychological distress, a factor that has been associated with a greater risk of developing diseases and death in adults (Somervell *et al.*, 1989). In those conditions, the character of the child may play an important role: those children who are more demanding and able to get attention may have better chances of surviving than those who are quiet.

Maternal factors

Maternal education

Several studies have linked the level of maternal education with child health and child mortality. In a review of available studies it was found that, for each one-year increase in education, there was an associated 7–9% decline of mortality in children under five years of age in developing countries (Cleland and van Ginneken, 1988). It is not clear how maternal education acts on child health. It probably functions as a proxy for several socio-economic advantages associated with better educated families (Desai and Alva, 1998), one of which could be access and utilization of health services (Cleland and Van Gineken, 1988). However, in statistical analyses controlling for wealth, mortality reduction is still strongly associated with educated mothers (Cleland and van Ginneken, 1989; Grosse and Auffrey 1989), suggesting that education itself could lead to improvements in child survival (Caldwell 1994). Education may also be associated with women having increased motivation and greater aspiration to improve their lives. Educated mothers may be more capable of surviving and fighting effectively for themselves and their families.

Some studies have tried to use maternal education as a public health intervention. Maternal education modified the effect of water and sanitation interventions in Malaysia (Esrey and Habicht, 1988). However, in a revealing prospective study done in Nicaragua, education seems to benefit mostly those individuals with lower intelligence scores, since those with higher intelligence levels have already acquired skills, values, knowledge, or attitudes related to improved child survival, even if they are not yet educated (Sandiford *et al.*, 1997).

Maternal self-esteem

As indicated earlier in this chapter, an important intervening variable may be maternal self-esteem. In developed countries, lower maternal self-esteem has been associated with poverty and lack of financial resources (Brody and Flor, 1997). Maternal stress and poor self-esteem is associated with spontaneous pre-term birth, with low birth weight (Edwards *et al.*, 1994; Copper *et al.*, 1996), and with post-partum depression (Hall *et al.*, 1996). Depression and low maternal self-esteem interfere with primary maternal attachment (Salzman, 1996), inducing poor maternal competence during infancy (Mercer and Ferketich, 1995), insufficient milk supply syndrome (Hill and Aldag, 1991), and infants with failure to thrive (Oates, 1984), and is thought to be a cause of child neglect and abuse (Christensen *et al.*, 1994; Lesnik-Oberstein *et al.*, 1995).

Few studies have evaluated these parameters in developing countries. In Jamaica, self-esteem was greater in women living in urban areas and in those with an adult male relative present at home, and there was less likelihood of unwanted pregnancy (Keddie, 1992). In Burkina Faso, low maternal self-esteem was associated with greater frequency of unwanted pregnancies in adolescents (Gorgen *et al.*, 1993). Poor maternal self-esteem is greater among adolescent pregnancies, a condition that is also associated with greater frequency of low birthweight and prematurity (Kessel *et al.*, 1985). More research is needed to understand the nature of maternal self-esteem in developing countries, to measure the magnitude of low maternal self-esteem in populations of low socio-economic conditions, and its relationship with maternal depression (see below), child health, and development.

Maternal depression

In recent years, it has been recognized that minor psychiatric illnesses and depression are a frequent condition in developing countries (see chapter 12, this volume). These conditions have been found in 30–50% of women in studies done in Brazil (Almeida-Filho, 1997) and other developing countries (Rahim and Cederblad, 1989; Reichenheim and Harpham, 1991), proportions that are under-represented or unrecognized in the official statistics of Ministries of Health in developing countries. Maternal depression is associated with urbanization (Ekblad, 1990; Harpham, 1990) and poverty (Reichenheim and Harpham, 1991; Bahar *et al.*, 1992; Saraceno and Barbui, 1997) and with recent immigrants who find difficulties in adapting to their new social environment (Coutinho *et al.*, 1996). It has been postulated that maternal depression mediates the link between childhood neglect and abuse, everyday stressors, and maternal self-esteem (Lutenbacher and Hall, 1998). Depressed mothers are less responsive to their children's needs, and less able to interact with them (Cox *et al.*, 1987). Children of depressed mothers have more emotional and behavioural disturbances as compared with those of non-depressed mothers (de Almeida Filho *et al.*, 1985; Cox *et al.*, 1987; Gross *et al.*, 1994; Cicchetti *et al.*, 1997). More importantly, children of depressed mothers (even from those who had a transient post-partum depression) have long-term consequences, possible to measure many years later (Murray and Stein, 1991). Non-psychotic post-partum depression seems to occur with a frequency of 10% of all deliveries in developed countries (Nott, 1987; Cooper *et al.*, 1988), and may be even higher in developing countries, as suggested by a study in Dubai, United Arab Emirates (Abou-Saleh and Ghubash, 1997). Post-partum depression has a negative influence on maternal role attainment and competence (Fowles, 1998), indicating its importance in child development.

Other maternal factors

The character and personality of the mother, as well as her life experience, may influence her capacity to raise her own children. In a study in Guatemala, women were classified into three behavioural styles: those who were proactive—action-oriented, taking the initiative; those who were reactive—tending to cope with their reality, responding to problems in a limited fashion; and those who were non-reactive—who were passive, and fatalistic about their future (Cosminsky, 1987; Scrimshaw MW and Scrimshaw SC, unpublished). The pattern of food distribution within the family may also be important. Some developing societies, such as Bangladesh, allocate the best quality foods and the greater amounts to the husbands, leaving children and women till last (Brown *et al.*, 1982; Abdullah and Wheeler, 1985), an issue taken up in chapter 16. Women's economic dependence and capacity to generate income may also be important. In single-parent families, employed mothers had more positive perceptions of their children, and provided more enriching home environments for their children, than unemployed mothers (Youngblut *et al.*, 1998). The age at first sexual encounter and marital status may also play a role, as may health status, since illnesses, particularly chronic illnesses such as tuberculosis, have a direct effect on ability to care for children. Finally, the way the family functions and interacts with each member may be very important. A US study showed that families that were classified as more cohesive and integrated had fewer health and social problems than those classified as disrupted and not integrated (Olson *et al.*, 1983).

Maternal–child interactions

Maternal and child characteristics play an important role in the quality, frequency, and intensity of the interactions between them and the type of care received by the child. These interactions, and the factors reviewed above, together with the prevailing cultural patterns, may determine the type and duration of breastfeeding, introduction of other dietary practices, health care utilization, and the care given to the child when ill. Care in terms of affection, emotional support, and effective allocation of resources, given in an atmosphere of stability and security, is very important for adequate child nutrition and development. It has been observed that those children living in hostile environments who grow better receive better-quality foods, have more physical interaction, affection, and praise from their mothers and relatives, and receive more verbal and environmental stimulation (Zeitlin, 1991). Children with better mental health in Salvador, Brazil, were those with better quality of family environment, who were better cared for, and who received good quality stimulation within the home environment (de Sousa Bastos and Almeida-Filho, 1990).

The type of early communication between mother and infant may be important for infant development, as indicated by a study on the infant cry characteristics and the mother's perception of the cry. Those mothers who were able adequately to identify the infant cry characteristics at one month of age, as measured in an acoustic laboratory, had infants with better language and cognitive performance at 18 months of age, as compared with those who did not (Lester *et al.*, 1995). The mother's ability to read her infant's cues was related to social support available to her and maternal self-esteem. Developmental and psychoanalytic studies have identified the importance of the early attachment between the parents (not just the mother) and the infant as essential for a normal child development (Brazelton and Cramer, 1991). Even before the child is born, parents go through a process of wishing for the baby and then establishing an early relationship during pregnancy, as a response to the growth of the child and the fetal movements that become increasingly obvious. Immediately after birth, there is a window of time in which early attachment is fostered by intimate contact between the newborn and the mother, a reaction that has been successfully used in the promotion of breastfeeding programmes in many developing countries. Later in life, the relationship between the child and the mother (parents) goes through a series of phases or characteristics (synchrony, symmetry, contingency, and entrainment) to allow the development of the needed security in the infant to be able later to move on to play games and became autonomous (Brazelton and Cramer, 1991). The child's character also seems to influence the mother's response and her self-perceived capacity and competence (Pridham *et al.*, 1994).

When children are raised in hostile and deprived environments, without adequate care and support from their parents, they often demonstrate behavioural problems and poor school performance at later stages. A study of children who were difficult to manage at school found links with maternal depression, parenting stress, and frequent family problems (Campbell, 1994). As mentioned earlier, those children at greater risk of dying became less active and remained silent in the presence of a hostile environment.

Child neglect and abuse

One of the consequences of poor maternal–child interaction is the neglect or the abuse of the child by their parents. Very few studies have been done of child abuse in developing countries. In one survey in India, physical abuse was found in families from middle-class professionals, where the majority (57%) reported using violence as a method to resolve conflict with their children (Segal, 1995). In Ghana, it was found that, in a community-based survey of childhood burns, 5% of cases were associated with evidence of deliberate child abuse (Forjuoh, 1995). In Nigeria, abandonment of normal infants by their parents (usually unmarried or very poor mothers in urban areas) was also reported (Okeahialam, 1984). These cases, however, may represent the extreme of an unrecognized global problem of child neglect and abuse in developing countries (Gelles and Cornell, 1983; Finkelhor and Korbin, 1988; Oyemade, 1991). The World Health Organization has estimated that the rate of child abuse and neglect could be between 13 and 20 per 100,000 live births (Belsey, 1993). In developed countries (Steinberg et al., 1981; Spearly and Lauderdale, 1983), child abuse and neglect is strongly associated with family income and job availability, and this may well be true in developing countries too.

Children with chronic illnesses or with congenital abnormalities are at greater risk of being neglected or even abused (Frodi, 1981; Jaudes and Diamond, 1986; Scheper-Hughes, 1990). Later in life, this becomes evident with the highly prevalent but frequently unrecognized sexual abuse of children, child labour, and other forms of child abuse. This may be one of the factors that explain the increasing number of street children seen in many large cities of developing countries (Segal and Ashtekar, 1994). These conditions are associated with higher childhood mortality, as explained earlier in this chapter. In developed countries, child abuse and neglect is considered as a possibility when a child is brought to an emergency service with an unexpected death (Christoffel et al., 1985). This pattern is just beginning to be recognized in developing countries, as documented in a study of 30 cases of childhood deaths caused by physical abuse in Kuala Lumpur, Malaysia (Kasim et al., 1995).

Surviving children who are abused are also affected for the rest of their lives. Verbal and sexual abuse appears to have a great impact on children's perception of themselves and the world (Ney et al., 1986). They will face similar difficulties to their parents when they constitute a family, repeating the same vicious circle of unwanted pregnancies, adolescent pregnancies, and single-parent families (Gara et al., 1996). Studies of children who were abused have not only identified deleterious developmental consequences to the child, but show that they maintain abuse in later life. It seems that the interaction between the abusive parent(s) and the child is such that both are involved in maintaining the situation (Crittenden, 1985; Augoustinos, 1987). In many cases, they are unable to break that circle without external help (Crittenden, 1985). In other cases, siblings are also involved in similar abusive behaviours to their parents, learning those behaviours from them, rather than in response to an infant's temperament (Crittenden, 1984).

The problems and consequences of child abuse and neglect are such that, in many developed countries, several intervention and prevention programmes have been launched (Krugman, 1991). It is expected that, in the future, this area will receive the attention it needs in developing countries, as an important strategy to reduce the social problems they are facing today.

Unwanted children

Many fertility surveys done in developing countries have indicated that the majority of pregnancies are unwanted, with higher prevalence in adolescents, and in poorer areas of countries going through an economic and fertility transition (Arancibia et al., 1989; Bongaarts, 1997; Pinto e Silva, 1998). Unwanted pregnancies are directly related to abortion practices that in developing countries may became complicated by infection and the death of the mother (Darney, 1988). Studies in developed countries have indicated that mothers of unwanted children have higher rates of anxiety and depression, as compared with those who wanted their pregnancies (Najman et al., 1991). Important information has been produced in these countries when children born to mothers who were denied an abortion were studied. Those children seem to do worse when compared with wanted children, and have lower skill development in childhood, less positive relationships with their mothers, greater fearfulness, and lower positive effect, as well as lower language developmental skills (Baydar, 1995). Unwanted boys seem to be at higher risk of developmental problems than unwanted girls (Dytrych et al., 1975). Unwanted children are also at higher risk for child abuse (Zuravin, 1991). Long-term follow-up studies of unwanted children have documented that there is a long-term impact on their self-esteem, even 23 years later (Axinn et al., 1998), and they have a higher rate of social and psychiatric problems even up to 35 years of age (Forssman and Thuwe, 1981). This higher risk of disease, and poor school and social performance could be explained, in part, by the self-selection of families with unwanted children that have less desire to improve their conditions, and probably greater social and psychological problems than their peers within the same social class (Rantakallio and Myhrman, 1980).

There is a need to do similar studies in developing countries, where the magnitude of the problem seems greater. An extreme of this range of unwanted children are those who are fostered. In a study in rural Sierra Leone, where a high proportion of children under three years of age are fostered and live away from their mothers, it has been observed that they are subject to nutritional problems due to intra-household discrimination in food allocation and access to medical treatment (Bledsoe et al., 1988).

Father's role

The presence of the father in the family is an important factor contributing to the well-being of children that is generally not recognized. Agencies involved with development projects in developing countries have only recently recognized the importance of involving both parents in their programmes. Some studies have found an association between childhood illnesses and mortality and the educational level of the father, as well as the stability of their presence in the home (Cutts *et al.*, 1996). Very few studies have focused on the role of fathers in the health of the family, and practically all have been carried out in developed countries.

Single parent families have a higher frequency of psychiatric disorders in their children, specially in those lacking a father during childhood (Moilanen and Rantakallio, 1988). In a study of twins raised by separate parents, children raised by their mothers developed tighter bonds with them inducing basic trust and better language development than twins raised by fathers, but had more neurotic symptoms in adolescence (Moilanen and Pennanen, 1997). In contrast, children raised by fathers were more frequently physical leaders, had fewer accidents, and were more independent than their twin brothers raised by mothers (Moilanen and Pennanen, 1997). In a study done in Hong Kong, paternal parenting was found to have a stronger influence on the adolescent psychological well-being than maternal parenting (Shek, 1999). These studies suggest not only that both parents are important but that the fathers are associated with facilitating the introduction of the child into society later in life. This is an area that requires further research in developing countries.

Social resources and networking

The performance of individuals in a particular society is regulated by their socio-cultural context. The existence of familial or social groups in developing countries is important for the function of families, particularly women. Social networks support and promote better mental and physical well-being of women in developing countries (Myntti, 1993) and have been used as a strategy to improve the self-esteem of women in these societies. Jobless, homeless women are at greater risk of psychological and mental problems, as are their families and children (Ensminger and Celentano, 1988; Winefield and Tiggemann 1990; Parker *et al.*, 1991). Women's groups in developing countries, like mothers' clubs or community kitchens, seem to self-select those women who are more proactive, energetic, and resourceful, leaving behind depressed women who are at greatest risk and need. More studies are needed to explore how to make these frequently available social networks more helpful to the women and families in greatest need.

Potential interventions

The health effects of the poor social and economic conditions that prevail in many communities in developing countries may seem so large that effective change in the quality of life of their inhabitants, particularly infants born to high-risk families, seems impossible without the overall economic development of the country. This may be quite true as a whole. However, since economic development requires many years of sustained economic growth, with adequate social policies, to be achieved, other strategies are needed while waiting for this long-term goal to occur.

No substantial research has been undertaken to investigate the potential contribution of interventions to reduce child neglect and abuse in developing countries. However, several reports suggest that this may be a fruitful area to explore. In developed countries, adolescents' knowledge of infant development affects their confidence in providing child care (Ruchala and James, 1997; Herrmann et al., 1998), increases their self-esteem, and prevents the development of child abuse and neglect (Marshall et al., 1991). Early recognition of high-risk pregnancies is feasible at prenatal care or in the post-partum period (Leventhal et al., 1989). Early interventions during the hospitalization period or soon after discharge from a maternity ward have been found to be effective in reducing maternal stress and promoting self-esteem (Fulton et al. 1991; Tucker et al., 1998). Community nursing visits to high-risk mothers improve their mental status and self-esteem (Vines and Williams-Burgess, 1994). Women-to-women programmes have increased maternal self-esteem and empowerment (McFarlane and Fehir, 1994), as observed by feminist groups in Peru (Galdos S, personal communication). Maternal employment improves child care in single parent families, even if the mother spends less time at home (Youngblut et al., 1998). In a recently published randomized, controlled study done in Zambia, home visits by midwives at 3, 7, 28, and 42 days after delivery were compared with no visits, both groups being offered regular care at the health clinic (Ransjo-Arvidson et al., 1998). There were fewer children with health problems, less perceived insufficient milk production, less early introduction of supplementary feedings, and mothers taking more action to solve infant health problems, in the group with home visits. Similar studies are needed in other developing countries, including the evaluation of the cost–benefits of these interventions.

Other interventions may also be available to modify some of the several variables that may be linked to socio-economic conditions, and which seem to be playing a role in the quality of care given to young children in developing countries (Fig. 7.2). Many of them are not amenable to public health or developmental interventions, but some could be the focus of specific interventions.

Several interventions are being delivered to improve the health status of children. Promotion of breast feeding and improvement of weaning foods should have an important impact on the nutritional status of children and on their

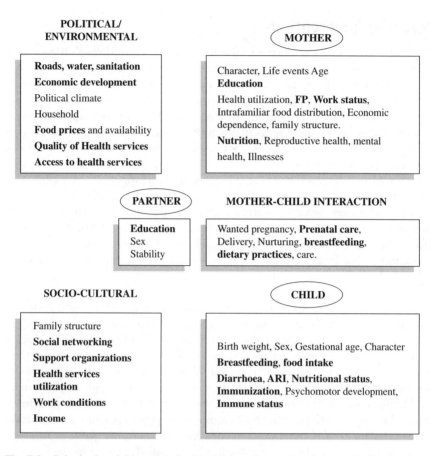

**POLITICAL/
ENVIRONMENTAL**

MOTHER

Roads, water, sanitation
Economic development
Political climate
Household
Food prices and availability
Quality of Health services
Access to health services

Character, Life events Age
Education
Health utilization, **FP, Work status,**
Intrafamiliar food distribution, Economic
dependence, family structure.
Nutrition, Reproductive health, mental
health, Illnesses

PARTNER   **MOTHER-CHILD INTERACTION**

Education
Sex
Stability

Wanted pregnancy, **Prenatal care,**
Delivery, Nurturing, **breastfeeding,**
dietary practices, care.

SOCIO-CULTURAL   **CHILD**

Family structure
Social networking
Support organizations
Health services
utilization
Work conditions
Income

Birth weight, Sex, Gestational age, Character
Breastfeeding, food intake
Diarrhoea, ARI, Nutritional status,
Immunization, Psychomotor development,
Immune status

Fig. 7.2 Principal variables related with child neglect and social marginalization in developing countries. Highlighted in bold letters are those that could be focus of public health and policy interventions

morbidity and mortality (Feachem and Koblinsky, 1984; Ashworth and Feachem, 1985). Prevention of infectious diseases through immunization (Lanata *et al.*, 1996*a*; 1996*b*), hygiene practices (Huttly *et al.*, 1994; 1997), adequate faeces disposal (Lanata *et al.*, 1998), and micro-nutrient supplementation (Zinc Investigators' Collaborative Group, in press), will have an important effect. On the maternal side, programmes that will improve the educational level of women, or promote family planning to increase birth-spacing, or improve the work status of women, and their nutritional status (including micro-nutrient deficiencies) are also important. Counselling and educational programmes on child care and infant feeding that could be applied during prenatal care programmes or after delivery could also be effective. Many developing countries are now promoting early skin-to-skin contact between the newborns and their mothers a few minutes after delivery to improve maternal attachment and to stimulate breastfeeding. In addition, the time that newborns spend separated from their mothers has been reduced with rooming-in programmes.

Little attention has been given to interventions that focus specifically on fathers. It is possible to conceive that programmes that offer education and counselling to fathers as well as those which allow them to be part of, and present during, the prenatal, labour, and post-partum periods, will have an important impact on their capacity to support their wives in the care of their children. The promotion of social networks and support organizations, with the aim of identifying and supporting women in greater need, will also be important. Health services need to explore how home visits by nurses or midwives, specially to high-risk women, would be a feasible intervention. On the macro level, the improvement of work conditions; water and sanitation programmes; economic development and improvement of salary scales; and greater availability of social systems like health and educational networks, with programmes that stimulate their improved quality, will always be important.

All these interventions, however, will most likely continue to benefit those women and individuals who are the less needy, at least at the beginning. This may be the price which has to be paid in order to make such interventions available to those individuals most at need (see chapter 1, this volume). Targeting programmes to high-risk groups may be an important strategy, but not at the expense of curtailing similar services to the population at large.

Conclusion

Communicable diseases, like diarrhoeal diseases in children from developing countries, are an important public health problem linked to poverty and other harsh socio-economic conditions affecting these populations. Traditional interventions against communicable diseases, like health care, immunization, improvement of nutritional status, and educational programmes, are important and needed, but they will have a limited success in poor peri-urban areas, because of the social marginalization that exists, associated with unwanted and neglected children. More studies are needed to describe the processes and factors that influence child neglect and abuse in developing countries. Interventions to promote maternal self-esteem, linked to prenatal care or the post-partum period, or with the utilization of community support networks, may be important and require further evaluation.

Acknowledgements

The author would like to thank Sarah Atkinson, Betzabe Butron, Oona Campbell, Simon Cousens, Patricia Davis, Wendy Graham, Trudy Harpham, Betty Kirkwood, Melissa Parker, and Steve Rogers for their contributions and insightful comments, and for encouragement to address this important topic.

Special thanks to the field workers and field co-ordinators from the Instituto de Investigación Nutricional, for their dedicated work with poor families in peri-urban Lima, and their initial recognition of, and attention to, this topic. This work was partially supported by the UK Overseas Development Administration (now the Department for International Development) by means of a grant for Dr Claudio F. Lanata to be a Visiting Research Fellow in the Maternal and Child Epidemiology Unit at the London School of Hygiene & Tropical Medicine.

REFERENCES

Abdullah M, Wheeler EF. Seasonal variations and the intra-household distribution of food in a Bangladeshi village. *American Journal of Clinical Nutrition*, 1985; **41**:1305–13

Abou-Saleh MT, Ghubash R. The prevalence of early postpartum psychiatric morbidity in Dubai: a transcultural perspective. *Acta Psychiatrica Scandinavica*, 1997; **95**:428–32

Almeida-Filho N, Mari J de J, Coutinho E *et al*. Brazilian multicentric study of psychiatric morbidity. Methodological features and prevalence estimates. *British Journal of Psychiatry*, 1997; **171**:524–9

Arancibia M, Vargas N, Calderon P *et al*. Unwanted children: incidence and characteristics among puerperal women in a hospital of Santiago. *Revista Chilena de Pediatria*, 1989; **60**:107–11

Ashworth A, Feachem RG. Interventions for the control of diarrhoeal diseases among young children: weaning education. *Bulletin of the World Health Organization*, 1985; **63**:1115–27

Augoustinos M. Developmental effects of child abuse: recent findings. *Child Abuse and Neglect*, 1987; **11**:15–27

Axinn WG, Barber JS, Thornton A. The long-term impact of parents' childbearing decisions on children's self-esteem. *Demography*, 1998; **35**:435–43

Bahar E, Henderson AS, Mackinnon AJ. An epidemiological study of mental health and socioeconomic conditions in Sumatera, Indonesia. *Acta Psychiatrica Scandinavica*, 1992; **85**:257–63

Barros FC, Huttly SR, Victora CG, Kirkwood BR, Vaughan JP. Comparison of the causes and consequences of prematurity and intrauterine growth retardation: a longitudinal study in southern Brazil. *Pediatrics*, 1992; **90**:238–44

Baydar N. Consequences for children of their birth planning status. *Family Planning Perspectives*, 1995; **27**:228–34, 245

Belsey MA. Child abuse: measuring a global problem. *World Health Statistics Quarterly*, 1993; **46**:69–77

Black RE, Lopez de Romaña G, Brown KH, Bravo N, Balazar OG, Kanashiro HC. Incidence and etiology of infantile diarrhea and major routes of transmission in Huascar, Peru. *American Journal of Epidemiology*, 1989; **129**:785–99

Bledsoe CH, Ewbank DC, Isiugo-Abanihe UC. The effect of child fostering on feeding practices and access to health services in rural Sierra Leone. *Social Science and Medicine*, 1988; **27**:627–36

Bongaarts J. Trends in unwanted childbearing in the developing world. *Studies in Family Planning*, 1997; **28**:267–77

Brazelton TB, Cramer BG. *The earliest relationship. Parents, infants and the drama of early attachment.* London: Karnac Books, 1991

Brody GH, Flor DL. Maternal psychological functioning, family processes, and child adjustment in rural, single-parent, African American families. *Developmental Psychology*, 1997; **33**:1000–11.

Brown KH, Black RE, Becker S, Nahar S, Sawyer J. Consumption of foods and nutrients by weanlings in rural Bangladesh. *American Journal of Clinical Nutrition*, 1982; **36**:878–89

Caldwell JC. How is greater maternal education translated into lower child mortality? *Health Transition Review*, 1994; **4**:224–9

Campbell SB. Hard-to-manage preschool boys: externalizing behaviour, social competence, and family context at two-year followup. *Journal of Abnormal Child Psychology*, 1994; **22**:147–66

Christensen MJ, Brayden RM, Dietrich MS, McLaughlin FJ, Sherrod KB, Altemeier WA. The prospective assessment of self-concept in neglectful and physically abusive low income mothers. *Child Abuse and Neglect*, 1994; **18**:225–32

Christoffel KK, Zieserl EJ, Chiaramonte J. Should child abuse and neglect be considered when a child dies unexpectedly? *American Journal of Diseases of Children*, 1985; **139**:876–80

Cicchetti D, Rogosch FA, Toth SL, Spagnola M. Effect, cognition, and the emergence of self-knowledge in the toddler offspring of depressed mothers. *Journal of Experimental Child Psychology*, 1997; **67**:338–62

Cleland JG, van Ginneken JK. Maternal education and child survival in developing countries: the search for pathways of influence. *Social Science and Medicine*, 1988; **27**:1357–68

Cleland J, van Ginneken J. Maternal schooling and childhood mortality. *Journal of Biosocial Science*, 1989; **10(suppl)**:13–34

Clemens J, Sack D, Rao M *et al.* The design and analysis of cholera vaccine trials: recent lessons from Bangladesh. *International Journal of Epidemiology*, 1993; **22**:724–30

Cooper PJ, Campbell EA, Day A, Kennerley H, Bond A. Non-psychotic psychiatric disorders after childbirth: a prospective study of prevalence, incidence, course and nature. *British Journal of Psychiatry*, 1988; **152**:799–806

Copper RL, Goldenberg RL, Das A, *et al.* The preterm prediction study: maternal stress is associated with spontaneous preterm birth at less than thirty–five weeks' gestation. National Institute of Child Health and Human Development Maternal–Fetal Medicine Units Network. *American Journal of Obstetrics and Gynecology*, 1996; **175**:1286–92

Cosminsky S. Women and health care in a Guatemalan plantation. *Social Science and Medicine*, 1987; **25**:1163–73

Coutinho E da S, de Almeida Filho N, Mari J de J, Rodrigues L. Minor psychiatric morbidity and internal migration in Brazil. *Social Psychiatry and Psychiatric Epidemiology*, 1996; **31**:173–9

Cox AD, Puckering C, Pound A, Mills M. The impact of maternal depression in young children. *Journal of Child Psychology and Psychiatry and Allied Disciplines*, 1987; **28**:917–28

Crittenden PM. Sibling interaction: evidence of a generational effect in maltreating infants. *Child Abuse and Neglect*, 1984; **8**:433–8

Crittenden PM. Maltreated infants: vulnerability and resilience. *Journal of Child Psychology and Psychiatry and Allied Disciplines*, 1985; **26**:85–96

Cutts FT, Dos Santos C, Novoa A, David P, Macassa G, Soares AC. Child and maternal mortality during a period of conflict in Beira City, Mozambique. *International Journal of Epidemiology*, 1996; **25**:349–56

Darney PD. Maternal deaths in the less developed world: preventable tragedies. *International Journal of Gynaecology and Obstetrics*, 1988; **26**:177–9

Das Gupta M. Death clustering, mother's education and the determinants of child mortality in rural Punjab, India. *Population Studies*, 1990; **44**:489–505

de Almeida Filho N, Santana V de S, de Souza AL, Jacobina RR. Relation between the parents' mental health and the mental health of children in an urban population of Salvadore–Bahia. *Acta Psiquiatrica y Psicologica de America Latina*, 1985; **31**:211–21

de Sousa Bastos AC, de Almeida-Filho N. Socioeconomic variables, family milieu, and child mental health in an urban area of Salvador (Bahia), Brazil. *Acta Psiquiatrica y Psicologica de America Latina*, 1990; **36**:147–54

Desai S, Alva S. Maternal education and child health: is there a strong causal relationship? *Demography*, 1998; **35**:71–81

Dytrych Z, Matejcek Z, Schuller V, David HP, Friedman HL. Children born to women denied abortion. *Family Planning Perspectives*, 1975; **7**:165–71

Edwards CH, Cole OJ, Oyemade UJ, *et al.* Maternal stress and pregnancy outcomes in a prenatal clinic population. *Journal of Nutrition*, 1994; **124**:1006S–21S

Ekblad S. Family stress and mental health during rapid urbanization. The vulnerability of children in growing third world cities. In: Nordberg E, Finer D (eds) *Society, environment and health in low-income countries.* Stockholm: Karolinska Institute, 1990, pp 113–27

Ensminger ME, Celentano DD. Unemployment and psychiatric distress: social resources and coping. *Social Science and Medicine*, 1988; **27**:239–47

Esrey SA, Habicht JP. Maternal literacy modifies the effect of toilets and piped water on infant survival in Malaysia. *American Journal of Epidemiology*, 1988; **127**:1079–87

Fauveau V, Koenig MA, Wojtyniak B. Excess female deaths among rural Bangladeshi children: an examination of cause-specific mortality and morbidity. *International Journal of Epidemiology*, 1991; **20**:729–35

Feachem RG, Koblinsky MA. Interventions for the control of diarrhoeal disease among young children: promotion of breast-feeding. *Bulletin of the World Health Organization*, 1984; **62**:271–91

Finkelhor D, Korbin J. Child abuse as an international issue. *Child Abuse and Neglect*, 1988; **12**:3–23

Forjuoh SN. Pattern of intentional burns to children in Ghana. *Child Abuse and Neglect*, 1995; **19**:837–41

Forssman H, Thuwe I. Continued follow-up study of 120 persons born after refusal of application for therapeutic abortion. *Acta Psychiatrica Scandinavica*, 1981; **64**:142–9

Fowles ER. The relationship between maternal role attainment and postpartum depression. *Health Care for Women International*, 1998; **19**:83–94

Frodi AM. Contribution of infant characteristics to child abuse. *American Journal of Mental Deficiency*, 1981; **85**:341–9

Fulton AM, Murphy KR, Anderson SL. Increasing adolescent mothers' knowledge of child development: an intervention program. *Adolescence*, 1991; **26**:73–81

Gara MA, Rosenberg S, Herzog EP. The abused child as parent. *Child Abuse and Neglect*, 1996; **20**:797–807

Gelles RJ, Cornell CP. International perspectives on child abuse. *Child Abuse and Neglect*, 1983; **7**:375–86

Gorgen R, Maier B, Diesfeld HJ. Problems related to schoolgirl pregnancies in Burkina Faso. *Studies in Family Planning*, 1993; **24**:283–94

Gross D, Conrad B, Fogg L, Wothke W. A longitudinal model of maternal self-efficacy, depression, and difficult temperament during toddlerhood. *Research in Nursing and Health* 1994; **17**:207–15

Grosse RN, Auffrey C. Literacy and health status in developing countries. *Annual Review of Public Health*, 1989; **10**:281–97

Hall LA, Kotch JB, Browne D, Rayens MK. Self–esteem as a mediator of the effects of stressors and social resources on depressive symptoms in postpartum mothers. *Nursing Research*, 1996; **45**:231–8

Harpham T. Urbanization and mental disorder. In: Leff J, Bhugra D (eds) *Principles of social psychiatry*. London: Blackwell Scientific Publications, 1990

Herrmann MM, Van Cleve L, Levisen L. Parenting competence, social support, and self-esteem in teen mothers case managed by public health nurses. *Public Health Nursing*, 1998; **15**:432–9

Hill PD, Aldag J. Potential indicators of insufficient milk supply syndrome. *Research in Nursing and Health*, 1991; **14**:11–9

Huttly SR, Lanata CF, Gonzales H *et al.* Observations on handwashing and defecation practices in a shanty town of Lima, Peru. *Journal of Diarrhoeal Diseases Research*, 1994; **12**:14–8

Huttly SR, Morris SS, Pisani V. Prevention of diarrhoea in young children in developing countries. *Bulletin of the World Health Organization*, 1997; **75**:163–74

Huttly SR, Lanata CF, Yeager BA, Fukumoto M, Del Aguila R, Kendall C. Feces, flies, and fetor: findings from a Peruvian shantytown. *Revista Panamericana de Salud Publica*, 1998; **4**:75–9

Jaudes PK, Diamond LJ. Neglect of chronically ill children. *American Journal of Diseases of Children*, 1986; **140**:655–8

Kasim MS, Cheah I, Shafie HM. Childhood deaths from physical abuse. *Child Abuse and Neglect*, 1995; **19**:847–54

Keddie AM. Psychosocial factors associated with teenage pregnancy in Jamaica. *Adolescence*, 1992; **27**:873–90

Kessel E, Sastrawinata S, Mumford SD. Correlates of fetal growth and survival. *Acta Paediatrica Scandinavica Supplementum*, 1985; **319**:120–7

Krugman RD. Child abuse and neglect: critical first steps in response to a national emergency. The report of the US Advisory Board on Child Abuse and Neglect. *American Journal of Diseases of Children*, 1991; **145**:513–5

Lanata CF, Black RE, Del Aguila R *et al.* Protection of Peruvian Children against Rotavirus diarrhea of specific serotypes by one, two, three doses of the RIT 4237 attenuated bovine Rotavirus vaccine. *Journal of Infectious Diseases*, 1989; **159**:452–9

Lanata CF, Black RE, Gilman RH, Lazo F, Del Aguila R. Epidemiologic, clinical and laboratory characteristics of acute *vs* persistent diarrhea in periurban Lima, Peru. *Journal of Pediatric Gastroenterology and Nutrition*, 1991; **12**:82–8

Lanata CF, Black RE, Maurtua D *et al.* Etiologic agents in acute vs. persistent diarrhea in children under three years of age in peri-urban Lima, Peru. *Acta Paediatrica Supplementum*, 1992; **381**:32–8

Lanata CF, Black RE, Flores J *et al.* Immunogenicity, safety and protective efficacy of one dose of the rhesus rotavirus vaccine and serotype 1 and 2 human–rhesus rotavirus reassortants in children from Lima, Peru. *Vaccine*, 1996a; **14**:237–43

Lanata CF, Midthum K, Black RE *et al.* Safety, immunogenicity and protective efficacy of one or three doses of the Rhesus tetravalent rotavirus vaccine in infants from Lima, Peru. *Journal of Infectious Diseases*, 1996b; **174**:268–75

Lanata CF, Huttly SR, Yeager BA. Diarrhoea: whose feces matter? Reflections from studies in a Peruvian shanty town. *Pediatric Infectious Disease Journal*, 1998; **17**:7–9

Lesnik-Oberstein M, Koers AJ, Cohen L. Parental hostility and its sources in psychologically abusive mothers: a test of the three-factor theory. *Child Abuse and Neglect*, 1995; **19**:33–49

Lester BM, Boukydis CF, Garcia-Coll CT *et al.* Developmental outcome as a function of the goodness of fit between the infant's cry characteristics and the mother's perception of her infant's cry. *Pediatrics*, 1995; **95**:516–21

Leventhal JM, Garber RB, Brady CA. Identification during the postpartum period of infants who are at high risk of child maltreatment. *Journal of Pediatrics*, 1989; **114**:481–7

Lopez de Romaña G, Brown K, Black RE. Health and growth of infants and young children in Huascar, Peru. *Ecology of Food and Nutrition*, 1987; **19**:213–29

Lutenbacher M, Hall LA. The effects of maternal psychosocial factors on parenting attitudes of low–income, single mothers with young children. *Nursing Research*, 1998; **47**:25–34

McFarlane J, Fehir J. De madres a madres: a community, primary health care program based on empowerment. *Health Education Quarterly*, 1994; **21**:381–94

Madise NJ, Diamond I. Determinants of infant mortality in Malawi: an analysis to control for death clustering within families. *Journal of Biosocial Science*, 1995; **27**:95–106

Marshall E, Buckner E, Powell K. Evaluation of a teen parent program designed to reduce child abuse and neglect and to strengthen families. *Journal of Child and Adolescent Psychiatric Mental Health Nursing*, 1991; **4**:96–100

Mercer RT, Ferketich SL. Experienced and inexperienced mothers' maternal competence during infancy. *Research in Nursing and Health*, 1995; **18**:333–43

Miller BD. Female infanticide and child neglect in rural North India. In: Scheper-Hughes N (ed). *Child Survival*. Dordrecht: D. Reidel, 1987, 95–112

Moilanen I, Pennanen P. 'Mother's child' and 'father's child' among twins. A longitudinal twin study from pregnancy to 21 years age, with special reference to development and psychiatric disorders. *Acta Geneticae Medicae et Gemellologiae Roma*, 1997; **46**:219–30

Moilanen I, Rantakallio P. The single parent family and the child's mental health. *Social Science and Medicine*, 1988; **27**:181–6

Murray L, Stein A. The effects of postnatal depression on mother–infant relations and infant development. In: Woodhead M, Carr R, Light P (eds). *Becoming a person. Child development and social context*, Vol. 1. London: Routledge, 1991, pp 142–66

Myntti C. Social determinants of child health in Yemen. *Social Science and Medicine*, 1993; **37**:233–40

Najman JM, Morrison J, Williams G, Andersen M, Keeping JD. The mental health of women 6 months after they give birth to an unwanted baby. A longitudinal study. *Social Science and Medicine*, 1991; **32**:241–7

Ney PG, Moore C, McPhee J, Trought P. Child abuse: a study of the child's perspective. *Child Abuse and Neglect*, 1986; **10**:511–8

Nott PN. Extent, timing and persistence of emotional disorders following childbirth. *British Journal of Psychiatry*, 1987; **151**:523–7

Oates RK. Child abuse and non-organic failure to thrive: similarities and differences in the parents. *Australian Paediatric Journal*, 1984; **20**:177–80

Okeahialam TC. Child abuse in Nigeria. *Child Abuse and Neglect*, 1984; **8**:69–73

Olson DH, Russell CS, Sprenkle DH. Circumplex model of marital and family systems: VI. Theoretical update. *Family Process*, 1983; **22**:69–83

Oyemade A. Child abuse and neglect: a global phenomenon. *African Journal of Medicine and Medical Sciences*, 1991; **20**:5–9

Parker RM, Rescorla LA, Finkelstein JA, Barnes N, Holmes JH, Stolley PD. A survey of the health of homeless children in Philadelphia shelters. *American Journal of Diseases of Children*, 1991; **145**:520–6

Penny ME, Peerson JM, Marin RM *et al.* Randomized, community-based trial of the effect of zinc supplementation, with and without other micronutrients, on the duration of persistent childhood diarrhea in Lima, Peru. *Journal of Pediatrics*, 1999; **135**:208–17

Pinto e Silva JL. Pregnancy during adolescence: wanted vs. unwanted. *International Journal of Gynaecology and Obstetrics*, 1998; **63**:S151–S156

Pridham KF, Chang AS, Chiu YM. Mothers' parenting self-appraisals: the contribution of perceived infant temperament. *Research in Nursing and Health*, 1994; **17**:381–92

Rahim SI, Cederblad M. Epidemiology of mental disorders in young adults of newly urbanised area in Khartoum, Sudan. *British Journal of Psychiatry*, 1989; **155**:44–7

Ransjo-Arvidson AB, Chintu K, Ng'andu N *et al.* Maternal and infant health problems after normal childbirth: a randomised controlled study in Zambia. *Journal of Epidemiology and Community Health*, 1998; **52**:385–91

Rantakallio P, Myhrman A. The child and family eight years after undesired conception. The child and family after undesired conception. *Scandinavian Journal of Social Medicine*, 1980; **8**:81–7

Reichenheim ME, Harpham T. Maternal mental health in a squatter settlement in Rio de Janeiro. *British Journal of Psychiatry*, 1991; **159**:683–90

Ruchala PL, James DC. Social support, knowledge of infant development, and maternal confidence among adolescent and adult mothers. *Journal of Obstetric, Gynecologic and Neonatal Nursing,* 1997; **26**:685–9

Salzman JP. Primary attachment in female adolescents: association with depression, self-esteem, and maternal identification. *Psychiatry*, 1996; **59**:20–33

Sandiford P, Cassel J, Sanchez G, Coldham C. Does intelligence account for the link between maternal literacy and child survival? *Social Science and Medicine*, 1997; **45**:1231–9

Saraceno B, Barbui C. Poverty and mental illness. *Canadian Journal of Psychiatry*, 1997; **42**:285–90

Sazawal S, Black RE, Menon VP *et al.* Effect of zinc and mineral supplementation in small for gestational age infants on growth and mortality. *FASEB J*, 1999; **13**:A376

Scheper-Hughes N. Difference and danger: the cultural dynamics of childhood stigma, rejection, and rescue. *Cleft Palate Journal*, 1990; **27**:301–10

Scheper-Hughes N. Social indifference to child death. *Lancet*, 1991a; **337**:1144–7

Scheper-Hughes N. *Death without weeping: the violence of everyday life in Brazil.* California: University of California Press, 1991b

Segal UA. Child abuse by the middle class? A study of professionals in India. *Child Abuse and Neglect*, 1995; **19**:217–31

Segal UA, Ashtekar A. Detection of intrafamilial child abuse: children at intake at a children's observation home in India. *Child Abuse and Neglect*, 1994; **18**:957–67

Shek DT. Parenting characteristics and adolescent psychological well-being: a longitudinal study in a Chinese context. *Genetic, Social and General Psychology Monographs*, 1999; **125**:27–44

Somervell PD, Kaplan BH, Heiss G, Tyroler HA, Kleinbaum DG, Obrist PA. Psychologic distress as a predictor of mortality. *American Journal of Epidemiology*, 1989; **130**:1013–23

Spearly JL, Lauderdale M. Community characteristics and ethnicity in the prediction of child maltreatment rates. *Child Abuse and Neglect*, 1983; **7**:91–105

Steinberg LD, Catalano R, Dooley D. Economic antecedents of child abuse and neglect. *Child Development*, 1981; **52**:975–85

Thein MM, Goh LG. The value of the girl child in Singapore. *Journal of the Singapore Paediatric Society*, 1991; **33**:107–16

Tucker S, Gross D, Fogg L, Delaney K, Lapporte R. The long-term efficacy of a behavioral parent training intervention for families with 2-year-olds. *Research in Nursing and Health*, 1998; **21**:199–210

Vines SW, Williams-Burgess C. Effects of a community health nursing parent–baby (ad)venture program on depression and other selected maternal–child health outcomes. *Public Health Nursing*, 1994; **11**:188–94

Winefield AH, Tiggemann M. Length of unemployment and psychological distress: longitudinal and cross-sectional data. *Social Science and Medicine*, 1990; **31**: 461–5

WHO/CHD Immunization-Linked Vitamin A Supplementation Study Group. Randomised trial to assess benefits and safety of vitamin A supplementation linked to immunisation in early infancy. *Lancet*, 1998, **352**:1257–63

Yeager BAC, Lanata CF, Lazo F, Verástegui H, Black RE. Transmission factors and socioeconomic status as determinants of diarrhoeal incidence in Lima, Perú. *Journal of Diarrhoeal Disease Research*, 1991; **9**:186–93

Youngblut JM, Singer LT, Madigan EA, Swegart LA, Rodgers WL. Maternal employment and parent–child relationships in single-parent families of low-birth-weight preschoolers. *Nursing Research*, 1998; **47**:114–21

Zeitlin M. Nutritional resilience in a hostile environment: positive deviance in child nutrition. *Nutrition Reviews*, 1991; **49**:259–68

Zinc Investigators' Collaborative Group. Prevention of diarrhea and acute lower respiratory infection by zinc supplementation in developing country children: pooled analysis of randomized controlled trials. *Journal of Pediatrics* (in press)

Zuravin SJ. Unplanned childbearing and family size: their relationship to child neglect and abuse. *Family Planning Perspectives*, 1991; **23**:155–61

8 Accounts of social capital: the mixed health effects of personal communities and voluntary groups

Stephen J. Kunitz

A spectre is haunting public health—the spectre of communitarianism, to paraphrase Marx (1996). Among many epidemiologists and public health workers, the idea of communitarianism—now known as social capital, is gaining considerable currency. '"Social capital"', writes Robert Putnam, 'refers to features of social organization such as networks, norms, and social trust that facilitate co-ordination and co-operation for mutual benefit' (Putnam, 1995). Social capital originates in membership in voluntary associations, and in dense networks of such organizations in any community, because it is in such setting that people learn to trust, to reciprocate, and to act in concert to demand public services and good government (Putnam et al., 1993). Its appeal derives from its critique of the growing inequalities that have been documented in a number of societies and from attempts to severely diminish if not dismantle the welfare state.

Putnam credits James Coleman with having first clearly developed the social capital theoretical framework. Coleman in his turn has written of social capital that it:

> [I]s defined by its function. It is not a single entity but a variety of different entities, with two elements in common: they all consist of some aspect of social structures, and they facilitate certain actions of actors—*whether persons or corporate actors*—within the structure. Like other forms of capital, social capital is productive, making possible the achievement of certain ends that in its absence would not be possible. Like physical capital and human capital, social capital is not completely fungible but may be specific to certain activities. A given form of social capital that is valuable in facilitating certain actions may be useless or even harmful for others. (Coleman, 1988, emphasis added.)

And he goes on to say that, 'Unlike other forms of capital, social capital inheres in the structure of relations between actors and among actors. It is not lodged either in the actors themselves or in physical implements of production.' The idea of social capital, according to Coleman, is meant to integrate two streams in social thought, the radical individualism of the economic notion of rational man, and the 'oversocialized' view of man characteristic of much sociology (Coleman, 1988).

Putnam's use of social capital seems to be somewhat different. Social capitalists, called 'the new republican theorists' by Putnam, stand in opposition to 'the defenders of classical liberal individualism' (Putnam *et al.*, 1993). They champion the importance in public policy of co-operation, community, equality, and inclusiveness as means of achieving a more just and humane society. Eva Cox has written, 'When Margaret Thatcher said there's no such thing as society, she lost the plot. Society is the myriad of ways people connect, linked by some common interests or characteristics.' And she goes on to speak of the 'often forgotten but powerful forces that connect us as social beings. These forces—trust, reciprocity and mutuality—survive in our everyday lives but are not reflected in public policy and therefore are losing ground' (Cox, 1995).

Social capital is often thought of as a societal phenomenon, reflected in such measures as degree of income equality or membership in secondary groups such as sports clubs, choirs, Rotary, and so on. As Cox's comment suggests, primary group ties—that is, relationships with kith and kin—are taken for granted. That, I think, is a mistake. Social capital is also produced by primary groups, and individuals may or may not possess it. That is a point made by Portes (1998), who writes that 'Social capital stands for the ability of actors to secure benefits by virtue of membership in social networks or other social structures.' And Coleman (1988) in the passage quoted above, and his own study of high school drop-outs, makes a similar point, for he measures social capital within the family and social capital outside the family. The former is measured by the presence of both parents and the strength of relationships among members; the latter by geographic mobility, which attenuates ties with other families and with the school. Thus high school students may possess social capital, or they may not, and its possession diminishes the probability of dropping out of school. That is, social capital is not simply produced by, and reflected in membership in secondary groups, which are measures of civic culture. It is also reflected in the structure and function of primary groups, or as I have called them, following Wellman, 'personal communities' (Wellman *et al.*, 1988).

Many of these ideas of social capital have found their way into epidemiology, public health, and health care policy (e.g. Kawachi *et al.*, 1997*a*) where they have mingled with and provided a new vocabulary for ideas that have long existed. In this chapter, I consider some of the studies which show positive associations between social capital and health (measured primarily as life expectancy), and some others which show no such association. I argue that the failure to show positive results is not necessarily methodological but has to do with the ambiguous nature of social capital itself. I describe some of the roots of the idea of social capital in nineteenth-century sociology, and I suggest that it is the very power of those ideas that has kept us from seeing just how mixed the effects of social capital can be. I consider primarily the work of Alexis de Tocqueville and Emile Durkheim, for they are the writers most commonly cited by contemporary commentators and investigators. My point is that at the level of both primary and secondary groups, that is to say, at the level of kinship and friendship networks and at the level of voluntary associations, social capital is a highly ambiguous concept. Under some circumstances the health effects may be beneficial. Under others they may be neutral or even detrimental.

Ecological studies of social capital

Most ecological studies are of high- or upper middle-income countries and use degree of income equality as the measure of the extent of social capital (Lynch and Kaplan, 1997). The results of many of them are strikingly consistent, whether at the national (Wilkinson, 1996), state (Kaplan et al., 1996; Kennedy et al., 1996; Kawachi et al., 1997b), or municipal level (Lynch et al., 1998). They show that the greater the income equality in the population, the higher the life expectancy. To explain these observations, Wilkinson (1996) has proposed that after the epidemiological transition to the stage of man-made and chronic diseases has been achieved, further increases in GNP per capita cease to be associated with increased life expectancy. Instead, an increasingly equal income distribution is associated with further increases in life expectancy.

Similar observations had been made previously by authors who have suggested that the explanation of the positive association between income inequality and mortality has a mathematical basis (Preston, 1976; Rodgers, 1979). This does not explain, however, why there is a graded relationship between income level and other measures of stratification on the one hand, and mortality on the other, even in high-income, low mortality societies. Absolute deprivation is not a sufficient explanation, and as a result various explanations based upon relative deprivation have been invoked (Adler et al., 1994; Wilkinson, 1996; Marmot et al., 1997). Rather than review those studies, I should like to turn instead to a consideration of other measures that have been said to represent the presence or absence of social capital.

Racial segregation may be considered a measure of social capital, or its absence, for it is a measure of lack of inclusiveness and of inequality. A number of studies of the association of segregation and mortality have been done in the US. For example, Hart and colleagues (1998) used data from metropolitan areas of the US to show that racial segregation was associated with increased mortality among African Americans but not whites.

In addition to segregation, a variety of other measures have been found to be associated both with income inequality and with mortality. In a study of the 50 states of the United States of America, Kaplan and colleagues (1996) have shown that income inequality is associated with lower levels of spending on education and other social infrastructure, and with high rates of homicide. Using data from 39 states, Kawachi et al. (1997b) showed that interpersonal

trust, membership in voluntary associations, and income equality were correlated, and all showed the expected relationship to life expectancy. On the basis
of path analysis, they argued that group membership was the intermediating
variable between income equality and life expectancy. But the situation is more
ambiguous than these observations suggest, as the following example illustrates.

The dialectics of social capital

When Alexis de Tocqueville, beloved of social capitalists, visited the US in 1831,
he observed profound differences between the people who had settled the New
England colonies and those who had settled the southern colonies. The men
who initially settled the South were adventurers who came without families in
search of wealth. They were followed by 'a more moral and orderly race of men'
who were, however, 'nowise above the level of the inferior classes in England.'
And of course the introduction of slavery exercised a 'prodigious ... influence
on the character, the laws, and all the future prospects of the South'
(Tocqueville, 1961).

These settlers compared unfavourably with those who settled the North. The
people who settled in the North 'belonged to the more independent classes of
their native country.' They were 'neither rich nor poor.' All were educated, and
in proportion to their number possessed 'a greater mass of intelligence than is
to be found in any European nation of our own time.' They were sober, moral,
family men who were accompanied by their wives and children (Tocqueville,
1961). They were, he continued, Puritans, and 'Puritanism was not merely a
religious doctrine, but it corresponded in many points with the most absolute
democratic and republican theories' (Tocqueville, 1961).

Other observers noted that southerners had come from the Celtic fringe of the
British Isles and brought with them an entirely different culture than the Puritans. It was a culture that was kin-based, and that emphasized the importance
of family and personal honour, the spoken over the written word, agrarian over
business values, and leisure over enterprise (McWhiney, 1989).

Many of these cultural differences persisted as Northerners and Southerners
pushed westward. People from New England tended to remain in the northern
tier of states, while southerners moved along the southern tier into the American
Southwest. One preacher wrote of the Yankee settlers in the Upper Midwest,
'[They] naturally unite themselves into corporate unions, and concentre their
strength for public works and purposes. They have the same desire for keeping
up schools, for cultivating psalmody, for settling ministers, and attending upon
religious worship; and unfortunately the same disposition to dogmatize, to
settle not only their own faith, but that of their neighbor, and to stand
resolutely, and dispute fiercely, for the slightest shade of difference of religious
opinion.' And he contrasted the Yankee settlers in Ohio who, 'in the strong exercise of social inclination, expressing itself in habits of neighborhood, [formed]
villages, and live[d] in them, ... to that sequestered and isolated condition, which

a Kentuckian, under the name of "range," considers as one of the desirable circumstance of existence' (McWhiney, 1989).

Reflecting the cultural differences between North and South were the political differences observed by Tocqueville. He wrote:

> Townships and a local activity exist in every State; but in no part of the confederation is a township to be met with precisely similar to those of New England. The more we descend towards the South, the less active does the business of the township or parish become; the number of magistrates, of functions, and of rights decreases; the population exercises a less immediate influence on affairs; town-meetings are less frequent, and the subjects of debate less numerous. The power of the elected magistrate is augmented, and that of the elector diminished, whilst the public spirit of the local communities is less awakened and less influential. (Tocqueville, 1961.)

That is to say, Tocqueville was describing variations in what is now called 'civic culture' every bit as profound as those described by Putnam in northern and southern Italy (Putnam *et al.*, 1993).

With this brief background in mind, we may recall some of the studies to which I have already referred of the association between social capital and mortality among American states and metropolitan areas. If one inspects the data displayed in those studies, they indicate that southern states have the lowest levels of social capital, the lowest levels of education, the highest levels of income inequality, and the highest levels of homicide and of overall mortality of all the states (see also Lester, 1994). Indeed, the southern predilection for homicide has been observed for well over a century (Gastil, 1971) and is high for both African Americans and whites (Lester, 1994).

Clearly, the legacy of the civic cultures implanted in the North and South in the seventeenth century continue to have profound consequences right down to the present, and at the state level the advantage seems to be to the North, where social capital is higher and mortality lower than in the South. At the metropolitan level, however, a paradox emerges. Our study of the impact of racial segregation on mortality in metropolitan regions indicated that, even adjusting for latitude and longitude, segregation was associated with an increase in deaths among African Americans but not among whites (Hart *et al.*, 1998). But we also observed that the most racially segregated metropolitan regions were in the Northeast and Upper Midwest, the very areas in which the civic culture which so impressed Tocqueville had taken deepest root. The two are not unrelated.

These cities were America's industrial heartland, and the relatively unskilled jobs available in their factories and mills provided economic opportunities for vast numbers of immigrants. In the nineteenth century, cities in the Northeast grew by annexation. They were able to acquire territory at the fringes and incorporate them within a larger city. This was to everyone's advantage. People in the annexed territory were glad to have city services such as water, sewers, paved roads, and trolley lines, and the city acquired an expanding tax base (Jackson, 1985).

In the late nineteenth and early twentieth centuries, however, as immigrants from Eastern and Southern Europe, and African Americans from the deep South, began flooding these cities, the older inhabitants moved to the suburbs and began erecting barriers that would prohibit annexation without their consent. They drew on the tradition of local community government to protect their economic, ethnic, and racial exclusivity, and they still do. As a result, these cities became the most racially segregated in the country, as well as the least elastic. That is, they are cities that have failed to expand their geographic boundaries to capture suburban growth. Consequently, the metropolitan areas of which they are a part are divided into many different municipalities with their own taxing authorities, school systems, and exclusionary zoning practices. The effect has been to create relatively affluent homogeneous suburbs and poverty-stricken inner cities, populated disproportionately by poor African Americans.

Thus the civic culture which impressed so many observers has also worked to strangle solutions to problems that were never anticipated when the colonies were established. And this suggests that local government and voluntary associations may cause as many problems as they solve, for they may introduce rigidity into social structures that require flexibility (Olson, 1982). To recognize the complex nature of civic culture and secondary associations requires more than ecological correlations of national and international data. It requires that we think about the history and culture of specific peoples and places. We see something similar when we turn to a consideration of primary groups and personal communities.

Social capital and primary groups

Just as social capital is fast becoming a paradigm with which to explain inequalities in health at the societal level, so in the form of social support and integration has it become important in studies of the health of individuals.[1] For investigators who write on the association between health and the social support provided by kin and friends have begun to draw on the literature on social capital as well. And as in studies at the societal level, so too at the individual level are there anomalous results that should encourage a more nuanced way of thinking about the processes at work.

The studies of social support and integration on the one hand, and subsequent mortality on the other, have shown that when support is high, the risk of mortality tends to be reduced, even after controlling for various measures of health status. The effects are particularly strong for white males. They are much weaker or non-existent for women and for non-whites, including African Americans (Schoenbach et al., 1986), Japanese-Americans (Reed et al., 1984), and Navajo Indians (Kunitz and Levy, 1988), primarily in rural populations.[2] One commentator has suggested that such anomalies:

have to do with the extent to which women and blacks are deeply integrated into stable, rural communities ... Under such circumstances, if these groups routinely obtain large doses of social support, specific measures tapping frequency of contact and size of network may be less differentiating than in less well-integrated communities. Furthermore, these sources of support may be so much a part of the normal daily lives of these people that they commonly go un-noticed and, as a result, are underreported in surveys of this sort. In urban areas, where people are more mobile, their awareness of sources of support and frequency of contact may be heightened. (Berkman, 1986.)

Indeed, it may well be that the differences are simply the result of methodo-logical difficulties, and that the instruments that have been used to measure inte-gration and support are too blunt to dissect subtle distinctions among populations where support is generally high. On the other hand, the notion that these anomalous results may be explained by the pervasiveness of social support rather than by its absence assumes that which must be demonstrated. It may be that there are true differences in the structure, meaning, and functioning of social networks in different populations and settings. For example, in a study in one southern community it was found that African Americans had lower levels of support than whites (Strogatz and James, 1986), rather than higher levels as suggested in the previous quotation. Moreover, while family networks have been shown to be important sources of support among African Americans, the con-flictual and non-supportive side of such networks has also been noted (Williams and Fenton, 1994).

Furthermore, in a variety of studies, women are found to report higher use of support than men, but they are also more likely than men to provide support. 'Thus, women may be more likely to be exposed to negative social outcomes regarding both themselves and others than is true for men. Women with larger networks may be more involved in dealing with the stresses of others and thus experience more stress than women with smaller networks or than men' (Sarason *et al.*, 1997).

Finally, living in poverty, living in a rural area, or living in a poor country means that informal social networks and primary groups are called upon to provide a broader range of services than they are in settings where the avail-ability of, and access to, formal services are greater (Wellman and Wortley, 1990). Without an infrastructure of public health services, widely accessible health care, public schools, a legal justice system, and other formal institutions, the establishment and maintenance of personal networks are a matter of survival (Granovetter, 1983). But social networks may also impose heavy burdens, for example when reciprocity is required by other members, or when gossip and other forms of coercion are used to control behaviour. That, of course, is one of the reasons people have fled small towns for large cities. The point is that kinship and friendship networks are not unambiguously support-ive and may exact very high costs. This is especially true where poverty and the absence of formal institutions force people to depend upon informal networks for all forms of assistance both large and small. This can impose intolerable burdens even as it makes some burdens tolerable.

Not only are different contexts associated with differences in the services provided by personal networks, but the structure of networks is different as well. In general:

> studies in several Western countries show that close relatives, especially parents, continue to be of central importance in personal networks. There are, however, differences between rural and urban populations and between social strata in the importance of extended kin as compared to friends and acquaintances. In larger cities as well as in middle classes, relations with extended kin become looser, while those with friends and acquaintances gain in importance. (Hollinger and Haller, 1990; Wellman, 1992.)

And network structure has profound consequences, even among social strata in the same society. For example, in secure settings such as those in which the middle and upper classes in developed countries live, loose networks based upon friendship are particularly well suited to obtaining jobs as well as needed services from a broad array of formal organizations (Granovetter, 1983). In contrast, dense networks in urban ghettos in the US isolate people from information about the availability of jobs and services elsewhere in the city (Wilson 1987).

Some of the complexities of the associations between social context and the structure, function, and effectiveness of social networks are suggested by the results of several studies among Navajo Indians in the American Southwest. Indian reservations like the Navajo's are generally very rural and characterized by high rates of poverty and unemployment. Traditionally, extended families have been both a common as well as the ideal form of social organization and in many instances still are because they are adaptive to the prevailing unstable economic conditions (Aberle, 1969; Kunitz, 1983). This pattern is changing substantially, however, as people move to towns on and off the reservation.

In a study of social integration and subsequent mortality among Navajo men and women 65 years of age and above, we found that only marital status was significantly associated with an increased risk of death, and only among men over the age of 75. No other measures of isolation or integration were significant (Kunitz and Levy, 1991). This was because in the Navajo context social integration meant that the family had to carry a heavy burden. For instance, a significant number of our elderly informants lived with adult children with physical or psychological disabilities for whom no institutional or day care services were available, and for whom the elderly parent was a major source of financial and other support. Rates of depression were significantly higher among these respondents than among people without such burdensome responsibilities.

We also observed that among women of childbearing age, use of contraception was more likely by those who were not living with their kin than among those who were, even adjusting for parity and education. This was because, in a generally pronatalist setting, women of childbearing age who lived in extended family arrangements were subjected to intense social pressure, and sometimes physical coercion, from their mothers and husbands not to use contraception, whereas those living neolocally were more autonomous and able to exercise choice (Kunitz and Tsianco, 1981).

But the freedom associated with neolocality is a mixed blessing. Young people who grew up in extended families learned to use alcohol in settings that emphasized responsibilities to kin and therefore shaped their careers as drinkers. While heavy drinking often led to serious difficulties, it was generally outgrown before catastrophe occurred (Kunitz and Levy, 1994). However, as the livestock economy has declined, people have left rural areas and residence within extended families and moved to reservation towns where they live neolocally, near unrelated neighbours, and attend school with non-relatives. In these new settings, the cross-generational fabric has been torn and a youth culture has emerged which, at the extremes, is characterized by gangs, violence, and highly risky drinking.[3] As a result, the homicide rate has tripled since the 1960s. Thus the same freedom from kin which has increased the likelihood of contraceptive use has also resulted in the creation of social networks that encourage destructive and self-destructive behaviour.

These brief examples illustrate some of the ways in which the larger context may influence the structure, functions, and effectiveness of social networks, and how these may in turn influence various dimensions of peoples' health and use of services. That is to say, social relations are not always supportive and may be damaging. This is particularly so when poverty, unemployment, insecurity, and inadequate infrastructure of formal organizations are prevalent. Under such conditions, people have little choice in those upon whom they must depend, and the consequences of enforced dependence on kinsmen may be quite mixed, for they may be oppressive as well as supportive. This is unlike the situation of the well-to-do in developed countries, where a good deal of freedom may be exercised in the choice of network members, where networks are looser, and where in any event the need for support from informal sources is less than in many other parts of the world. It is this sort of complexity that explains why social relations which are often assumed to be a form of social capital and of positive value may be of little value or actually harmful.

Conclusion

The use of inequality and social capital to explain contemporary mortality patterns represents a co-mingling of two intellectual traditions. The concern with income inequality is part of the long-running Standard of Living debate that has preoccupied historians and economists for many years (Engerman, 1994; 1997). One side of the debate—the optimists—has argued that economic development may benefit people unevenly, but in general everyone benefits: a rising tide lifts all ships. The other side—the pessimists—argues that not only do people not benefit equally, but that it is widening gaps between strata that have deleterious consequences, even as GNP per capita is increasing.

The idea of social capital draws upon a related tradition. Some of the most powerful themes running through the social thought of the past almost two centuries—community, alienation, authority—have represented attempts to come to terms with the consequences of the democratic revolution in France and the Industrial Revolution which began in England (Nisbet, 1996). For some, like Herbert Spenser and William Graham Sumner, the freeing of individuals from the bonds of community and kin, the evolution of nuclear families, and the emergence of *laissez-faire* capitalism were at once welcome and inevitable (Bramson, 1961; Peel, 1971). Others were at least ambivalent if not hostile. A widely shared view of thinkers as different as Engels, Marx, and Tocqueville was that the two revolutions had destroyed aristocratic institutions and local communities which had mediated between individuals and the state.

The result was mass society, alienation, and overwhelmingly powerful central governments with no intermediating institutions between them and their citizens. Social capital is in this tradition: for the answer to the individualism, atomism, and alienation of contemporary society—civic cultures woven together by networks of voluntary—is not so different from the answers given by many of our nineteenth-century intellectual ancestors.

Thus when Tocqueville went to America, it was to study the most democratic nation of his day. What he found, especially in New England, was municipal governments which were just the sort of intermediating institutions whose absence he feared would lead to despotism in France. He thought other forms of association could also serve the same function as aristocracy had. He wrote:

> An association for political, commercial, or manufacturing purposes, or even for those of science and literature, is a powerful and enlightened member of the community, which cannot be disposed of at pleasure, or oppressed without remonstrance: and which, by defending its own rights against encroachments of the government, saves the common liberties of the country. (Tocqueville, 1961.)

Durkheim, whose name and study of suicide are cited and recited like a mantra in virtually every article in the field of social epidemiology, made similar observations. The two forms of suicide which he thought were most important in his time were egoistic and anomic. The egoistic type was the result of loss of cohesion, particularly in religious society (Durkheim, 1951). That is why he claimed that rates among Protestants were higher than among Catholics. Anomic suicide was the result of loss of restraint, prompted by the growth of industrial society (Durkheim, 1951). Rates and patterns of suicide were, he argued, just one instance of 'the whole of our historical development,' the 'chief characteristic [of which] is to have swept cleanly away all the older forms of social organization.' He continued; 'The great change brought about by the French Revolution was precisely to carry this leveling to a point hitherto unknown ... Only one collective form survived the tempest: the State ...

[I]ndividuals are no longer subject to any other collective control but the State, so it is the sole organized collectivity' (Durkheim, 1951). And he used the same metaphor of mass society used by many of his contemporaries. 'Individuals', he said, 'tumble over one another like so many liquid molecules' (Durkheim, 1951; Kunitz, 1971).

He dismissed the solution proposed by other writers: 'the restitution of local groups of something of their old autonomy', and advocated instead a different sort of intermediating institution: corporatism. 'The only decentralization which would make possible the multiplication of the centers of communal life without weakening national unity is what might be called *occupational decentralization*' (Durkheim, 1951, emphasis in original). His diagnosis of the problem of his age, his solution to it, and his ambivalence about democracy, could have been Tocqueville's.

I have stressed the importance of the historical processes to which Tocqueville in the first half of the nineteenth century and Durkheim in the second were responding, because their understanding of their world has shaped our understanding of ours. To be sure, we have inherited their world, but precisely because their insights are so powerful and their writing so persuasive, we run the risk of allowing them to overdetermine how we understand our world. Durkheim's study of suicide, for instance, has been so influential and is so frequently cited not because his analyses were valid. Indeed, they probably were not (Day, 1987; van Poppel and Day, 1996). But validity is not the point. His work continues to be so influential because he addressed concerns that we share and provided answers to which we resonate. The same is true of our response to Tocqueville.

But our world is different from theirs. Local governments may involve their citizens in civic life, as Tocqueville suggested, but they may also promote exclusivity and protect citizens from integration into larger regional structures that may be widely beneficial. Associations 'for political, commercial, or manufacturing purposes' may protect their own interests, as Tocqueville and Durkheim both suggested, but in the process may be harmful to the health and well-being of the public. This is amply demonstrated by the opposition of the tobacco industry trade association to limitations on cigarette advertising and sales, and by the destruction of President Clinton's plan for health care reform by a coalition of voluntary associations including the National Rifle Association, the Christian Coalition, the National Federation of Independent Businesses, and the Health Insurance Association of America (Johnson and Broder, 1996).

Churches may be the most integrative institutions in Hispanic and African-American communities, but their deep conservatism prevented them from acting early in the AIDS crisis and has contributed to its severity (Perrow and Guillen, 1990). And kinship and friendship networks may provide support to their members but may also exact high costs, resulting in resentment and stress as well as delinquency and criminal behaviour. Social capital may be valuable in facilitating certain actions, as James Coleman wrote, but 'may be useless or even harmful for others' (Coleman, 1988).[4]

The quest for community has been a recurring theme in social and political thought. Certainly in the US, perhaps the most individualistic of nations, it has been significant from the nineteenth century to the present in the form of utopian communities and encounter and support groups.[5] Such communities generally represent a withdrawal from civil society rather than engagement with it, and for this reason, the new republican theorists distance themselves from communitarianism. Nonetheless, they share common concerns and insights. Most importantly, both abjure *laissez-faire* individualism in favour of the beneficial effects of association. (Bellah *et al.*, 1985). I have argued that whatever other benefits may derive from association—and I believe them to be both real and significant—improved health is not invariably one of them, for social ties may bind us together, but they may also imprison us.

Acknowledgements

Theodore M. Brown, William T. Bluhm, Stanley L. Engerman, David Leon, John Lynch, and Simon Szreter commented on various early versions of this manuscript.

Notes

1. Some of the articles which address this issue are: Cassel, 1976; Cobb, 1976; Broadhead *et al.*, 1983; Thoits, 1982; 1995.
2. Some of the relevant publications are: Berkman and Syme, 1979; Blazer, 1982; Zuckerman *et al.*, 1984; Seeman *et al.*, 1987; House *et al.*, 1988; Hanson *et al.*, 1989; Welin *et al.*, 1992.
3. The results of these studies are as yet mostly unpublished. See Kunitz *et al.*, 1998; 1999; and Henderson *et al.* (in press).
4. Since completing the penultimate draft of this chapter, I have been referred to an article by Alejandro Portes (1998) which makes a number of points very similar to those made here. I am grateful to Simon Szreter for the citation.
5. A number of relevant citations include: Hine, 1953; Noyes, 1961; Holloway, 1966; Bestor, 1970; Nordhoff, 1970; Kanter, 1972; Roberts, 1972; Wuthnow, 1994.

REFERENCES

Aberle DF. A plan for Navajo economic development. In: *Toward economic development for Native American communities.* A compendium of papers submitted to the Sub-Committee on Economy in Government of the Joint Economic committee of the Congress of the United States. Washington, DC: US Government Printing Office, 1969

Adler NE, Boyce T, Chesney MA *et al.* Socioeconomic status and health: the challenge of the gradient. *American Psychologist*, 1994; **49**:15–24

Atkinson AB, Rainwater L, Smeeding TM. *Income distribution in OECD countries: evidence from the Luxembourg Income Study*. OECD Social Policy Studies No. 18. Paris: Organization for Economic Co-operation and Development, 1995

Bellah RN, Sullivan WM, Tipton SM. *Habits of the heart: individualism and commitment in American life*. Berkeley: University of California Press, 1985

Berkman LF. Social networks, support, and health: taking the next step forward. *American Journal of Epidemiology*, 1986; **123**:559–62

Berkman LF, Syme SL. Social networks, host resistance, and mortality: a nine-year follow-up study of Alameda County Residents. *American Journal of Epidemiology*, 1979; **109**:186–204.

Bestor, A. *Backwoods utopias: the sectarian origins and the Owenite phase of Communitarian Socialism in America 1663–1829*, (2nd edn). Philadelphia: University of Pennsylvania Press, 1970

Blazer DG. Social support and mortality in an elderly community population. *American Journal of Epidemiology*, 1982; **115**:684–94

Bott E. *Family and social network: roles, norms and external relationships in ordinary urban families*. London: Tavistock, 1957

Bramson L. *The political context of sociology*. Princeton: Princeton University Press, 1961

Broadhead WE, Kaplan BH, James SA et al.. The epidemiologic evidence for a relationship between social support and health. *American Journal of Epidemiology*, 1983; **117**:521–37

Cassel J. The contribution of the social environment to host resistance. *American Journal of Epidemiology*, 1976; **104**:107–23

Cobb S. Social support as a moderator of life stress. *Psychosomatic Medicine, 1976*; **38**:300–14

Coleman JS. Social capital in the creation of human capital. *American Journal of Sociology*, 1988; **94(Suppl)**:S95–S120

Cox E. *A truly civil society*. Sydney: ABC Books, 1995

Day LH. Durkheim on religion and suicide—a demographic critique. *Sociology*, 1987; **21**:449–61

Durkheim E. *Suicide: a study in sociology*, (trans. JA Spaulding and G Simpson). New York: The Free Press, 1951

Engerman SL. Reflections on the Standard of Living debate: new arguments and new evidence. In: James JA, Thomas M (eds) *Capitalism in context. Essays on economic development and cultural change in honor of R M Hartwell*. Chicago: University of Chicago Press, 1994, pp 50–82

Engerman SL. The Standard of Living debate in international perspective: measures and indicators. In: Steckel RH, Floud R (eds) *Health and welfare during industrialization*. Chicago: The University of Chicago Press, 1997, pp 17–45

Gastil RD. Homicide and a regional culture of violence. *American Sociological Review,* 1971; **36**:412–27

Geertsen R, Kane RL, Klauber MR, Rindflesh M, Gray R. A reexamination of Suchman's view of social factors in health care utilization. *Journal of Health and Social Behavior*, 1975; **16**:226–37

Granovetter M. The strength of weak ties: a network theory revisited. In Collins R (ed) *Sociological theory*. San Francisco: Jossey-Bass, 1983

Hanson BS, Isacsson SO, Janzon L, Lindell SE. Social network and social support influence mortality in elderly men. *American Journal of Epidemiology,* 1989; **130**:100–11

Hart K, Kunitz SJ, Mukamel D, Sell R. Metropolitan governance, residential segregation, and mortality among African Americans. *American Journal of Public Health,* 1998; **88**:434–8

Henderson EB, Kunitz SJ, Levy JE. The origins of Navajo Youth Gangs. *American Indian Culture and Research Journal* (in press)

Hine RV. *California's Utopian Communities.* New Haven: Yale University Press, 1953

Hollinger F, Haller M. Kinship and social networks in modern societies: a cross-cultural comparison among seven nations. *European Sociological Review,* 1990; **6**:103–24

Holloway M. *Heavens on Earth: utopian communities in America 1680–1880.* New York: Dover Publication, Inc., 1966

House JS, Landis KR, Umberson D. Social relationships and health. *Science,* 1988; **241**:540–5

Inter-American Development Bank. *Facing up to inequality in Latin America.* Baltimore: The Johns Hopkins University Press, 1998

Jackson KT. *Crabgrass Frontier.* New York: Oxford University Press, 1985

Johnson H, Broder DS. *The System: the American way of politics at the breaking point.* Boston: Little, Brown and Co., 1996

Kanter RM. *Commitment and community: communes and utopias in sociological perspective.* Cambridge: Harvard University Press, 1972

Kaplan GA, Pamuk ER, Lynch JW, Cohen RD, Balfour JL. Income inequality and mortality in the United States. *British Medical Journal,* 1996; **312**:999–1003

Kawachi I, Kennedy BP, Lochner, K. Long live community: social capital and public health. *The American Prospect,* 1997*a*; **35(November–December)**:56–9

Kawachi I, Kennedy BP, Lochner K, Prothrow-Stith D. Social capital, income inequality and mortality. *American Journal of Public Health,* 1997*b*; **87**:1491–8

Kennedy BP, Kawachi, I, Prothrow-Stith, D. Income distribution and mortality: cross sectional ecological study of the Robin Hood Index in the United States. *British Medical Journal,* 1996; **312**:1004–7

Kunitz SJ. The Social Philosophy of John Collier. *Ethnohistory,* 1971; **18**:213–29

Kunitz SJ. *Disease change and the role of medicine.* Berkeley: University of California Press, 1983

Kunitz SJ, Levy JE. A prospective study of isolation and mortality in a cohort of elderly Navajo Indians. *Journal of Cross-Cultural Gerontology,* 1988; **3**:71–85

Kunitz SJ, Levy JE. *Navajo aging: the transition from family to institutional support.* Tucson: University of Arizona Press, 1991

Kunitz SJ, Levy LE. *Drinking careers: a twenty-five year follow-up of three Navajo populations.* New Haven: Yale University Press, 1994

Kunitz SJ, Tsianco MC. Kinship dependence and contraceptive use among Navajo Women. *Human Biology,* 1981; **53**:439–52

Kunitz SJ, Gabriel KR, Levy JE *et al.* Alcohol dependence and conduct disorder among Navajo Indians. *Journal of Studies on Alcohol,* 1998; **60**:159–67

Kunitz SJ, Gabriel KR, Levy JE. Risk factors for conduct disorder among Navajo men and women. *Social Psychiatry and Psychiatric Epidemiology,* 1999; **34**:180–9

Lester D. *Patterns of suicide and homicide in America.* New York: Nova Science Publisher, Inc., 1994

Litwak E, Messeri, J, Wolfe S, Gorman S, Silverstein M, Guilarte M. Organization theory, social supports, and mortality rates: a theoretical convergence. *American Sociological Review*, 1989; **54**:49–66

Lynch JW, Kaplan GA. Understanding how inequality in the distribution of income affects health. *Journal of Health Psychology*, 1997; **2**:297–314

Lynch JW, Kaplan GA, Pamuk ER *et al.* Income inequality and mortality in metropolitan areas of the United States. *American Journal of Public Health*, 1998; **88**:1074–80

Marx K. Capital. *A critique of political economy*. London: Penguin, 1996

McKinlay JB. Social networks, lay consultation and help-seeking behavior. *Social Forces*, 1973; **51**:275–92

McWhiney G. *Cracker culture: Celtic ways in the Old South*. Tuscaloosa: The University of Alabama Press, 1989

Marmot M, Ryff CD, Bumpass LL, Shipley M, Marks NF. Social inequalities in health: next questions and converging evidence. *Social Science and Medicine,* 1997; **44**:901–10

Nisbet RA. *The Sociological Tradition*. New York: Basic Books, 1996

Nordhoff B. *The communistic societies of the United States*. New York: Schocken Books, 1970

Noyes JH. *History of American socialisms*. New York: Hillary House Publishers, Ltd., 1961

Olson, M. *The rise and decline of nations: economic growth, stagflation, and social rigidities*. New Haven: Yale University Press, 1982

Peel JDY. *Herbert Spencer: the evolution of a sociologist*. London: Heinemann Educational, 1971

Perrow C, Guillen MF. *The AIDS disaster: the failure of organizations in New York and the nation*. New Haven: Yale University Press, 1990

Portes A. Social capital: its origins and applications in modern sociology. *Annual Review of Sociology*, 1998; **24**:1–24

Preston SH. *Mortality patterns in national populations: with special reference to recorded causes of death*. New York: Academic Press, 1976

Putnam RD. Bowling alone: America's declining social capital. *Journal of Democracy*, 1995; **6(1)**:65–78

Putnam RD, Leonardi I, Nanetti RY. *Making democracy work: civic traditions in modern Italy*. Princeton: Princeton University Press, 1993

Reed D, McGee D, Yano K. Psychosocial processes and general susceptibility to chronic disease. *American Journal of Epidemiology*, 1984; **119**:356–70

Roberts RE. *The new communes: coming together in America*. Englewood Cliffs, NJ: Prentice-Hall, 1972

Rodgers GB. Income and inequality as determinants of mortality: an international cross-section analysis. *Population Studies*, 1979; **33**:343–51

Salloway JC, Dillon PB. A comparison of family networks and friend networks in health care utilization. *Journal of Comparative Family Studies*, 1973; **4**:131–42

Sarason BR, Sarason IG, Gurung RAR. Close personal relationships and health outcomes: a key to the role of social support. In: Duck S (ed) *Handbook of personal relationships: theory, research, and interventions*, (2nd edn). Chichester: John Wiley and Sons, 1997

Schoenbach VJ, Kaplan BH, Fredman, L, Kleinbaum DG. Social ties and mortality in Evans County, Georgia. *American Journal of Epidemiology*, 1986; **123**:577–91

Seeman TE, Kaplan GA, Knudsen L, Cohen R, Guralnik J. Social network ties and mortality among the elderly in the Alameda County Study. *American Journal of Epidemiology*, 1987; **126**:714–23

Strogatz DS, James SA. Social support and hypertension among blacks and whites in a rural, southern community. *American Journal of Epidemiology*, 1986; **124**:949–56

Suchman EA. Sociomedical variations among ethnic groups. *American Journal of Sociology*, 1964; **70**:319–31

Suchman EA. Social patterns of illness and medical care. *Journal of Health and Human Behavior*, 1965; **6**:2–16

Thoits PA. Conceptual, methodological and theoretical problems in studying social support as a buffer against life stress. *Journal of Health and Social Behavior,* 1982; **23**:145–59

Thoits PA. Stress coping, and social support processes: where are we? what next? *Journal of Health and Social Behavior*, 1995; **(Extra Issue)**:53–79

Tocqueville, A de. *Democracy in America*, (2 vols), (trans. H Reeve). New York: Schocken Books, 1961

van Poppel F, Day LH. A Test of Durkheim's Theory of Suicide—without committing the 'ecological fallacy'. *American Sociological Review*, 1996; **61**:500–7

Welin L, Larsson B, Svardsudd K, Tibblin B, Tibblin G. Social network and activities in relation to mortality from cardiovascular diseases, cancer and other causes: a 12 year follow-up of the Study of Men Born in 1913 and 1923. *Journal of Epidemiology and Community Health*, 1992; **46**:127–32

Wellman B. Which types of ties and networks provide what kinds of social support? *Advances in Group Processes*, 1992; **9**:207–35

Wellman B, Wortley S. Different strokes from different folks: community ties and social support. *American Journal of Sociology*, 1990; **96**:558–88

Wellman B, Carrington PJ, Hall A. Networks as personal communities. In: Wellman B, Berkowitz SD (eds) *Social structures: a network approach.* Cambridge: Cambridge University Press, 1988, pp 130–84

Wilkinson RG. *Unhealthy societies: the afflictions of inequality.* London: Routledge, 1996

Williams DR, Fenton TB. The mental health of African-Americans: findings, questions, and directions. In: Livingston IL (ed) *Handbook of Black American health: the mosaic of conditions, issues, policies, and prospects.* Westport, CT: Greenwood Press, 1994

Wilson WJ. *The truly disadvantaged: the inner city, the underclass and public policy.* Chicago: The University of Chicago Press, 1987

World Bank. *From plan to market: World Development Report 1996.* New York: Oxford University Press, 1996

Wuthnow R. *Sharing the journey: support groups and America's new quest for community.* New York: The Free Press, 1994

Zuckerman DM, Kasl SV, Ostfeld AM. Psychosocial predictors of mortality among the elderly poor. *American Journal of Epidemiology*, 1984; **119**:410–23

9 Do health care systems contribute to inequalities?

Maureen Mackintosh

This chapter considers the implications for health care policy—and specifically for models and processes of health sector reform—of the role that health care systems play in generating poverty and inequality.[1] That exclusionary and inequitable health care systems form an element of wider social inequality, and reinforce other sources of poverty, is well understood.[2] However, this aspect of health care systems is curiously underplayed in the current health policy literature. Current debate in the literature focuses on the impact of health care systems on health outcomes (arrow A in Fig. 9.1) and on the impact of social inequality on health outcomes (B). It does not pay anything like the same attention to the direct interaction between social inequality and health care systems themselves (C).

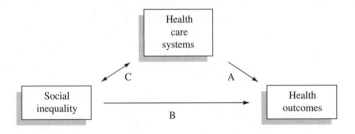

Fig. 9.1 Health/inequality interactions

This chapter seeks to contribute to redressing this situation. It analyses health care systems as a core element of social inequality in any society, in the sense that unequal legitimate claims upon a health care system, and unequal experiences of seeking care, are important elements of poverty and social inequality in people's experience. It argues that health care systems, as social institutions, are built out of the existing social structure, and carry its inequalities within them. However, health care systems are *also*, and at the same time, a key site for contestation of existing inequality: they offer a representation back to us of our societies' capacities for care, and a public space for reworking those capacities.

Effective health sector reform, that seeks to revise the social institutions of health care in more equitable directions, needs to draw on an effective theory of health care system/inequality interaction. At present health sector reform models tend to be prescriptive in content, which implies, as argued below, that they tend to disguise or mis-specify the links between the reforms and inequality. Building on more adequate concepts of institutions and of the nature of claims (outlined later), it is possible to rework health sector reform proposals to address the need for greater institutional inclusiveness and more spaces for public contestation of inequality and exclusion.

Prescriptive health sector reform models

If the health care system were widely understood among health care policy makers as a core element and institutional expression of social inequality, then one would expect the policy literature, including the large literature on health sector reform models, to address this problem conceptually as well as prescriptively. That is, it would analyse health care systems as embedded social and cultural institutions, changes to which interact with wider social, economic, and institutional change.

In practice, however, the health policy and management literature of the 1980s and 1990s on health sector reform displays—with exceptions—a prescriptive cast.[3] It has three predominant characteristics. First, it has a technocratic bent. That is, it proposes structural change in pursuit of aims that are cast as self-evidently desirable and technical (as opposed to political) in nature, such as more efficient use of capped resources and better allocative efficiency or 'responsiveness'. Second, the structural proposals mix market mechanisms (including privatization) with decentralization of public management and regulation of health care. And third, reform is also given an equity objective, stated usually in terms of more progressive targeting of public funding on the poor.

This literature treats the government as the decision maker. The health care system itself often seems oddly 'transparent': a set of rules and formal organizations that can be rewritten, reorganized, and redirected, given the political will. To the extent that social inequality enters directly into these models, it is chiefly in terms of the difficulties of building a political coalition for reform at government level.[4] The health sector reform documents of the World Bank, notably the 1993 *World Development Report: investing in health* (World Bank, 1993), display a characteristic mix of technocratic prescription and equity theme, often propounding health sector reform in low-income countries as an application of (a particular interpretation of) reform in high income contexts:

> Probably the most important [OECD health care] reforms of the 1980s involved the introduction of improved incentives and regulations for providers and

insurers, with the aim of raising the productivity of rationed resources . . . the United Kingdom has moved away from its integrated National Health Service and toward more autonomous and competitive physicians and hospitals. (World Bank, 1993.)

The Bank goes on to specify an aim of reform in low income contexts as '. . . freeing resources to target the poor'(World Bank, 1993).

This mix of technocratic presentation and equity theme characterizes the official, semi-official, health management-oriented, and economic literature on reform in the two areas used to develop the argument in the rest of this chapter. In the UK, often seen (as above) as a health sector reform pioneer among OECD countries, management academics, economists, and (in the 1980s and early 1990s) politicians have presented the reforms as an application of 'new public management' ideas to the search for better health care with rationed resources.[5] In the UK, the purchaser/provider split instituted by the reforms was associated with an equity theme, in that the purchasers were given a duty to assess local needs.

In Eastern and Southern Africa, from which my other examples are drawn, the research literature confirms that health sector reform is strongly driven by donors' models of reform, not by reform proposals emanating from within the local health care systems, despite the leverage exercised by local Ministries of Health once the reform process is under way (Mogedal *et al.*, 1995).[6] The reform models combine (a) a strong emphasis on cost-effectiveness analysis of alloca-tional problems, pointing to a public sector focus on primary care; with (b) the introduction of market mechanisms in the form of public sector charging and privatization, plus decentralization of public sector provision and funding (Gilson and Mills, 1995; Leighton, 1996; World Bank, 1996; Gilson and Travis, 1998). In this context, the donors' objectives explicitly include targeting public sector resources to where they will most reduce the disease burden, and filling gaps in the primary and preventative care system for the poor in order to do this.

Improving the allocation of health care resources and improving equity are both highly desirable objectives. However, the prescriptive approach—and a widespread willingness to accept the reformers' stated intentions at face value— have obscured both the mixed objectives being pursued in practice, and the problematic implications of context and institutional process for the outcomes of the reforms in the health sector.

Unequalizing reforms

There is a curious dissociation between the cast of thought in the health sector reform literature, and the social, economic, and political *context* of reform, as reflected in broader socio-economic research on social sector and welfare state issues. Both in the UK and in Eastern and Southern Africa—for example—the health sector reforms have formed part of broader *unequalizing*[7] social and economic reform processes. In both areas, the broader reforms associated with economic liberalization have been widely understood, within government and in public debate, as intentionally promoting greater social and economic inequality.

The UK National Health Service (NHS) reforms

The UK NHS reforms were thought up, pursued, and fought over in an intensely unequalizing context: one of widening income inequality, rising poverty, unequalizing welfare regime changes, and cultural and ideological changes legitimating greater inequality. The 'Big Bang' in the City of London, privatization of the utilities, the emergence of mass structural unemployment associated with the collapse of much heavy manufacturing, mining, and ship-building, the rise in part-time employment and the decline in wages at the bottom of the scale: the interaction of all this drove an enormously sharp rise in inequality and poverty in the UK in the 1980s and the first half of the 1990s (Hills, 1995; 1996; Goodman *et al.*, 1997; Atkinson, 1999).

In the welfare system, the context was a sharp decline in the relative value of universal benefits (such as pensions), and a shift from universal towards means-tested benefits, bringing, in the UK context, social stigma and contested individualized decision making to many more people. Young people were very hard hit. In this unequalizing context, the shift to higher and more widespread individual fee payment—especially flat rate payment—that occurred in social care, nursing home and home nursing care, health care (higher prescription and dental charges), social and public housing (higher rents), and education (payment by parents for a wide range of activities and services and for uniforms) all exacerbated inequality.

The final aspect of the unequalizing context united a deliberate squeeze on public spending with an ideological and institutional emphasis on privatization and mixed public/private provision. The effects were to encourage and force some people out into private and non-profit provision in pensions, social and nursing care, education, social housing, dentistry, transport, and some aspects of health care (such as certain surgical interventions).

In this context the NHS reforms were not—and were not seen as—simply technical reforms to improve health care. They were *also* understood, with government encouragement, as ways of bringing private sector management, financial incentives, private funding, and competition into a health service the government perceived as monolithic and resistant to change (Timmins, 1995). The 'internal market' reforms opened up scope for privatization of parts of the system. The government floated proposals to provide tax incentives—even opt outs—for private medical insurance[8] (Timmins, 1995). The government quite explicitly sought a more diverse—that is, more unequal—health service. As Margaret Thatcher put it in 1989: 'Those who can afford to pay for themselves should not take up beds from others' (Timmins, 1995).

This was a period of constant discursive emphasis on wealth generation and individual self-support; of the politically-driven language of scrounging; of public denigration of the poor and of notions of care and solidarity. The (short-lived and dishonourable) NHS management catch-phrase of 'treatment not care'[9] is of a piece with the period's political emphasis on individual responsibility and competition as drivers of economic growth and social improvement.

The 'market-like' NHS reforms of the 1980s and early 1990s were thus not a separate category of public action, somehow outside the general drive towards greater inequality. The potential and actual unequalizing effects of the NHS reforms were deeply contested in the UK, and are being partly reversed; further-more, the reforms themselves have opened up new possibilities and spaces for contestation (see below). However, the lessons drawn from the UK experience in, particularly, the World Bank's health sector reform literature largely ignore the contestation, seeking instead to associate the proposed structural changes with socially equitable purposes the original reformers did not share.

This is the more curious in that resistance to health care commercialization has been in no way special to the UK. The World Bank (1993) noted rather dis-appointedly that in the (non-US) OECD countries, 'Despite widespread calls for privatization of finance, no country has reduced its commitment to public coverage.'

Eastern and Southern African health sector reforms

The context of reforms elsewhere has been comparably unequalizing. In Eastern and Southern Africa (ESA) the context of broader social sector reform has included colonial and military misrule and war, as in Mozambique, Zimbabwe, and Uganda, and severe economic crisis in most of the region, also including Zambia, Malawi, Tanzania, and Kenya. The crises have brought declining formal sector employment, widening income distributions, increasing poverty, and fiscal deficits. The timing of economic crisis has varied greatly between countries, but in much of the region[10] the 1980s and early 1990s were a time of crisis associated with 'adjustment' measures including privatization, fiscal squeeze, and economic liberalization. (Cornia et al., 1987; Hanlon, 1991; Semboja and Thirkildsen, 1995; Gibbons, 1996; Raikes and Gibbons, 1996; Kalumba, 1997).

This economic context was experienced locally as a crisis of extended family support systems, a crisis to which social sectors were unable to respond.[11] Education and health care deteriorated in quality and availability throughout the region as public expenditure on services fell (Dodge and Wiebe, 1985; Hanlon, 1991; Woelk, 1994; Semboja and Thirkildsen, 1995; Kalumba, 1997; Tibandebage, 1999). There was a rise in informal charging in the public sector, encouraged by a dramatic decline in public sector wages and salaries in those countries worst affected (Doriye, 1992; McPake et al., 1999). The effect was to exacerbate social division between those who could pay and those who were increasingly excluded because they could not. Morbidity and mortality worsened in many countries (Mogedal *et al.*, 1995).

In this context, the effect of the social sector reform programmes on inequality is much debated. The ESA structural reforms of health care systems have had three main elements, though details and processes differ: liberalization and privatization (including increasing NGO provision), the charging of user fees for public services, and decentralized public sector management (Gilson and Mills, 1995; Mogedal *et al.*, 1995; Leighton, 1996; Beattie *et al.*, 1998). Behind these structural prescriptions lie models of reform strongly propounded by donor governments and the World Bank: the privatization of secondary and tertiary care perceived as primarily serving the middle class; the separation of regulation (and some funding) from management of remaining public sector provision; and a mix of user fees and decentralized accountability to make primary provision more locally responsive. The reforms are locally managed, and driven in many countries by fiscal crisis; but their form—and especially the emphasis on decentralization—owes a great deal to donor pressure (Mogedal *et al.*, 1995; Gilson and Travis, 1998).

These reforms are widely seen by local commentators and professionals, and by field researchers, as unequalizing in content and effect, despite the prior (if patchy) experience of informal charges. There are three main reasons for that perception. One is that formal charges *legitimate* exclusion and unequal access. Fees for public sector primary and secondary education, and for different levels of health care, impact most severely on the poor, and research shows them to have exclusionary effects. Exemption mechanisms work poorly (Gilson *et al.*, 1995; Oyugi, 1995; McPake *et al.*, 1999; Tibandebage, 1999).

Second, the reform models entrench unequalizing processes, intentionally, within the institutions of the system. The *aim* is separate systems for the middle classes and those in formal employment, through the privatization of such provision; public primary provision for the poor is intentionally gap-filling, notably primary care in rural areas. Decentralization in this economic context also generally means—initially at least—better-off districts doing better, since many countries do not have equalizing grant systems (Gilson and Travis, 1998).

Finally, many local commentators worry about the thin conception of the public sector in health care in these reforms. One doctor and academic recently summarized the reforms as privatizing middle class provision so that there will be more public funds available for the poor,[12] and wondered why reformers expect the public sector suddenly to become more progressive in an increasingly unequal context? Doctors and health planners share the fears expressed in the UK that legitimating commercialism and dividing the system will simply increase unequalizing pressures within the state itself.

In summary, health sector reform models, in the UK and Eastern and Southern Africa, have been presented in policy documents as equalizing in intent. Yet they have also been locally understood, for good reason, as deliberately unequalizing in health system terms: as reforms that seek to embed and legitimize existing and emerging structural market-based inequity within the health care institutions. This contradiction has bred, in both areas, some new spaces for contestation of inequality and exclusion. The rest of this paper outlines a conceptual framework for health sector reform that grasps this contradiction, with the aim of assisting better institutional design.

Health care institutions and 'social settlements'

A more adequate characterization of health care systems for policy purposes would not disguise unequalizing processes, but would build an understanding of inequality into the framework of policies designed to combat it. To achieve this requires a 'thicker' and more culturally rooted concept of health care institutions that understands them as always embodying inequality within unequal societies.

Conceptualizing 'institutions'

A relevant definition of 'institution' can be drawn from the anthropological literature. Mary Douglas's (1987) analysis of institutions starts from the idea that an institution is, 'minimally ... a convention'. This resembles the economic institutionalists' definitions of institutions (North, 1990) in terms of norms, habits, and conventions of behaviour. It locates formal rules and organizations as just one element of the full institutional context, along with informal understandings, including norms of market behaviour.

Douglas is particularly interested in the *legitimation* of institutions: the way in which patterns of behaviour come to seem natural and proper. So a deeper definition of institution in her work is a 'legitimised social grouping' such as 'a family, a game, or a ceremony'. Legitimation, in Douglas' view, typically involves both reasoned justifications of patterns of behaviour and the invoking for this purpose of 'naturalising' analogies. An example of the latter can be drawn from the writings of economic institutionalists. Oliver Williamson (1975), justifying his use of markets as a standard of comparison for other institutional forms, writes: 'In the beginning was the market.' He invokes by this phrase—how ironically it is hard to tell—existence before sin, natural creation and evolution without human intervention. Similar comparisons between the assumed normality of market exchange and the process of administrative (bureaucratic) service delivery—the latter a last resort when markets 'fail'—carry motivational weight in the social sector reform policy documents.

In Douglas's view of institutions, naturalizing cognitive conventions arise and stabilize (or not) over time through the interaction of discourse and experience. 'Discourse' here refers to shared meanings and ideas that form the basis of communication. Mutual feedback between behaviour, experience, and ideas can create an institution that in a recognizable sense 'works'.[13] Once an institution has become 'naturalized' and legitimate, it 'makes' big decisions for us. People think and act 'within the scope of institutions they build' (Douglas, 1987).

'Social settlements' in health care systems

This type of institutional analysis leads us to consider health care, not as an integrated system in the functional sense, but as an overlapping group of social institutions that are cross-cut by institutions wider than health care, such as kinship and gender. The patterns of inequality in any society are framed by strong legitimizing conventions of thought: from caste-based social distinctions carrying religious significance, via deeply embedded assumptions of gender inequality, to shared expectations that the more educated should receive higher incomes. Major social institutions such as health care systems build on many of these shared assumptions, and are themselves bearers of broader social inequality and privilege.

The health care systems of both the UK and Eastern and Southern Africa illustrate the point. The design of the UK NHS embodied an explicit compromise with the organized medical professions. Internal inequalities established from the beginning included steep status hierarchies and strong privileges for consultants in terms of earnings from private practice (Timmins, 1995). Professional hierarchies initially strongly reflected inequalities in the wider society, with consultants largely male and from the upper middle classes, and nursing being a largely working-class female profession including increasing numbers of Afro-Caribbean nurses; this social hierarchy has been changing, but only slowly (Langan, 1998). Funding has long favoured hospital treatment and curative care over home-based and chronic care, in ways that respond to medical hierarchy and that disadvantage in particular the poor elderly and their carers. There is strong though debated evidence that variability in access and quality of curative care favours the middle classes.[14]

In Eastern and Southern Africa, parallel inequalities structure health care institutions. The demands and costs of medical training—as well as the financial rewards—imply that doctors tend to be drawn from more privileged social groups. Nursing is a problematic profession for its members. In many countries, nursing was one of the few professions open to African people before Independence. Caught between doctors and patients within a deteriorating health care system, nurses have seen their working conditions, pay, and social status decline sharply since Independence, reflecting the general decline in public services.[15] Despite major efforts by governments to develop primary care, big differences remained before reform between urban and rural access and service quality. Subsidy patterns that focused on treatment for public servants and the military and supported urban secondary and tertiary care tended to favour the better off. Once economic deterioration set in, informal charging and falling quality in primary care reinforced the existing inequalities.

The pre-reform health services in both areas carried these inequalities while, at the same time, they also embodied 'universalist' principles that explicitly sought to redress other existing inequalities, notably exclusion of would-be patients from health care through inability to pay. In the UK after 1945, the NHS expressed a commitment to universal access in time of need. This universalism was rooted in a process of post-war reconstruction that rejected certain aspects of social inequity and created new rights of citizenship (Timmins, 1995; Hughes, 1998).

The ESA post-Independence governments saw their health services, in parallel fashion, as key elements of the construction of new states and of new relations between states and citizens, and all attempted greatly to expand access. The Frelimo government in Mozambique in the late 1970s was particularly explicit about this aspect of health services: 'It is often in the hospital that the people see reflected the organisation of our state.'[16] In Tanzania, the 1970s saw a big shift in policy away from hospital building towards construction of rural health centres and dispensaries, and the training of suitable staff; Mozambique was notably successful in making the same shift soon after independence (Hanlon, 1991; Tibandebage, 1999). The self-help movement in post-Independence Kenya generated health facilities that were taken over by the state in the 1970s (Oyugi, 1995). Comparable policies and initiatives can be documented across the region.

This mix of embedded inequalities, shaped by unequal citizenship, and redistributive attack on specific forms of exclusion, has been labelled in the UK social policy literature a 'social settlement' (Williams, 1989; Hughes, 1998). The 'settlement' has proved remarkably stable because it has offered—like other Western European health care systems—insurance against the risk of needing health care (and against the risk of being unable to pay for it), plus perceived opportunities for relative privilege for the better off, combined with substantial redistribution towards those on low incomes. Institutional inequality can, in this way, actually *stabilize* highly redistributive health care provision (Barr, 1994; Besley *et al.*, 1994).

Health care reform, in this framework, should thus be understood as a breaking up and reworking of the compromises between inequality and redistribution embedded in the health care system (Mackintosh, 1996; Hughes, 1998). In Douglas's framework, people think and act for themselves, but work inevitably with the ideas and experiences they share with others. The remaking of those shared meanings recreates institutional culture in new forms. This analytical framework thus internalizes the point frequently made in the literature that health care systems are embedded within distinct cultural contexts, and not 'transferable' in any simple way.[17]

During the reform process, we would expect to find competing discourses, seeking to legitimate and contest the new inequalities embedded within reformed systems. These discourses embody competing notions of right and wrong, of priorities and principles, of who can do what, what can be discussed and what will be suppressed.[18] The UK reforms were marked by such contested discursive change, as public service was reworked in market language (Mackintosh, 1997).

In health in particular, this change was much resented.[19] The market language sought to 'naturalise' the commodification of health services, including higher regressive charges for previously low-priced or free care and treatment, by invoking familiar and powerful images of customers and consumer rights. The 'contracting' language also operated to obscure the re-embedding of social class hierarchy within the new managerial forms of organization (Mackintosh, 1999; Towers *et al.*, 1999).

Presentation of the reforms in Eastern and Southern Africa has also sought to legitimize market-based inequalities, with considerable emphasis on 'willingness to pay' for health care. Institutional processes in public sector institutions that charge fees tend in practice to prioritize financial stability over access, and hence to legitimize exclusion of those who cannot pay (Mackintosh and Gilson, 1999; Tibandebage and Mackintosh, 1999). Reform models also present market segmentation as a rational response to restricted public funding, despite the evidence that excluding the poor from out-patient public hospital care at a time when urban primary care is becoming predominantly private (and only the formally employed have insurance) can be highly regressive.

Poverty, claims and representations in health care

If inequality is institutionally embedded in health care systems, then so is effective contestation and redistribution. If reformed health care systems are to be genuine new settlements, embodying new forms of redistribution, then the capacity and commitment to redistribute have to be built into the institutions of the system. This involves the creation of a legitimate basis for the poor to claim health care, and a strengthening of institutional capacities to make, and the commitment to respond to, such claims.

Poverty and health care claims

Health care systems that do not offer care—that take a narrow or an abusive view of their duties—thereby contribute profoundly to people's experience what it is to be poor. To face abuse or to have fear cumulated when at one's most vulnerable—to be denied care—is an element of what poverty is as it is experienced (Tibandebage and Mackintosh, 1999). The failure of care is a core element of social exclusion: Kaijage and Tibaijuka (1996) place exclusion in the failure of access to 'economic and cultural resources', including land and cash, education, and family, kinship, and community support systems, and also in the failure of government social sectors, including health care, to sustain and supplement such community support systems in times of crisis.

A growing literature on poverty and vulnerability focuses, not just on income, but on the tangible and intangible assets of the poor. However, these studies underplay the asset value of effective claims to health care. Moser (1998), for example, defines potential assets to include 'health status', skills and education, and household relationships and networks of mutual support. Some networks, such as pooled savings schemes and reciprocal lending, assist access to health care. Relationships *with* the health care system are not considered assets, except for credit from private practitioners. Carter and May (1999), in a study of class and poverty in South Africa, treat claiming systems for cash (pensions and disability allowances) as assets—but not claims to health care or education. Comparably, both the 'capabilities' and the 'basic needs' approach to poverty centre on health status, and neither treat *care* as a need in itself (Drèze and Sen, 1989; Doyal and Gough, 1991). However, effective care in response to need and vulnerability strengthens people's agency and self respect, as well as increasing physical well-being.

Legitimate claims to health care should therefore be considered as social assets for the poor, and institutional design of health care reform should seek to strengthen effective legitimate claims.[20] A 'claim', in this analysis, is the duty owed to an individual that they should have a good or service (Broome, 1989; Mooney and Jan 1997). Claims may be of different strengths—they are not 'absolute' in the sense that rights are often considered to be. Concepts of fairness prescribe 'how far each person's claim should be satisfied *relative* to the satisfaction of other people's claims. Stronger claims require more satisfaction . . .' (Broome, 1989).

Claims in health care are rooted in needs, and the formulation and agreement upon the strength of health care claims is necessarily an institutional process (Mooney, 1998). In unequal societies, some people's claims will be denied legitimacy, and some legitimated claims are likely to remain unfulfilled. Decision-making responds to institutionalized understandings of priorities and principles and also on institutional experiences of active claiming. Hence the culture and operation of the health care system (as a whole, public and private) *is* the way in which claims are established, legitimated, and denied or fulfilled by 'society'.

The implication is that health care claims are *relational*; they are shaped by the norms and experiences governing patients' relations to providers. The literature on sustainable primary care (e.g. LaFond, 1995) emphasizes its relational nature and its roots in trust and shared understandings; and studies of health system collapse demonstrate how people try to re-establish—sometimes in perverse ways—control over risk (for example, Birungi, 1998).

Claiming greater equality within unequal systems

The UK reform experience suggests two important elements that interact to sustain legitimate claims to care within unequal systems. The first is 'universals': shared and stated general commitments that form a principled basis for claims. The second is organized support for making claims.

The UK reforms opened up new spaces for claims by the disadvantaged and excluded. The shift to 'consumerist' notions of provision invited demands for more respect for and communication with patients. The 'purchasers'' duty to define local needs similarly opened up political spaces for interest groups to contest professional definitions of need, for example of the needs of people with disabilities. And individual needs-assessment for domiciliary and nursing care—intended by the reformers to assist rationing—gave campaigning groups a new handle for contesting failure to meet need. In this context, the 1970s and 1980s social movements' history of organizing could be put to good effect in establishing new effective claims (Harrison and Mort, 1998; Barnes, 1999). In sum, the consumerist orientation opened up, in some unforeseen ways, spaces for new *collective* definition of needs and collective and individual claims for resources.

This history suggests that more attention may need to be paid to strengthening the claiming process in the Eastern and Southern African health sector reforms. Those reforms too potentially create new spaces for contesting inequity and exclusion. Some donors and local officials see the entrenching of a culture of official payment not only as aimed at raising funds, but also as stimulating and legitimizing activism by patients around quality of care. They believe that people will more readily defend and contest services they pay for, and many user fee financing models build in community participation or community management. Officializing payment within a decentralized planning context can also stimulate experiments in pre-payment systems, and these in turn can provide a site for community organizing around health care issues, including exemptions for the indigent (Gilson *et al.*, 1995; Mackintosh and Gilson, 1999).

Furthermore, open and official payment in the public sector makes comparison with the NGO and private sectors in terms of value for money a natural progression.[21] Best provision in each sector can be used as a benchmark to exert pressure on others. Private and NGO competition can provide alternative styles of care, and in some contexts offer an escape from punitive cultures in public sector health care, thus helping to force change. A regulatory duty on government, established by the reforms, can also force governmental providers to meet common quality standards and to provide information to patients.

But all this change requires a confident, well-informed, and indeed organized public. While many local health officials are eloquent about the importance of people developing confidence to complain and to express needs, the current health sector reform models pay little attention to such relational issues. While the reform models promote an essential package of care, this is as an aspiration, a package to be delivered. Londoño and Frenk (1997) point out, in a critique of segmented Latin American health care systems, that such a package should rather be institutionally and discursively construed not as a 'minimum' but as a 'nucleus of universality'. The authors reconceptualize the package as a 'social commitment based on citizenship principles' and argue that it should be a key focus for social mobilization and participation, promoted and encouraged by the public sector. Most health sector reform models ignore this analytical link between 'universal' commitments and the promotion of activism in claiming care, a link which draws—like this chapter—on 'a conceptualization of health systems in terms of the *relationships* between populations and institutions' (Londoño and Frenk, 1997).

Conclusion: poverty, inequality, and health care policy

This paper has argued that social inequality directly shapes inequitable health care systems, and that the failure of legitimate claims to health care is a core element of poverty as it is experienced. It follows that commitments to redistributive health care, and notions of the public good that sustain those commitments, have to be actively constituted and sustained within unequal health care institutions. Local policy debate on reform frequently recognizes this. A Zambian health policy maker, for example, writes of the need for a 'negotiated health order' (Kalumba, 1997), and discusses the tension in the reform process between 'needing popular legitimacy as a basis for authority' and 'meeting the state's need to make the administrative structures for resource allocation coincide with the social balance of power'.

The 'social settlement' approach to institutional design in health care, put forward here, is aimed not at accepting inequality for its own sake, but at employing particular inequalities to help to stabilize and sustain institutional commitment to particular forms of redistribution. The approach to conceptualizing health sector reform implied by this paper might be summarized as follows.

- Begin by accepting the relational nature of health care, and focus attention on strengthening the capacity of the poor to make claims. Seek to strengthen in particular effective interaction between non-state public action to support claims and responses from the health care system.

- Establish some principled universal commitments—such as an essential package of care—as a basis for claims, and focus institutional design around ensuring that all sectors of health care fulfil the commitments. Consider both medical treatments and also care and respect for patients, when formulating universal principles.

- Decide what inequalities to live with within the system and be open about them. Seek to associate middle-class reliance on privilege with middle-class acceptance of duty to others, drawing on their experience of health care institutions. Do not allow the better off to segregate themselves institutionally.

- Concentrate on improving information about health care in the public domain, including information about governmental facilities, and on strengthening the capacity of the public—better off and poor—to organize around health care.

- Seek to shape the private sector through negotiation and public pressure, as well as formal regulation. Influence the private sector institutional culture by blurring boundaries, using a mixture of incentives, demands, and professional pressure. Publicize bad practices, kite mark. Try to avoid the creation of powerful private sector lobbies against socially inclusive institutions: try not to create active *enemies* of the poor.

- Take discourse seriously. The public representations of the health care system are important. Health care systems shape how we learn who we are in society, what we can expect, how we may behave.[22] They help to create a more individualist or a more mutual society, they polarize or string links of solidarity across divides. Ethical and redistributive commitments in health care are *both* a set of principles *and* an institutional construction in the form of a set of working understandings. Such commitments have to be constantly reconstructed in a market-dominated or market-pressured system.

Notes

1. I owe a great deal of my understanding of these issues to research, writing, and discussion over the last two years with Paula Tibandebage and Lucy Gilson, and over a much longer period with Pam Smith. Continuing research with Paula Tibandebage is financed by the UK Department of International Development (DFID), whose support is gratefully acknowledged. However, the contents of this chapter are the sole responsibility of the author, and do not reflect the policies and practices of the DFID. This chapter began life as a talk, and the style (including the rather sweeping approach to a very large and necessarily less than fully referenced literature) continues to reflect that origin.

2. The understanding is implicit, of course, in the 'targeting' literature which proposes to concentrate public health care resources on primary care for the poor, and underlies government policies seeking to universalise health care access. The literature on 'safety nets' in the adjustment process is rooted in the 'basic needs' approach to poverty, including access to basic health care (Cornia *et al.,* 1987; Vivian, 1995), and the 'public action' literature, rooted in the capabilities approach to poverty, similarly sees health care as an important focus (for example, Drèze and Sen, 1989; 1995).

3. In place of a very long but necessarily incomplete set of references, this argument is *illustrated* below using the literature on two case study areas. Counter-examples from the literature are also considered below.

4. Political coalition building is important, but not my topic here; from an extensive literature see, for example, Jeffrey, 1988; Reich, 1995; Chiang, 1997. The World Bank (1993; 1997) tends to see political issues in terms of 'removing obstacles to reform'; for a research paper along the same lines, see Leighton, 1996.

5. Department of Health, 1989 and HMSO, 1990 are the key official documents. Much economic commentary has taken the objectives of the reforms at face value, and evaluated them in their own terms; for example, Robinson and Le Grand, 1994; Flynn and Williams, 1997. The classic 'new public management' text is Osborne and Gaebler, 1992; see also Pollitt, 1993; Clarke and Newman, 1997.

6. The discussion draws examples from Tanzania, Malawi, Kenya, Mozambique, Zambia, and Zimbabwe, and to a lesser extent from Botswana and South Africa, where the social, economic, and political pressures surrounding health care reform are each very different.

7. I am using 'unequalizing' throughout as shorthand for 'promoting or resulting in greater social and economic inequality', understanding inequality in a broad sense to include income inequality, rising social division and exclusion, and rising inequality in capabilities, access to services, and quality of life.

8. Only tax relief on premiums for the elderly was ever introduced—for a time.

9. Source: fieldwork; see Mackintosh and Smith, 1996.

10. Botswana went through a recession and severe drought in the early 1980s, but has escaped economic crisis of the severity faced by much of the rest of the region and has experienced substantial economic growth.

11. Kaijage and Tibaijuka (1996) and Tibaijuka (1997) make this argument for Tanzania.

12. The source for this paragraph is recent fieldwork in Tanzania—see Mackintosh and Tibandebage, 1998. The summary echoes Margaret Thatcher's formula quoted above—a formula that was resisted in the UK.

13. For an example of field research addressing these feedbacks during reform, see Mackintosh (1997; in press).

14. Le Grand, 1982; Goodin and Le Grand, 1987. For critiques see O'Donnell and Propper, 1991; Powell, 1995.

15. Jewkes et al., 1998; the authors note that the situation of nurses and quality of nursing in the region is under-researched.

16. Speech by President Samora Machel, 1979, quoted in Walt and Melamed, 1983.

17. For example, Fuchs (1993) makes this point for Canada and the US.

18. Dryzek (1996) analyses competing discourses in the process of institutional design; Mackintosh (in press) uses the framework in more detail in the context of health care reform.

19. In 1989 William Waldegrave, then Secretary of State for Health, acknowledged this resentment and anxiety, noting that the public 'think we do not know the difference between a hospital and a supermarket' (quoted in Butler, 1994).

20. I owe my introduction to the 'claims' literature and its application to health care to Lucy Gilson.

21. In recent research in Tanzania (see Tibandebage and Mackintosh, 1999), a clear finding was that patients and would-be patients from all social backgrounds had no difficulty in understanding and responding to a question asking which type of facilities offered best value for money.

22. This is also of course an old argument; see for example Titmuss, 1970.

REFERENCES

Atkinson AB. Income inequality in the UK. *Health Economics*, 1999; **8**:283–8
Barnes M. Users as citizens: collective action and the local governance of welfare. *Social Policy and Administration*, 1999; **33**:73–90

Barr N. *The Economics of the Welfare State*, (2nd edn). Oxford: Oxford University Press, 1994

Beattie A, Doherty J, Gilson L, Lanmbo E, Shaw P (eds). *Sustainable health care financing in Southern Africa*. Washington DC: World Bank, 1998

Besley T, Gouveia M, Drèze J. Health care. *Economic Policy*, 1994; **19**:199–258

Birungi H. Injections and self-help: risk and trust in Ugandan health care. *Social Science and Medicine*, 1998; **47**:1455–62

Broome J. What's the good of equality? In: Hey JD (ed) *Current issues in micro-economics*. Basingstoke: Macmillan, 1989

Butler J. Origins and early development. In: Robinson R and Le Grand J (eds) *Evaluating the Health Service Reforms*. London: King's Fund Institute, 1994, pp13–23

Carter MR, May J. Poverty, livelihood and class in rural South Africa. *World Development*, 1999; **27**:1–20

Chiang TL. Taiwan's 1995 health care reform. *Health Policy*, 1997; **39**:225–39

Clarke J, Newman J. *The managerial state: power, politics and ideology in the remaking of social welfare*. London: Sage, 1997

Cornia GA, Jolly R, Stewart F (eds). *Adjustment with a human face. Vol. 1: protecting the vulnerable and promoting growth.*Oxford: Clarendon Press, 1987

Dodge CP, Wiebe PD (eds). *Crisis in Uganda: the breakdown of health services*. Oxford: Pergamon, 1985

Doriye J. Public office and private gain: an interpretation of the Tanzanian experience. In: Wuyts M, Mackintosh M, Hewitt T (eds) *Development policy and public action*. Oxford: Oxford University Press, 1992

Douglas M. *How institutions think*. London: Routledge and Kegan Paul, 1987

Doyal L, Gough I. *A theory of human needs*. Basingstoke: Macmillan, 1991

Drèze J, Sen A (eds). *Hunger and public action*. Oxford: Clarendon Press, 1989

Drèze J, Sen A. *India: economic development and social opportunity*. Delhi: Oxford University Press, 1995

Dryzek J. The informal logic of institutional design. In: Goodin RE (ed) *The theory of institutional design*. Cambridge: Cambridge University Press, 1996

Flynn R, Williams G (eds). *Contracting for health: quasi-markets and the National Health Service*. Oxford: Oxford University Press, 1997

Fuchs VR. *The future of health policy*. Cambridge, MA: Harvard University Press, 1993

Gibbons P. Zimbabwe 1991–4. In: Engeberg-Pedersen P, Gibbons P, Raikes P, Udshalt L (eds) *Structural adjustment in Africa: a survey of the evidence*. Oxford: James Currey, 1996

Gilson L, Mills A. Health sector reforms in sub–Saharan Africa: lessons of the last ten years. *Health Policy*, 1995; **32**:215–43

Gilson L, Travis P. *Health system decentralisation in Africa: an overview of experiences in eight countries*. Mimeo, January 1998

Gilson L, Russell S, Buse K. The political economy of user fees with targeting: developing equitable health financing policy. *Journal of International Development*, 1995; **7**:369–402

Goodin RE, Le Grand J. *Not only the poor: the middle classes and the welfare state*. London: Allen and Unwin, 1987

Goodman A, Johnson P, Webb S. *Inequality in the UK.* Oxford: Oxford University Press, 1997

Great Britain Department of Health. *Working for patients.* Presented to Parliament by the Secretaries of State for Health, Wales, Northern Ireland and Scotland by Command of Her Majesty, January 1989. Cmnd 555. London: HMSO, 1989

Hanlon J. *Mozambique: who calls the shots?* London: James Currey, 1991

Harrison S, Mort M. Which champions, which people? Public and user involvement in health care as a technology of legitimation. *Social Policy and Administration*, 1998; **32**:60–70

Hills J. *Inquiry into income and wealth.*York: Joseph Rowntree Foundation, 1995

Hills J (ed). *New inequalities: the changing distribution of income and wealth in the United Kingdom.* Cambridge: Cambridge University Press, 1996

HMSO. *NHS and Community Care Act.* London: HMSO, 1990

Hughes G. Picking over the remains: the welfare state settlements of the post-Second World War UK. In: Hughes G, Lewis G. *Unsettling welfare: the reconstruction of social policy.* London: Routledge, 1998

Jeffrey R. *The politics of health in India.* Berkeley: University of California Press, 1988

Jewkes R, Abrahams N, Mvo Z. Why do nurses abuse patients? Reflections from South African obstetric services. *Social Science and Medicine*, 1988; **47**:1781–95

Kaijage F, Tibaijuka A. *Poverty and social exclusion in Tanzania.* Geneva: International Institute for Labour Studies, 1996

Kalumba K. *Towards an equity-oriented policy of decentralisation in health systems under conditions of turbulence: the case of Zambia.* WHO Forum on Health Sector Reform Discussion Paper 6 [WHO/ARA/97.2]. Geneva: World Health Organization, 1997

LaFond A. *Sustaining primary health care.* New York: St Martin's Press, 1995

Langan M. The restructuring of health care. In: Hughes G, Lewis G. *Unsettling welfare: the reconstruction of social policy.* London: Routledge, 1998

Le Grand J. *The strategy of equality: redistribution and the social services.* London: Allen and Unwin, 1982

Leighton C. Strategies for achieving health financing reform in Africa. *World Development*, 1996; **24**:1511–25

Londoño J-L, Frenk J. Structured pluralism: towards an innovative model for health system reform in Latin America. *Health Policy*, 1997; **41**:1–36

Mackintosh M. Introduction: the public good. *Soundings*, 1996; **4**

Mackintosh M. Economic culture and quasi-markets in local government: the case of contracting for social care. *Local Government Studies*, 1997; **23**:80–102

Mackintosh M. Public management for social inclusion. In: Minogue M, Polidano C, Hulme D (eds) *Beyond the new public management: changing ideas and practices in governance.* Aldershot: Edward Elgar, 1999

Mackintosh M. Flexible contracting? Economic cultures and implicit contracts in social care. *Journal of Social Policy*, 2000; **29** (in press)

Mackintosh M, Gilson L. *Non-market relationships in health care.* Paper for WIDER workshop on group behaviour and development. Helsinki: September 1999

Mackintosh M and Smith P. Perverse incentives: an NHS notebook. *Soundings*, 1996; **4**

Mackintosh M and Tibandebage P. Economic analysis of an emerging mixed health care system, and implications for management and regulation: initial themes and issues of research design. ESRF Discussion Paper. Dar es Salaam: April 1998

McPake B, Asiimwe D, Mwesigye F *et al.* Informal economic activities of public health workers in Uganda: implications for quality and accessibility of care. *Social Science and Medicine*, 1999; **49**:849–65

Mogedal S, Steen SH, Mpelumbe G. Health sector reform and organisational issues at the local level: lessons from selected African countries. *Journal of International Development*, 1995; **7**:349–68

Mooney G. 'Communitarian claims' as an ethical basis for allocating health care resources. *Social Science and Medicine*, 1998; **47**:1171–80

Mooney G, Jan S. Vertical equity: weighting outcomes or establishing procedures? *Health Policy*, 1997; **39**: 79–87

Moser CON. The asset vulnerability framework: re-assessing urban poverty reduction strategies. *World Development*, 1998; **26**:1–19

North DC. *Institutions, institutional change and economic performance.* Cambridge: Cambridge University Press, 1990

O'Donnell O, Propper C. Equity and the distribution of UK National Health Service resources. *Journal of Health Economics*, 1991; **10**:1–19

Osborne D, Gaebler T. *Reinventing Government: how the entrepreneurial spirit is transforming the public sector.* Reading, Massachussetts: Addison-Wesley, 1992

Oyugi WO. Service provision in rural Kenya: who benefits? In: Semboja J, Therkildsen O (eds) *Service provision under stress in East Africa. The state, NGOs and people's organizations in Kenya, Tanzania and Uganda.* London: James Currey, 1995

Pollitt C. *Managerialism and the public services: cuts or cultural change in the 1990s?*, (2nd edn). Oxford: Blackwell, 1993

Powell M. The Strategy of Equality revisited. *Journal of Social Policy*, 1995; **24**:163–85

Raikes P, Gibbons P. Tanzania 1986–94. In: Engeberg-Pedersen P, Gibbons P, Raikes P, Udshalt L (eds) *Structural adjustment in Africa: a survey of the evidence.* Oxford: James Currey, 1996

Reich MR. The politics of health care reform in developing countries: three cases of pharmaceutical policy. *Health Policy*, 1995; **32**:47–77

Robinson R, Le Grand J (eds). *Evaluating the NHS Reforms.* London: Kings Fund Institute, 1994

Semboja J, Therkildsen O. A new look at service provision in East Africa. In: Semboja J, Therkildsen O (eds) *Service provision under stress in East Africa. The state, NGOs and people's organizations in Kenya, Tanzania and Uganda.* London: James Currey, 1995

Tibaijuka A. AIDS and economic welfare in peasant agriculture: case studies from Kagabiro village, Kagera Region, Tanzania. *World Development*, 1997; **25**:963–75

Tibandebage P. Charging for health care in Tanzania: official pricing in a liberalised environment. In: Mackintosh M, Roy R (eds) *Economic decentralization and public management reform.* Aldershot: Edward Elgar, 1999

Tibandebage P, Mackintosh M. *Institutional cultures and regulatory relationships in a liberalising health care system: a Tanzanian case study.* ESRF Discussion Paper for WIDER workshop on 'Group behaviour and development'. September, 1999

Timmins N. *The Five Giants: a biography of the Welfare State.* London: Harper Collins, 1995

Titmuss RM. *The Gift Relationship: from human blood to social policy.* London: Allen and Unwin, 1970

Towers B, Smith P, Mackintosh M. Dimensions of class in the integration of health and social care. *Journal of Interprofessional Care*, 1999; **13**:219–28

Vivian J (ed). *Adjustment and social sector restructuring*. London: Frank Cass, 1995

Walt G, Melamed A (eds). *Mozambique: towards a people's health service*. London: Zed Books, 1983

Williams F. *Social policy, a critical introduction—issues of race, gender and class*. Cambridge: Polity Press, 1989

Williamson OE. *Markets and hierarchies*. New York: Free Press, 1975

Woelk GB. Primary health care in Zimbabwe: can it survive? *Social Science and Medicine*, 1994; **39**:1027–35

World Bank. *World Development Report 1993: investing in health*. Washington DC: Oxford University Press

World Bank. *Health policy in Eastern Africa: a structural approach to resource allocation*, (Vols I–IV). Eastern Africa Department, Africa Region, World Bank, 1996

World Bank. *World Development Report 1997: the State in a changing world*. New York: Oxford University Press, 1997

10 Measuring health inequality: challenges and new directions

Christopher J. L. Murray, Julio Frenk, and
Emmanuela E. Gakidou

> It really boils down to this: that all life is interrelated. We are all caught in an inescapable network of mutuality, tied into a single garment of destiny. Whatever affects one directly, affects all indirectly. (Martin Luther King, Jr. 1968.)

Inequalities in health, both across and within populations, are a major public concern. Building on a long-standing tradition (e.g. Antonovsky, 1967), there has been a remarkable increase in interest in health inequalities and social group health differences since the early 1980s (Whitehead, 1992; Feinstein, 1993; Marmot *et al.*, 1997; Beaglehole and Bonita, 1998). This interest has been expressed in the political arena in many countries and international organizations as well as through the volume of scientific papers on the subject (Kaplan and Lynch, 1997; Acheson, 1998).

In this chapter we will discuss two topics related to health inequalities. Our goal is to bring attention to the issues and feed into the current debate in the literature. First, we will address the measurement of health inequality; second, we will discuss social inequalities as determinants of health status. We are approaching health inequalities from a new perspective which we hope will provide additional insight into determinants and implications for policy.

Current perspectives

Before proposing a new framework for the measurement of health inequality it will be useful to review the current approaches in a structured way. This section begins with a typology of existing measures and proceeds to the proposed new framework for measuring health inequality among individuals in a population.

Figure 10.1 depicts the current analytical perspectives in the measurement of health-related inequalities. The three major types of analyses are discussed in more detail below. The current literature is predominantly focused on measur-

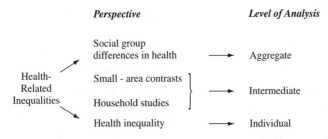

Perspective   *Level of Analysis*

Fig. 10.1 Analytical perspectives in the study of health-related inequalities

ing social group differences in health, by categorizing individuals into groups defined by characteristics such as education, income, and occupational class, and comparing average levels of health across these groups. Small-area contrasts are less prominent in the existing research, but should be given special consideration, as they are a form of social group analysis, using location as the variable by which they categorize individuals. These studies are at an intermediate level of analysis, being more refined than social groups, and closer to the individual level. The smaller the area of analysis and the more homogeneous the population in each area, the closer the analysis gets to the individual level. We define health inequality to be differences in health across individuals in a population. This type of analysis is underutilized, despite the fact that it is very powerful and has fundamental policy implications (Murray *et al.*, 1999).

Social group differences in health

There is a vast amount of literature on studies of social group differences in health which has brought a lot of attention to health inequalities in the last decade. An attempt to summarize the field is beyond the scope of this chapter. However, we want to draw attention to the remarkable results that have been published. This body of work has been crucial to the placement of inequalities in health in the agenda of health policy makers and has also indicated areas where more research is needed. We would like to highlight three challenges that this approach of measuring health inequalities is faced with.

Definition of social group

One of the most long-lasting debates in the social sciences has been concerned with the way in which individuals should be categorized. In light of the universal presence of stratification in all societies, it is not surprising that all major sociological traditions have attempted to capture the key dimensions along which social groups can be differentiated. Figure 10.2 attempts to summarize the main traditions in this respect, especially those that have been applied to the health field.

'Social class' is a concept that is often applied without rigorous limits. Yet two

Construct	Approach to Measurement
Social class (K. Marx)	Relationship to the means of production
Social class (M. Weber)	Market capacity and life-chances
Socio-economic status (Multiple authors)	Income, education and occupation Prestige Gender, ethnicity
Social position (K. Davis)	Status Office

Fig. 10.2   Major traditions in defining social groups

classical social scientists, Karl Marx and Max Weber, both gave it a central role in their respective theoretical frameworks, although each conceptualized it in very different ways. In the Marxist tradition, the key criterion to define social class is the relationship to the means of production. Although not a dominant perspective in the study of social group differences in health, it is possible to find some epidemiological studies that are based on the Marxist concept of social class. (For a rigorous attempt at operationalizing this concept, see Bronfman and Tuiran, 1984).

Weber moved beyond the polarized Marxist categorization in order to account for other dimensions of social stratification. He introduced the notion of market capacity, as determined not only by capital ownership but also by skill and education, which generates different 'life-chances' for individuals to receive rewards. The limitations of defining social groups mostly along economic dimensions led many sociologists, especially in the US, to substitute social class with the broader construct of 'socio-economic status'. Many different variables have been used in the literature to operationalize this concept, although the most common approach is to use a combination of income, education, and occupation. The multidimensionality of social stratification has led many authors to base their measures on broader notions of prestige. Likewise, key elements of social identity, such as gender and ethnicity, have also been used extensively.

Recently, some authors working on social differences in health have adopted the notion of 'social position' as the underlying construct that would account for the pervasive inequalities seen even in affluent societies (Gregorio et al., 1997; Wilkinson, 1997). This notion was originally introduced by Kingsley Davis in 1949. To the elements of status, social position adds those of office, i.e. a position in a specific organization. The concept is therefore very broad.

Despite the wealth of theoretical elaborations produced by social scientists to justify a particular approach to categorizing social groups, epidemiological studies often use measures interchangeably, without seriously considering the theoretical implications. Indeed, very often the choice of a particular catego-

rization in social epidemiological studies seems to depend more on the availability of data than on an explicit theoretical framework. This has led to a great
heterogeneity in the concepts and measures found in the literature.

Comparability and generalizability of results
Even if we assume that for each population individuals have been categorized
appropriately into social groups, the issue of comparing results across countries
still remains a significant drawback of this type of analysis. The most significant
use of the measurement of health inequalities is the comparison across populations of the magnitude of inequalities observed and the study of their determinants. Meaningful comparisons may not be feasible across countries when
different social groups are used to categorize the population. This challenge is
well recognized in the literature on socio-economic inequalities in health.

An example of social group differences comes from studies of self-assessed
health in the Netherlands and Australia. Both studies used the question 'Do you
rate your health as excellent, good, fair, or poor?' and compared the percentage
of the population in each country who rated their health as less than good, using
two different categorical variables. The social group variable used in the case of
the Netherlands was educational attainment, while in Australia it was ethnicity.
It is interesting to see that in the Netherlands the subgroup with the lowest education had the highest percentage of individuals reporting that their health as
less than good, while the more educated reported themselves to be in better
health. As is shown in Fig. 10.3, in Australia, it was the aboriginal population
who reported themselves as healthier than the general Australian population,
despite the fact that they are certainly the more disadvantaged on both socio-
economic measures (such as income or education) and health measures (such as
life expectancy).

This example highlights two important issues. First, the measure of health
used is self-reported health status, which may not be comparable across countries.
Second, it is difficult to draw meaningful comparisons across countries when the
variable used to categorize individuals into social groups is not the same. Both
these issues are relevant to the literature on socio-economic inequalities in
health, in which numerous studies report differences across social groups on
self-reported health status, often including comparisons across countries. Even
though these challenges have been well recognized in the literature, the lack of
concrete solutions suggests that alternative approaches to the measurement of
health inequalities need to be developed.

Study of determinants of health inequalities
An additional challenge to the analytical framework of social group differences is
revealed when one pursues the study of the determinants of health inequalities.
When the primary analysis is undertaken by calculating differences in health
across social groups, the results are already confounded by the choice of social
variable. The variable used to categorize individuals into groups is pre-supposed

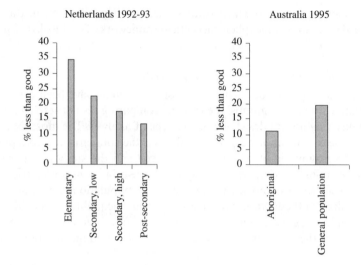

Fig. 10.3   Social group differences in self-assessed health

to be the one with the major effect. Further analysis of other determinants is most often not undertaken precisely because the assumption made at the onset of the study is that the major determinant of the differences across individuals is the factor used to categorize them. Analysis of other determinants could be conducted within groups. However, this set-up does not allow us to study other variables at the population level; we can only look at their effects across individuals in the same social group.

Despite the fact that studies of social group differences have brought remarkable attention to the field of health inequalities, the challenges to this approach described above indicate that alternative ways of analysing health inequalities should be examined. Since this is a topic with fundamental policy relevance, its measurement and the study of its determinants should be vigorously pursued. We describe two additional approaches; small-area analyses, which can also be considered as a subgroup of social group analyses, and individual health inequality analyses.

Small-area analyses

Analyses of inequalities in health which categorize the population by location deserve special note. Small geographical areas can be considered a type of social group. When the geographical areas used to categorize the population are small and represent relatively homogeneous groups, they provide a more refined categorization of the population than characteristics like race or occupation. As demonstrated by the few small-area analyses that have looked at health inequality, the magnitude of variation that is revealed in this type of analysis is much greater than differences across social groups. A study of patterns of mortality in US counties (Murray *et al.*, 1998) has revealed remarkable differences in life expectancy at birth across geographically defined groups of population. Life expectancy at birth for males in 1990 has a range of 16.5 years, from 61 to 77.5 years, and for females has a range of 13 years, from 70.5 to 83.5 years. When the population is further divided into race groups, the range observed becomes even larger. The lowest life expectancy (56.5 years) occurs among American Indian and Alaskan Native males in six counties in the state of South Dakota. On the other end of the range are Asian and Pacific Islander females in Bergen county in the state of New Jersey, with a life expectancy at birth of 97.8 years. The difference in life expectancy between the highest and lowest populations is 41.3 years, which is similar to the range observed across the world (Murray *et al.*, 1998).

This range is much larger than other differences in life expectancy reported from social group analysis. The power of the small-area analyses is that they approximate household- or individual-level analysis, under the assumption that populations in the same age–sex–race group within the same counties are similar. In the study of social group differences, the implicit assumption is that within social groups there is little variation across individuals. For many examples, the assumption of homogeneity in small areas is more likely to hold than the assumption of homogeneity within social groups. One of the reasons is that in small-area analyses the grouping variable, location, has many more categories than any social variable. This attribute gives small-area analyses the ability to detect larger variations than are observed in the studies of social group differences in health.

Small-area analyses can provide us with enough observation points to be able to plot the distribution of life expectancy at birth and thus reach additional interesting conclusions. Figure 10.4 depicts the distribution of life expectancy at birth for males in US counties and county clusters for 1970, 1980, and 1990. On the horizontal axis is the value of life expectancy in years. The values on the vertical axis show the proportion of the population that corresponds to each value of life expectancy. The area under each curve is 1, i.e. 100% of the population. Average life expectancy increased for males between 1970 and 1980; it also increased from 1980 to 1990, but at a slower rate, as can be seen by the shift in the curves to the right. The range from lowest to highest narrowed from 1970 to 1980 from 16.0 years to 15.3 years, but widened again between 1980 and 1990 to 16.5 years. This indicates that inequality in life expectancy at birth decreased in the first decade, but increased during the second decade.

The importance of looking at the whole distribution rather than just average values for groups of the population is also emphasized by Fig. 10.5. This figure depicts the distribution of life expectancy at birth for males in Japan, Mexico, and the US, around 1990. The axes are the same as in Fig. 10.4, with life expectancy in years on the horizontal axis and percentage of the population on the vertical axis. In this figure we see that Japan has the highest average life

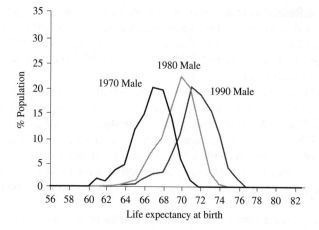

Fig. 10.4 US population distribution by life expectancy at birth for males in 2077 US counties and county clusters

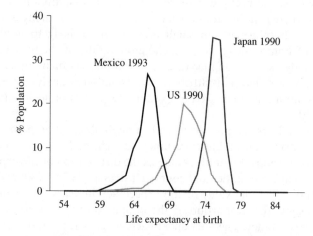

Fig. 10.5 Population distribution by average male life expectancy at birth

expectancy, followed by the US and then by Mexico. However, the distribution of life expectancy at birth in these three countries varies greatly. Japan appears to have the narrowest distribution, suggesting the lowest degree of inequality, as well as the highest average level.

The height of the peak corresponds approximately to the percentage of the population that are at the mean value. The higher the peak and the narrower the dispersion around it, the lower the inequality in life expectancy. Mexico, which has the lowest mean value, appears to have a narrower distribution than the US and also a higher peak, indicating that across geographical units the distribution of life expectancy is most unequal in the US. Even though the US has achieved a great shift in the distribution from 1970 to 1990, it has not made much progress in narrowing the gap between the highest and the lowest. This is a very important finding for policy makers, as it demonstrates the need to look at the entire distribution of health across the population as well as simply its average level—a point taken up by Gwatkin in chapter 11 (this volume).

Thus small-area analyses reveal a large variation in health status across geographical units. The extent of this variation is much greater than that revealed by other social group analyses. If we assume that individuals cluster in areas with individuals of similar risks and if the geographical areas across countries are of similar size, then the results from small-area analyses are comparable and meaningful. These assumptions will not always hold. Furthermore, because of aggregation, some of the true variation in health is still masked in the small-area analyses. Therefore, it is best to measure health inequality across individuals, as the problems of comparability and aggregation disappear and they are the entity we are interested in. Nonetheless, small-area analyses are a very useful analytical tool which, in conjunction with individual-level analyses, can help shape policy discussions.

A new approach to health inequality

We propose to use the term 'health inequality' to refer to the variation in health status across individuals in a population. This is a use that is quite distinct from the concept of inequalities in health as used in studies of health differences between social groups. Particular measures of health inequalities can reflect the range of variation from best to worst or the distribution of individuals within that range. This use of 'health inequality' to refer to a composite measure of individual-level variation is consistent with other disciplines studying inequality across individuals, as exemplified by the extensive literature on income inequality. For example, income inequality is frequently measured using the Gini coefficient, which is a function of the distribution of income across individuals or households. Measures of inequality of income or health are important because the same average level of income or health could correspond to vastly different distributions of these variables across individuals in a population. A concern for inequality is a concern for the distribution of attributes such as income or health across individuals.

Why should we measure health inequality?

Some authors argue that measuring health inequality across individuals is not interesting: '. . . the main problem is that such a measure [of individual inequality] answers a different—possibly rather uninteresting—question about generalized variability within a society distinct from systematic variability based on social stratification within society' (Wilkinson, 1997).

Variation across individuals in health can be attributed at the simplest level to four factors: chance, genes, the environment (broadly defined to include all physical and social factors), and the interaction between genes and the environment. The argument that individual variation is uninteresting must rest on the claim that the components of individual variation due to chance and perhaps genes are not important or are without normative significance (Murray *et al.*, 1999). It is highly unlikely that chance is responsible for the observed variation in the magnitude of health inequality across countries. Differences in health inequality across countries that can be attributed to genes, the environment, or the interaction between them have high normative significance and should not be ignored.

In the study of inequality, most of us are concerned with inequality of *risk* and inequality of *outcome*. Consider the analogy to income. If the government taxes every individual one dollar and then selects one individual through a lottery to receive all the proceeds, real income inequality would increase. But this is only due to chance; the expectation of income is equally distributed prior to the outcome of the lottery. In the case of income and health, risks and outcomes both matter. If all differences in health across individuals are simply due to chance then the degree of inequality across countries would be the same. The empirical results on health inequality across populations will resolve this concern.

Some researchers conducting analyses of social group differences argue that 'it clearly is a defect [of measures of individual inequality] if one takes the view—as many do—that what is interesting—and indeed worrying—about inequality in health is not that they exist, but that they mirror inequalities in socio-economic status' (Wagstaff *et al.*, 1991). This is not an empirical but strictly a normative argument, albeit a defensible normative argument (Wagstaff *et al.*, 1991; Valkonen, 1993), that only those health inequalities that correlate with other socio-economic inequalities are interesting. If health, as most would agree, is a critical component of human well-being, inequality of health should also be considered intrinsically important, independent of its correlation with other components of well-being, such as income or education.

The parallel argument for income, that income inequality is interesting only to the extent that it correlates with health or education inequality, would not be seriously entertained. Rather, it is clearly a conceptual and analytical strength to separate the measurement of health inequality from normative claims on the types of health inequalities that are considered inequitable and deserving of public action. We make the normative claim that health is a fundamental component of well-being and, as such, is important in its own right, independent of the associations between levels of health and levels of socio-economic variables.

If one is interested in health of populations, then the distribution of health is also of interest, since the same average level could correspond to very equitable or very inequitable distributions of health. Even though two populations may enjoy the same average level of health, the claim could be made that the population with the more unequal distribution is less desirable than the population with less inequality and therefore more public action should be taken in the population that has the higher level of inequality.

Social group inequalities in health do not convey the same picture as the individual-level inequality in health, as they assume that all individuals within the same subgroup of the population enjoy the same level of health. It is well established that there is a correlation between income and health. The magnitude of that correlation can only be determined by individual-level data and has not been studied extensively. The researchers that study social group differences in health make the implicit assumption that socio-economic status, approximated by a different variable in each country, is highly correlated with health. Therefore, one need only measure social group differences in health, as they adequately reflect health inequality. This claim is hard to defend. The counter argument from health researchers could be that one should measure health inequality in social groups, thereby making the analogous claim that health is the variable of interest and as such, it should be used to measure social inequality. Therefore rather than measuring Gini coefficients for income, we could measure health inequality and that would give us sufficient information for the inequality in social variables.

These arguments are not sustainable, as they are consistent with any degree of correlation between health and income. Figures 10.6 and 10.7 illustrate this point. They show a population in which income and health have a correlation of 1.0 (Fig. 10.6) and another population where that correlation is 0.5 (Fig. 10.7).

The three-dimensional graphs show how income and health are jointly distributed across the population. The bar charts show how health levels change across income deciles and how income levels change across health deciles. In both figures, health and income increase monotonically. We cannot draw the conclusion that because health status increases across income deciles and income increases across health deciles we only need to study one of the two variables and we will have sufficient information on the distribution of the other. By construction, there is a lot more variation within deciles in Fig. 10.6 than in Fig. 10.7 (since the correlation between income and health was much lower in Fig. 10.7). However, that is not apparent from the bar charts themselves and could only be seen if individual-level analyses where undertaken.

Therefore, even though income and health are correlated, there is a fundamental need to study the distribution of each independently. The study of health inequality should not be considered secondary, but rather complementary to the study of inequalities in social status. In addition, the determinants of health inequality are likely to be different from those of socio-economic inequalities and their analysis can only be performed if one uses the individual as the level of analysis.

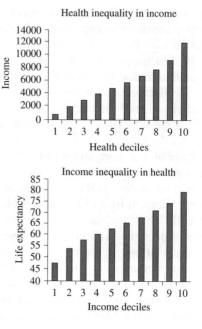

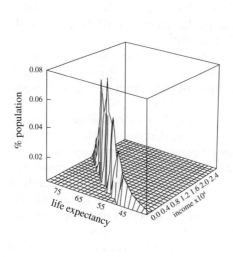

Fig. 10.6 Distribution of health and income

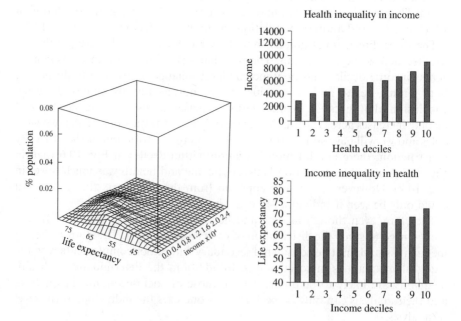

Fig. 10.7 Distribution of health and income

Measures of health inequality[1]

There has been little discussion in the health literature on measures to summarize the distribution of health across individuals in a population. Based on the wide array of measures used to summarize the distribution of income (Sen, 1997), and taking into account the fact that absolute, a nd not just relative, differences in health expectancies may matter, we propose two families of measures: individual–mean differences and inter-individual differences.

Individual-mean differences

Measures of individual-mean differences (IMD) compare each individual's health to the mean of the population. The general form is:

$$IMD(\alpha, \beta) = \frac{\sum_{i=1}^{n}|y_i - \mu|^\alpha}{n\mu^\beta}$$

where y_i is the health of individual i, μ is the mean health of the population, and n is the number of individuals in the population. The parameter α changes the significance attached to differences in health observed at the ends of the distribution, compared to differences observed near the mean of the distribution. The parameter β controls the extent to which the measure is purely relative to the mean or absolute. Common examples of individual–mean differences are the variance when $\alpha = 2$ and $\beta = 0$, and the coefficient of variation when $\alpha = 2$ and $\beta = 1$. However, many other individual-mean difference measures are possible. When $\beta = 1$, the measure is strictly relative and when $\beta = 0$ it is measuring absolute deviations from the mean but β could be any value between 0 or 1, reflecting some mix of concern between relative and absolute individual–mean difference.

Inter-individual differences

Another family of measures is based on comparing each individual's health (or income for that matter) to every other individual's health rather than comparing each individual to the mean of the population. We propose the general form of these measures inter-individual differences (IID) to be:

$$IID(\alpha, \beta) = \frac{\sum_{i=1}^{n}\sum_{j=1}^{n}|y_i - y_j|^\alpha}{2n^2\mu^\beta}$$

where y_i is the health of individual i and y_j is the health of individual j, μ is the mean health of the population, and n is the number of individuals in the population. The parameters α and β are the same as for the individual–mean measures described above. A well-known example of this family is the Gini coefficient often used to measure income distribution, where $\alpha = 1$ and $\beta = 1$. The Gini is often represented as being derived graphically from the Lorenz curve (Lorenz, 1905) of a population, but in fact is algebraically equal to the equation above. It is worth noting that when $\alpha = 2$ the individual–mean difference and the inter-individual difference for any given population distribution are identical. For any other values of α they are different.

Choosing a single index of health inequality

For standard comparisons we need to choose a single index of health inequality to summarize the distribution of health expectancy for a population. This choice requires the resolution of three fundamentally normative issues: which family of measures to use, what should be the value of α and what should be the value of β. These choices are normative choices, and individuals' preferences for these can be elicited through a series of questions that isolate the effect of each on the index of inequality.

We will provide illustrative examples of what these choices entail. For reasons of simplicity we will use a population of seven individuals (which can also be thought to be seven homogeneous groups of individuals). In each example we will transfer a specified number of years of health expectancy[2] from an individual who is better-off (i.e. higher health expectancy) to an individual who is worse-off. The transfers will be described in the text and are also depicted in Figs 10.8–10.10. There are three types of choices to be made. For each choice we will present two populations and the question will be 'Which represents a greater decrease in inequality: the transfer in population A or the transfer in population B?'

β: relative versus absolute inequality

One of the key choices that has to be explicitly made is whether we are more concerned about absolute differences in health, relative differences in health, or a mix of both with some weights, depending on our preferences. Figure 10.8 illustrates reductions of health inequality in two populations brought about by transferring equivalent years of health expectancy from the better off to the worse off. Using this example we can explore the extent to which individuals are concerned about relative inequality, absolute inequality, or some mixture of the two. The situation depicted in Fig. 10.8 is the following: populations A and B have similar distributions of life expectancy across the seven individuals, but at different levels. In population A the mean is 20 years, while in population B the mean is 60 years. In population A, 5 years of life expectancy are transferred from an individual whose life expectancy is 35 years to an individual whose life expectancy is 5 years. In population B, 5 years of health expectancy are transferred from an individual with health expectancy of 75 years (highest in the population) to an individual with health expectancy of 45 years (lowest in the population). Which of the two transfers results in a greater decrease of health

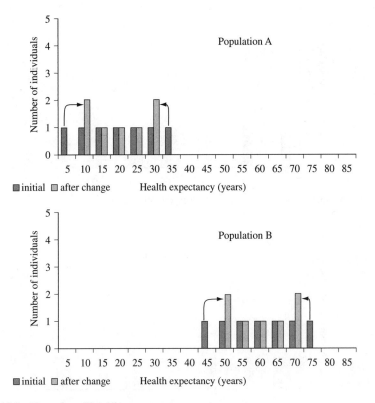

Fig. 10.8 Transfer of health expectancy

inequality? The answer people give to this question is informative about their preferences for the value of β (between 0 and 1).

α: intensity of health gain/loss

The second normative choice has to do with whether gains or losses of health that occur at the ends of the distribution should be treated differently from gains or losses of health that occur near the mean. Consider the two reductions in health inequality depicted in Fig. 10.9. Both populations are at the same level of health expectancy, with a mean value of 20 years. In population A, 5 years of health expectancy are transferred from the individual with the highest value (35 years) to the individual with the lowest value (5 years). In population B, 5 years of health expectancy are transferred from the individual with health expectancy of 30 years to the individual with a health expectancy of 10 years. Which of the two transfers represents a greater decrease in health inequality?

If scenario A is chosen, then the measure used would need to weigh more

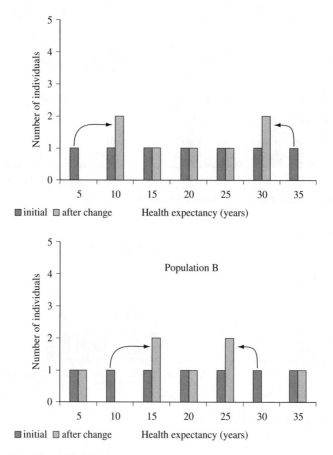

Fig. 10.9 Transfer of health expectancy

heavily transfers of health occurring at the ends of the distribution. If the respondent is indifferent, then all transfers of the same amount should be weighed equally, regardless of which part of the distribution they occurred in. If the choice is A, then α will be greater than one; if the respondent is indifferent between the two scenarios, then $\alpha = 1$. By constructing other questions where the amount of health expectancy that is transferred is different in magnitude, the exact value of α could be elicited.

Inter-individual versus individual–mean differences

The third choice refers to the family of measures: individual–mean or inter-individual comparisons. In the calculation of inequality in a population all measures include a difference between individual i and another entity. In Fig. 10.10, the two reductions in health inequality illustrate the choice. Both populations have the same mean value of health expectancy (both before and after

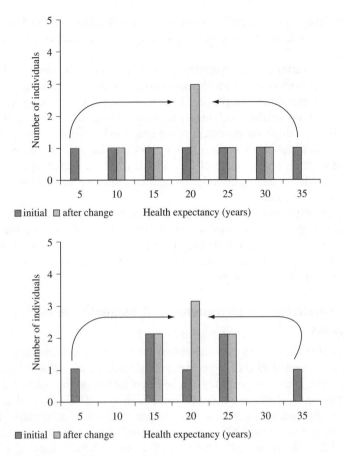

Fig. 10.10 Transfer to health expectancy

the transfer) and the exact same amount of health is transferred in both cases. The initial distribution of health is different in the two populations. In both populations 15 years of health expectancy are transferred from the individual in the upper end of the distribution (35 years) to the individual at the lower end of the distribution (5 years). The question again is 'which of the two scenarios represents a greater decrease in inequality?' Those who prefer A are expressing a view that what counts is not only where the individual starts and where they end up, but also where the rest of the population is. Those who are indifferent between A and B believe that what is really important is the absolute change achieved, regardless of where other people are in the distribution. In the first case, we would use a measure of inter-individual comparisons, while in the second case we would use a measure of individual–mean differences.

Because of the nature of the inter-individual comparison measures, the normative choices about the intensity of the transfer and about the family of measures are not completely separable. Inter-individual comparison measures, even when $\alpha = 1$, are more sensitive to equivalent transfers of risk farther from the mean.

Through a series of such questions, we could elicit individuals' values for the design of a summary index for the distribution of health expectancy. Population surveys or convenience samples could provide information from a wide range of individuals. How should such measurements be used to develop a WHO index of health inequality? We do not propose empirical ethics as a blind tool for resolution of normative choices; rather we believe that the results of measuring these values for a broad range of individuals will be a useful input to a deliberative process for choosing an index of health inequality for regular use by WHO in its work with countries.

Based on initial limited investigation, we suspect that most people will prefer a measure with a mix of absolute and relative inequality, with a bigger weight for differences farther from the mean, and with a consideration of intervening individuals. Yet these questions clearly require broader empirical assessment of the values held by different persons.

Operationalizing the measurement of inequality in health expectancy

We argue that the quantity of interest for measuring health inequality is the distribution of period health expectancy (Gakidou et al., 2000). How can this be measured? Health expectancy can be calculated from the risks of death or ill-health that individuals are exposed to at each age. Risk is not observed, only outcomes. An individual with a 10% chance of death is either alive or dead at the end of a time period; this fact provides us with no information as to what his/her risk of death actually was. Nevertheless, we believe that the distribution of health risks can be reasonably approximated through a variety of techniques. The combination of these techniques lays out a reasonable strategy to estimate the distribution of health expectancy. The strategy can be divided into four distinct approaches: measuring the distribution of child mortality risk, measuring the distribution of adult mortality risk, measuring the distribution of life expectancy and health expectancy directly through small-area analyses, and measuring the distribution of non-fatal health outcomes.

Child mortality risk

While we cannot observe child mortality risk, we can observe the variation in the proportion of a mother's children who have died, which provides information at a very fine level of aggregation (namely households) on the distribution of child death risk. Using simulation, we can evaluate the difference in the distribution of outcomes from that which would be expected based on a distribution of equal risk. Data on children ever born and children surviving for women of different ages are widely available from the Living Standards Measurement

Studies (LSMS) (Grosh and Glewwe, 1996), the Demographic and Health Surveys (DHS) (1999), and many censuses and surveys.

Adult mortality risk

For children, grouping data by mother provides fine grained information on the distribution of mortality risks in the population. Unfortunately, we have no such handle to measure the distribution of adult mortality. Similar information on the survivorship of siblings could in principle be used but it would refer to average mortality experience over decades and the technical challenges have yet to be solved. Other strategies need to be developed.

Distribution of life expectancy or health expectancy for groups

One method to approximate the distribution of health expectancy in the population is to divide the population into groups that are expected to have similar health expectancies and measure directly the health expectation for those groups. Inevitably, this will underestimate the distribution of health expectancy in the population even if the groups are perfectly non-overlapping in terms of their individual health expectancies. The more refined the groupings the more we will approximate the true underlying distribution of health expectancy. Small-area analyses hold out the promise of being one of the most refined methods for revealing the underlying distribution of health expectancy in a population. For example, a detailed age–sex–race group analysis of counties in the US has revealed a range in life expectancy across counties of 41.3 years (Murray et al., 1998). The smaller the level of aggregation we can achieve, the more likely we are to find groups of individuals with similar health risks. Results from small-area analyses can be fed into the estimation of individual health expectancy.

The distribution of non-fatal health outcomes

Measurement of non-fatal health outcomes on continuous or polychotomous scales provides more information from which to estimate the distribution of risk across individuals. Numerous surveys provide information on self-reported health status using a variety of instruments. The main problem to date with this information is the comparability of the responses across different cultures, levels of educational attainment, and incomes. For example, the rich often report worse non-fatal health outcomes than the poor (Murray and Chen, 1992; Australian Institute of Health and Welfare, 1996). Problems of comparability must be resolved before such datasets can be used to contribute to estimation of health expectancy in the population.

We need simultaneously to pursue the development of methods and datasets to measure these different dimensions of the distribution of health expectancy. We recognize there is a great need for new methods to integrate these different measurements into one estimation of the distribution of health expectancy in populations.

A focus on the inequality of age-specific health risks (inputs to the distribution of health expectancy) may re-invigorate interest in some health problems. For example, many specific occupational exposures are not major contributors to average levels of population health expectancy but they may contribute to markedly elevated risks for a small minority. Such increases in risks will contribute to the inequality of health expectancy. As we better quantify the distribution of health expectancy the role of occupational and local environmental exposures in contributing to risk inequality may become apparent. Interest in inequality in health risks in developed countries may also draw attention to the impressive inequality in adult male mortality risk. In a country like the US, there is considerably more inequality in adult male mortality risk than in child or adult female mortality risks (Murray *et al.*, 1998).

The task of measuring the distribution of health expectancy will need to make use of cross-sectional survey data on the prevalence of various non-fatal health outcomes. Measuring health inequality is fundamentally about comparing the distribution of the health status of individuals within populations and comparing distributions of different populations. If self-reported responses from the application of various health status surveys, using instruments such as SF-36, EUROQOL, or activities of daily living, are to be used in estimating health expectancy, special attention will need to be paid to the comparability of these responses across cultural groups. There is evidence that current instruments for measuring health status in surveys may not be comparable (Johansson, 1991; 1992; Murray and Chen, 1992). Hopefully the work on inequality will improve comparability of health status survey responses across cultural groups.

There is growing consensus that improvement in average levels of health is not a sufficient indicator of health system performance. The distribution of such improvement is an equally important dimension of performance. In order to

Environmental Determinants	*Inter-individual Determinants*	*Individual Determinants*

• Social environment
  + Inequality
  + Social capital
  + Health care
    system
	• Rank
	
	• Distance
	
	• Networks
		• Assets
		  + Wealth
		  + Knowledge
		  + Use of health
		    services

• Physical environment		• Behaviour
		  + Risk factors
		  + Health-care seeking

		• Physio-pathological mechanisms

Fig. 10.11 The causal web in health: a simplified view

place health inequality at the centre of the policy debate, we must develop better ways of measuring it. That will be the only way of ascertaining the true magnitude of the problem and of monitoring progress towards its solution.

Social inequalities as determinants of health

Figure 10.11 presents a simplified view of a possible explanatory framework for determinants of health. Each individual has a number of characteristics and attributes that affect his/her health status. These include their income and wealth, their educational level and knowledge on health issues, their use of health services, all of which can directly influence their health status. At the individual level there are also a number of behaviours that can directly enhance health—such as exercise, health care seeking—or directly harm health—such as smoking, alcohol abuse, and obesity. These factors are particular to each individual and, for the most part, do not have a health effect on those around them. At the other end of the spectrum there are the environmental determinants of health, defining the environment to encompass physical and social attributes. The effects of the physical environment on health have been studied extensively and we will not attempt to summarize them here. The social environment, which includes factors such as the structure of the health care system, social inequalities, and social capital, has also received great attention in the literature.

We would like to draw attention to a category of determinants that has not been discussed extensively, namely determinants of health that arise from inter-individual relationships. Inter-individual determinants refer to factors that affect health that are particular to the individual's position in society with respect to those around him. We address three types of such factors: rank, distance, and networks.

Rank is an individual's position in the social hierarchy. There have been a number of studies on social inequalities that have examined differences in health status with respect to rank. For example the Whitehall study examines differences in health across groups of individuals ranked by civil service grade (Marmot *et al.*, 1991). Rank is an absolute measure of position, as it is independent of how much better off those with higher ranks are. Picture a society in which individual A is ranked 500 out of 1000 with respect to income. If all individuals above A get a sudden doubling of their income while the income of A and all those below him remains the same, everybody's rank will remain the same, while the disparity between their incomes will have grown significantly.

Distance is a measure of how far individual A is from all those above him. We calculate distance from the top to be equal to the sum of the difference in income between individual A and all individuals above him divided by the mean. In the example above, A's rank would have remained the same, while the measure of distance would have increased significantly.

The following example is used to demonstrate the difference between rank, distance, and community-level inequality.

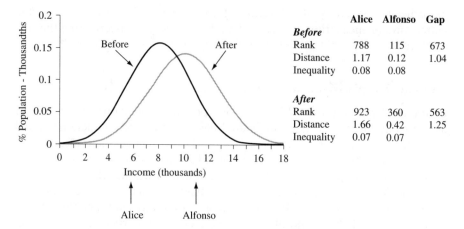

Fig. 10.12 Rank, distance, and inequality

We have two individuals in a population shown in Figure 10.12, Alice and Alfonso. The community-level inequality as measured by the Gini coefficient for income is 0.08. At the onset of our example, Alice has an income of 6000 while Alfonso has an income of 11,000. Within their community, Alice's rank is 788 while Alfonso's is 115, with an absolute difference in rank between them of 673. In terms of distance from the top, Alice is 1.17 and Alfonso is 0.12, with an absolute difference in distance between them of 1.04. Imagine an overall increase in the income level of the community while Alice's and Alfonso's incomes remain unchanged. The community-level inequality has decreased to 0.07. Their ranks have now fallen to 923 and 360 respectively, with a rank difference of 563. The distance from the top for Alice is now 1.66 while for Alfonso it is 0.42, with a difference between them of 1.25. So, in this example the answer to the question 'has inequality increased or decreased with the rise in income level?' depends on the measure chosen. The Gini coefficient has fallen, indicating an overall decrease in the community-level relative inequality. Between individuals, the rank difference between Alice and Alfonso has decreased, while the distance between them has increased. This indicates that the choice of measure affects how one perceived increases and decreases in inequality.

These inter-individual comparisons become particularly interesting in the context of the technological advances that change the networks of individuals. The definition of an individual's network has become more complex in the last decades. Relative deprivation, a concept originally formulated by Samuel Stouffer and colleagues (1949) related an individual's feelings to the perception of the condition of like-status others. In the present era of communications and travel, it is unclear how to identify the appropriate relative group of like-status others is. For example, in defining the network or interaction group of a computer programmer in Silicon Valley, should we include computer programmers in India or just the population in Silicon Valley? The term 'relative deprivation' is used arbitrarily in the literature; comparisons are made more on the basis of data availability than a thoughtful consideration of who the relevant network of individuals should be. The changing nature of individuals' networks poses an additional methodological challenge in the measurement of health inequality and of the effects of social inequalities on health status of populations.

Conclusion

Health inequality has become the focus of increasing attention on the part both of researchers and of policy makers. There is an urgent need for advancing our understanding in order to better orient policies towards improvements along this crucial dimension of health system performance. In this chapter we have suggested an alternative framework for studying health inequality. We are proposing it as a complementary approach to the valuable analyses that have been conducted to date. With continued research it can lead to better evidence on the magnitude and determinants of health inequality. Addressing the compelling problem of health inequality will no doubt be a major item on the analytical and policies agendas of the twenty-first century.

Notes

1. This section of the chapter has appeared in: Gakidou et al., 2000, and is reproduced by kind permission of the World Health Organization.

2. Health expectancy is considered to be the number of years in equivalent full health an individual born today can expect to live. For a more detailed explanation for this choice of health indicator see Gakidou et al., 2000.

REFERENCES

Acheson D. *Independent inquiry into inequalities in health*. London: The Stationery Office, 1998

Antonovsky A. Social class, life expectancy and overall mortality. *Milbank Memorial Fund Quarterly*, 1967; **45**:31–73

Australian Institute of Health and Welfare. *Australia's health: the fifth biennial report of the Australian Institute of Health and Welfare*. Canberra: AGPS, 1996

Beaglehole R, Bonita R. Public health at the crossroads: which way forward? *Lancet*, 1998; **351**:590–2

Bronfman M, Tuiran RA. La desigualdad social ante la muerte: clases sociales y mortalidad. *Cuadernos Medico Sociales*, 1984; **29–30**:53–75

Davis K. *Human society*. New York: Macmillan, 1949

Demographic and Health Survey. http://www.measuredhs.com, 15 August, 2000

Feinstein JJ. The relationship between socioeconomic status and health: a review of the literature. *Milbank Quarterly*, 1993; **71**:279–322

Gakidou EE, Murray CJL, Frenk J. Defining and measuring health inequality: an approach based on the distribution of health expectancy. *Bulletin of the World Health Organization*, 2000; **78**:42–54

Gini C. *Variabilita e mutabilita*. Bologna, 1912

Gregorio DI, Walsh SJ, Paturzo D. The effects of occupation-based social position on mortality in a large American cohort. *American Journal of Public Health*, 1997; **87**:1472–5

Grosh M, Glewwe P. *A Guide to Living Standards Surveys and Their Data Sets*. Washington, DC: The World Bank, 1995 (updated on March 1, 1996)

Johansson SR. The health transition: the cultural inflation of morbidity during the decline of mortality. *Health Transition Review*, 1991; **1**:39–68

Johansson SR. Measuring the cultural inflation of morbidity during the decline of mortality. *Health Transition Review*, 1992; **2**:78–89

Kaplan GA, Lynch JW. Whither studies on the socioeconomic foundations of population health? *American Journal of Public Health*, 1997; **87**:1409–11

Lorenz MO. Methods for measuring the concentration of wealth. *Journal of the American Statistical Association*, 1905; **9**

Marmot MG, Smith GD, Stansfeld S *et al*. Health inequalities among British civil servants: the Whitehall II study. *Lancet*, 1991; **337**:1387–93

Marmot M, Ryff CD, Bumpass LL, Shipley M, Marks NF. Social inequalities in health: next questions and converging evidence. *Social Science and Medicine*, 1997; **44**:901–10

Murray CJL, Chen LC. Understanding morbidity change. *Population and Development Review*, 1992; **18**:481–503

Murray CJL, Michaud C, McKenna M, Marks JM. *US patterns of mortality by county and race: 1965–1994*. Cambridge, MA: Harvard School of Public Health and National Center for Disease Prevention and Health Promotion, 1998

Murray CJL, Gakidou EE, Frenk J. Health inequalities and social group differences: what should we measure? *Bulletin of the World Health Organization*, 1999; **77**:537–43

Sen A. *On economic inequality*. Oxford: Clarendon Press, 1997

Stouffer SA *et al*. *The American Soldier: adjustment during army life*. Princeton, New Jersey: Princeton University Press, 1949

Valkonen T. Problems in the measurement and international comparisons of socio-economic differences in mortality. *Social Science and Medicine*, 1993; **36**:409–18

Wagstaff A, Paci P, van Doorslaer E. On the measurement of inequalities in health. *Social Science and Medicine*, 1991; **33**:545–57

Whitehead M. The concepts and principles of equity and health. *International Journal of Health Services*, 1992; **22**:429–45

Wilkinson RG. Socioeconomic determinants of health. Health inequalities: relative or absolute material standards? *British Medical Journal*, 1997; **314**:591–5

11 Poverty and inequalities in health within developing countries: filling the information gap

Davidson R. Gwatkin

The intense concern for the health of the poor frequently expressed in discussions of developing country health problems has, until very recently, failed to produce comparably significant efforts to collect the information needed to act upon this concern. As a result, there is little firm, systematic information about the health status and health service use by the impoverished, or about poor–rich health status or service use differentials within countries. Further, little use has been made of such information as does exist in the formulation of health policy objectives and in the design of health programmes. This chapter discusses the lack, and limited use of, data on poor–rich health inequalities and the health of the poor, especially within developing countries; summarizes what data do exist, and what efforts to produce additional information are under way; and suggests priorities for future investigation.

Traditional lack of attention to the collection of health inequality data

The claim that the collection of data about health inequalities has traditionally attracted little attention can most easily by supported through a contrast between data collection efforts in the health and economic development fields. The contrast is of particular interest because of the close relationship in thinking between poverty in the health and economic development fields during the late 1970s and early 1980s. During that period, the 'basic human needs' school, with its special focus on the poor, replaced the emphasis on society-wide economic growth in development thinking, and gave rise to publications like the 1980 *World Development Report* on poverty. In the health field, the philosophy of health for all and primary health care that emerged from the 1978 Alma Ata Conference was quite congruent with the basic human needs development school (World Health Organization, 1978). Yet while common in philosophy, the empirical *sequelae* of the two movements were quite different.

In the area of economic development, the concern for poverty that emerged in the 1970s gave rise to a determined effort to produce basic information. Prominent in this effort was the establishment of an international poverty line, defined as the amount of consumption needed to purchase a nutritionally adequate diet; and a vigorous programme of household data analysis to produce estimates of the number of people in each country and region whose consumption placed them below that line. A second, related line of activity was the compilation and periodic information about intra-country income inequalities, as measured by the well-known Gini coefficient.

As a result, the World Bank, which played a leading role in the effort just described, now regularly publishes sets of estimates about levels and trends of poverty in the world, and also sets of data about intra-country income inequality that permit an assessment of differences and trends. For instance, the 1998 edition of the Bank's *World Development Indicators* includes a table indicating the Gini coefficient and the percentage of national income going to each economically-defined quintile of the population for some 80 countries (World Bank, 1998). Another table indicates the percentage of the population below the poverty line in nearly 50 countries.

Nothing comparable was attempted in health. Thus, the 1998 *World Development Indicators* contain no information about intra-country differences in health conditions. Rather, all information relates to conditions in countries as a whole. For example, there is information about infant mortality in entire country populations, but not about infant mortality among the poorest 20% of the population, or among those in the population who subsist below a country's poverty line. One can find data about the percentage of births attended by trained health staff; but not about the percentage of births among the poor which receive such attention, or about how big a poor–rich difference exists in this regard. Figures are provided for overall government health expenditures, but not for how the beneficiaries of those expenditures are distributed across economic class.

The second point advanced in the opening paragraph—of the limited role that health conditions specific to the poor play in the health policy process—can also be illustrated through a contrast between the way in which economic development and health policy objectives are typically established. Take, for example, a particularly prominent set of development objectives: the year 2015 core targets developed from the 1995 Copenhagen Social Summit by the OECD's Development Assistance Committee (OECD, 1996). The economic target in the OECD set is framed in terms of conditions prevailing among the poor. That is, it does not follow the earlier practice in economic development planning of establishing a target annual rate of per capita income growth for the society as a whole. Rather, the target refers only to that segment of the society below the poverty line, saying 'the proportion of people living in extreme poverty in developing countries should be reduced by at least one-half by 2015.'

Contrast this with the health objectives set forth in this same set of targets. These say that: 'The death rate for infants and children under the age of five years should be reduced in each developing country by two thirds the 1990 level by 2015. The rate of maternal mortality should be reduced by three fourths during the same period.' These objectives are framed in terms of average societal mortality rates, without regard to how progress toward them might be distributed among different socio-economic classes within society.

It is certainly true that the focus on infant, child, and maternal mortality provides more of a poverty orientation than reliance on some other indicator like life expectancy since, as will be seen later, deaths at an early age or at childbirth are particularly frequent among the poor. However, the congruence even between infant and child mortality in society at large and health status among the poor is far from exact. This lack of congruence can be demonstrated with reference to infant and child mortality in the developing world as a whole. Take the figures in the right-hand column of Table 11.1, derived from the estimates of the global burden of disease in 1990. These show that infant and child deaths among the poorest 20% of the developing world's population represent about 35% of total infant and child deaths recorded in the developing countries. This 35 % is considerably higher than the 20% that would prevail were infant and child deaths spread evenly across all socio-economic classes. Also, in line with what was said above, the 35% figure is notably larger than the comparable percentages found among older age groups. Among people 60 years and older, for example, only around 20% of all developing-country deaths occur among the poorest 20% of the population—an indication that, unlike deaths at

Table 11.1 Deaths in the developing world, 1990

Age group	Number of deaths in entire developing world population	Deaths in poorest 20% of developing world population	Deaths in poorest 20% as percentage of deaths in entire population
0–4	12,539,000	4,931,000	**35.0%**
5–14	2,268,000	718,000	**31.7%**
15–29	2,808,000	911,000	**32.4%**
30–44	2,847,000	781,000	**27.4%**
45–59	4,478,000	1,039,000	**23.2%**
60+	14,614,000	2,879,000	**19.7%**

Sources: *Total number of deaths in the developing world*: Tabulated from data for India, China, Other Asia and Islands, Sub-Sahara Africa, Latin America and the Caribbean, and the Middle Eastern Crescent countries (Murray and Lopez, 1996 pp. 441–61
Number of deaths in the poorest 20% of the developing world's population: Unpublished tabulation by Patrick Heuveline of data for six regions referred to in preceing paragraph, as drawn from Murray and Lopez, *op. cit.*, and following procedure described in Gwatkin and Guillot, 1999

younger ages, mortality in this older age group does not affect the poor disproportionately.

However, the 35% figure also means that only slightly more than one-third of all deaths in the developing world occur among extremely poor population groups; the remaining 65% take place among the 80% of the world's population that is not so poor. Given that infant and child mortality rates are currently close to zero in developed countries (being around 6–7 deaths per 1000 live births), it would possible in principle to achieve close to a 65% improvement in global infant and child mortality through declines in the top 80% of the population alone. This means coming quite close to achieving the OECD objective of a two-thirds reduction without affecting conditions prevailing among the poorest 20%—and to attain that objective fully through a scenario involving only a minimal improvement in this group and through an increase in poor–rich inequalities.

Such a potential scenario argues against looking to societal averages as the basis for establishing health objectives relevant for the poor, since objectives expressed in terms of averages could be met through a strategy that ends up benefiting primarily the better off. The need, rather, is for health objectives expressed in terms analogous to those used in establishing the OECD economic goals: that is, in terms of health conditions prevailing among the poor alone, or in terms of the poor relative to the rich. There are several ways in which objectives of this sort could be framed. For example:

- an X-year increase in life expectancy among the poorest 20% of a country's population; or

- a reduction in the infant mortality ratio between the poorest and richest 20% of a country's population from Y:1 to Z:1.

Recent increase in attention to distributional information about health

The earlier-noted neglect of information about the distributional aspects of health status and health service use means that the lack of relevant data represents an important impediment to the establishment of health goals like those just described. However, the situation appears about to change. A recent renewal of concern for the health of the poor has given rise to a large number of investigations into the health status of different groups within developing countries. In addition to numerous individual country studies, over a dozen inter-country study projects on health equity and the health of the poor are under way (Carr et al., 1998). Among the inter-country projects are three initiatives that seek to provide basic information about health status and health service use among different people within countries.

The first of these to produce published results is a WHO exercise, whose initial findings (described further below) appeared in the 1999 *World Health Report*

(World Health Organization, 1999). This exercise draws on published country-level statistics for the percentage of people below the poverty line and for the health indicators of interest for each of some 40–50 countries. Through statistical analysis of these country-level data, it is possible to estimate the value of each health indicator among people above and below the poverty line in each of the countries covered.

The second exercise, undertaken in the World Bank, relies on household data from a series of Bank-supported living standards measurement studies (LSMS) carried out in approximately 25 developing countries. The LSMS studies are known for the careful attention paid to the collection of accurate household expenditure information. This, together with anthropometric and mortality data that the surveys also contain, makes it possible to produce estimates of health status by economic class. The first findings of data from this source were recently published (Wagstaff, 2000).

The third effort is also sponsored by the World Bank and it too relies on household data. The source of the data is the set studies executed in approximately 50 countries under the auspices of the USAID-assisted Demographic and Health Surveys (DHS) programme. These studies contain comparable information about a wide range of maternal and child health status and service use indicators. Unlike the LSMS studies, the DHS surveys do not cover expenditure. Economic status is defined instead in terms of wealth, as measured through an index based on responses to a series of household asset questions contained in the DHS survey instrument. For each country, the Bank has commissioned the DHS secretariat to produce tabulations, by wealth quintile of the population, for approximately 30 health status and health service utilization indicators.

Initial findings from initiatives like these are already beginning to produce results that are likely to be found surprising and that might well force significant modifications in the way that health inequalities are viewed. An example is the set findings in the paper that presents the first results from the second of the three initiatives just described (Wagstaff, 2000). The paper presents estimates about infant and child mortality inequalities among economic quintiles (defined in terms of consumption) in nine developing countries. Not surprisingly, the estimates point toward large differences in the degree of health inequalities that exist within the countries covered, suggest that such inequalities are more or less positively related to the severity of income inequality that exists within those countries, and indicate that health inequalities tend to be larger in Latin American countries than elsewhere. But there is at least one finding that is less intuitively obvious: in three of the nine countries (Ghana, Pakistan, Vietnam) infant mortality inequalities are so small that the value of the statistical inequality measure used does not differ significantly from zero or total equality. Should further research confirm and extend this finding to other countries, the conclusion would be that there are no significant inequalities among economic quintiles in a third or so of the world's developing countries—a conclusion that one can probably describe with some assurance as departing markedly from the current conventional wisdom.

Findings like this lie largely in the future, however. In the meantime, the information available about poor–rich differences in health status deal primarily with such non-economic dimensions of poverty as educational status, occupation, and place of residence (urban-rural). Such information is quite useful as a reminder that there is much more to poverty than a lack of financial resources, and it provides insights that can usefully complement those resulting from an economic perspective. However, as discussed in chapter 10, these sorts of data also have important technical limitations. An example is the relatively small number of categories used, and the unequal number of people within each category, both within and across countries. Education status can serve as an illustration. In sub-Saharan Africa, one-half to three-quarters of the population has had either no education or an incomplete primary education; and the numbers of people with a secondary or higher education will be quite small. In Latin America, only a third or so of the population will have not completed primary school. The number of people with a university education will be very large. This being the case, the same gap in health status between uneducated and highly educated in the two regions— say, a 10-year difference in life expectancy—could produce very different results if presented as a difference between the poorest and richest quintiles of the population.

Much of the systematically-compiled information available about differences by education, occupation, and place of residence comes from DHS survey data, thanks to a series of cross-country summary reports that DHS has published over the years. For this reason, DHS data will figure prominently in what follows, although information from other sources will be drawn upon as well.

The impressions produced by the currently-available information can be grouped in the five categories listed below:

• Poor–rich differences in mortality;

• Differences between poor and rich with respect to self-assessed health status;

• Health service use by poor and rich;

• Poor–rich variations in the use of government and private health services; and

• the extent to which the financial resources that governments devote to health services benefit the poor relative to the rich.

Poor–rich mortality differences

It will come as no surprise to find that death rates among the poor are higher than among the rich. The poor–rich differences are considerably larger at younger ages with respect to communicable diseases than with respect to non-communicable diseases. Whether the differences are widening or narrowing is not clear.

Differences at younger ages

In the developing world as a whole, infant and child mortality appears to be of the order of two to three times as high among the lowest and highest population groups as measured by poverty status, mother's education, or father's occupation. Rural–urban differences are less marked.

Mother's education

As shown in Table 11.2, under-five mortality was, on average, 2.3 times as high among children born to women without any education, compared with children of women with secondary and higher education in the 20 countries in Africa,

Table 11.2 Under-five mortality according to mother's education (expressed in terms of the number of deaths per 1,000 live births)

Country	Mother's educational status		No education as a multiple of Secondary Higher education
	No education	Secondary/ Higher education	
Asia/Near East/North Africa			
Indonesia	111	51	**2.2**
Morocco	91	22	**4.1**
Pakistan	128	65	**2.0**
Philippines	152	42	**3.6**
Turkey	109	30	**3.6**
Latin America/Caribbean			
Colombia	(74)	25	**3.0**
Dominican Republic	91	31	**2.9**
Peru	150	45	**3.3**
Sub-Saharan Africa			
Burkina Faso	212	87	**2.4**
Cameroon	198	80	**2.5**
Ghana	166	69	**1.7**
Kenya	100	54	**1.9**
Madagascar	223	114	**2.0**
Malawi	255	127	**2.0**
Namibia	97	76	**1.3**
Niger	334	106	**3.2**
Nigeria	211	113	**1.9**
Rwanda	177	94	**1.9**
Senegal	171	52	**3.3**
Zambia	204	135	**1.5**
Unweighted Average	164	71	**2.3**

Notes: The figures are under-five mortality rates as reported on Demographic and Health Surveys undertaken between 1990 and 1994. All rates are for the ten years preceding the survey. Figure in parenthesis is based on fewer than 500 (but more than 250) births.
Source: Bicego and Ahmad, 1996, p 38

Asia, and Latin America covered by the DHS programme during the period 1990–4. In all but one case, the ratio was 1.5 or more; in several countries, it was above 3.0. In 17 of the 20 countries, the decline in infant mortality levels between the lowest and highest educational levels was steady or monotonic.

Father's occupation

In the same 20 countries, under-five mortality among children whose fathers worked in agriculture averaged 1.9 times as high as among those whose fathers had professional, technical, or clerical occupations. As shown in Table 11.3, the range was from roughly 1.3 to 2.9. But when middle occupational groups—blue

Table 11.3   Under-five mortality according to father's occupation

Country	Father's occupation		Agricultural as a multiple of Prof., Tech., or Clerical
	Agricultural	Professional, Technical, or Clerical	
Asia/Near East/North Africa			
Indonesia	110	49	**2.2**
Morocco	92	48	**1.9**
Pakistan	142	90	**1.6**
Philippines	79	37	**2.1**
Turkey	114	44	**2.6**
Latin America/Caribbean			
Colombia	36	17	**2.1**
Dominican Republic	97	33	**2.9**
Peru	131	49	**2.7**
Sub-Saharan Africa			
Burkina Faso	213	(89)	**2.4**
Cameroon	178	83	**2.1**
Ghana	156	92	**1.7**
Kenya	106	60	**1.8**
Madagascar	190	91	**2.1**
Malawi	257	180	**1.4**
Namibia	91	70	**1.3**
Niger	345	144	**2.4**
Nigeria	218	131	**1.7**
Rwanda	168	(132)	**1.3**
Senegal	191	84	**2.3**
Zambia	211	116	**1.8**
Unweighted Average	156	82	**1.9**

Notes: The figures are under-five mortality rates as reported on Demographic and Health Surveys undertaken between 1990 and 1994. All rates are for the ten years preceding the survey. Figure in parenthesis is based on fewer than 500 (but more than 250) births
Source: Bicego and Ahmad, 1996, p 45

collar, and sales/service—are also taken into consideration, the picture becomes considerably more complicated, since the decline from lowest to highest occupation is steady or monotonic among only half of the countries.

Rural–urban residence

The rural–urban differences in under-five mortality in these 20 countries showed a somewhat smaller variation. As shown in Table 11.4, at one end of the range was Colombia, where mortality was about 10% higher in urban than in rural areas. At the other was Peru, where it was nearly twice as high in the countryside as in the cities. On average, as shown in Table 11.4, rural mortality was 45% higher than urban.

Table 11.4   Under-five mortality according to place of residence

Country	Place of residence		Rural as a multiple of Urban
	Rural	Urban	
Asia/Near East/North Africa			
Indonesia	106	59	**1.8**
Morocco	98	59	**1.7**
Pakistan	132	94	**1.4**
Philippines	73	53	**1.4**
Turkey	99	67	**1.5**
Latin America/Caribbean			
Colombia	33	36	**0.9**
Dominican Republic	84	47	**1.8**
Peru	131	67	**2.0**
Sub-Saharan Africa			
Burkina Faso	214	148	**1.4**
Cameroon	159	120	**1.3**
Ghana	149	90	**1.7**
Kenya	96	75	**1.3**
Madagascar	183	142	**1.3**
Malawi	N.A.	N.A.	**N.A.**
Namibia	96	86	**1.1**
Niger	347	210	**1.7**
Nigeria	208	130	**1.6**
Rwanda	163	155	**1.1**
Senegal	184	102	**1.8**
Zambia	201	151	**1.3**
Unweighted Average	145	100	**1.5**

Notes: The figures are under-five mortality rates as reported on Demographic and Health Surveys undertaken between 1990 and 1994. All rates are for the ten years preceding the survey. N.A. means 'not available'
Source: Bicego and Ahmad, 1996, p 30

Differences at older ages

Two types of information are available concerning poor–rich mortality differences at older age levels. One type of information is the previously-noted set of WHO country-level data concerning mortality differences between those members of the population below and above the absolute poverty line. The other type consists of data from a pair of burden-of-disease studies that covered age of death as well as cause. Both types of information suggest considerably smaller differences at older than at younger ages. The WHO data are available for 46 developing countries, and for age groups 0–4 and 15–59 (WHO, 1999). In 41, or all but five of the countries covered, poor/non-poor differences are larger in the age group 0–4 than in the age group 15–59. The unweighted average poor/non-poor ratio for all 46 countries at ages 0–4 is 4.6:1. At ages 15–59, the average poor/non-poor ratio is 3.2:1.

The burden-of-disease studies permit a considerably more detailed disaggregation of the population groups by age, and also comparisons of mortality levels in smaller, comparably-sized groups at either end of the economic spectrum, rather than simply between those above or below the poverty line. Perhaps not surprisingly in light of such differences, the burden-of-disease studies produce a much stronger impression concerning the larger size of poor–rich differences among infants and children.

The first of the burden-of-disease exercises is a simple simulation exercise for two hypothetical populations: one characteristic of a high-mortality population, with the demographic features of a typical sub-Sahara African country in the late 1980s; and one representing a low-mortality population, with demographic characteristics typical of a Latin American society at that same time (Gwatkin, 1993). The starting point for the simulation was the determination of the average life expectancy for the region concerned from standard demographic sources. This turned out to be around 55.0 years for Sub-Sahara Africa and 67.5 years for Latin America. Then, on the basis of information drawn from 14 developing countries, the life expectancy of the poorest 10–20% of the population was set at 7.5 years below the mean; and that of the richest 10–20% of the population was set at 7.5 years above the mean—so that there is a 15-year life expectancy difference between the poor and rich groups. In all cases, it was assumed that age-specific mortality patterns corresponded to those of the Coale–Demeny West model life tables; and the values of the mortality rates at each age were read off from those tables for the levels of life expectancy concerned: i.e. 47.5 and 62.5 years for the high mortality population; and 60.0 and 75.0 years for the low-mortality society.

The results are reproduced in Fig. 11.1. Not surprisingly, in each society the ratio is always greater than one, indicating a higher probability of death among the poor than among the rich at every age level. But the size of the poor–rich difference varies greatly among age groups, following a similar pattern in each

(Mortality among poorest 10-20% of population as a multiple of mortality among the richest 10-20%)

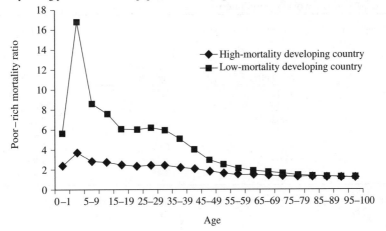

Fig. 11.1   Poor–Rich differences in mortality at different ages in typical high- and low mortality developing countries

society. In each, the ratio is fairly high at ages 0–1, peaks at ages 1–4, then declines more or less steadily thereafter.

The relative poor–rich differences are particularly marked in the lower-mortality society, where child (age 1–4) mortality is over 15 times as high in the poor population group as in the rich one. Thereafter, the differential declines rapidly, so that by middle age (45–49 years), it is only three times; and among the elderly (60 years and above) it is below two.

Such findings are reinforced by their similarity with findings of a second exercise: a comparison of the age of death among people living the poorest and richest 20% of the world's countries in 1990 (Gwatkin and Guillot, 1999; Gwatkin *et al.*, 1999). This exercise employed the same approach that Christopher Murray and Alan Lopez developed, in their well-known global burden-of-disease study (Murray and Lopez, 1996), in order to estimate the cause and age patterns of illness and death among the population of the world as a whole. The results of the exercise, reproduced in Table 11.5, showed that mortality in the poor population group is 9–10 times that of the rich at ages 0–14. The ratio drops sharply to around 4:1 at ages 15–29, and continues to decline so that it is under 1.5:1 at age 70 and above.

Differences by cause of death

Poor–rich differences by cause of death are considerably more difficult to measure than are comparable differences with respect to age, simply because so much

Table 11.5   Differences in mortality at different ages between the richest and poorest 20% of the world's population

Age group	Age-specific death rates		Poor–Rich ratio
	Poorest 20% of the global population	Richest 20% of the global population	
0–14	38.45	4.27	**9.0**
5–14	3.47	0.35	**10.0**
15–29	3.62	0.92	**3.9**
30–44	6.00	1.75	**3.4**
45–59	13.09	6.02	**2.2**
60–69	33.69	17.35	**1.9**
70+	96.05	68.45	**1.4**

Source: Unpublished calculations by Michel Guillot, made in course of preparing Gwatkin and Guillot, 1999

less attention has thus far been paid to them. However, it is possible to provide illustrations with reference to the two exercises employed in the preceding section. A variant of the approach applied there to estimate poor–rich differences with respect to the age of death can be employed to approximate poor–rich variations in the cause of death.

The first illustration, for poor–rich differences in low- and high-income developing countries, starts with the same life expectancies at birth as in the exercise described earlier (Gwatkin, 1993). (That is, 47.5 and 62.5 years for the poorest and richest 10–20% of the population, respectively, in a typical low-income (Sub-Sahara African) country; as 60.0 and 75.0 years for the poorest 10–20% of the population, respectively, in a high-income (Latin American) developing country.) Once the life expectancy is specified, it is possible to draw on findings from a well-established tradition of empirical research (Preston, 1976; Hakulinen et al., 1986; Bulatao, 1993), which has determined that the relative importance of different causes of death varies systematically with the level of death from all causes together. Thus, once one knows the overall level of mortality in a population group—indicated in this illustration by life expectancy—statistical relationships established through prior analyses of countries with reliable data make it possible to produce at least a crude estimate of the distribution of death by cause.

The summarized results of applying this approach to the poor and rich groups in the two hypothetical societies that are the subject of this section appear in Figure 11.2. For each of six major causes of death, the figure shows the ratio of mortality among the poorest to the richest section of the population of a high-mortality and a low-mortality developing country. These ratios have been standardized for inter group differences in age structure.

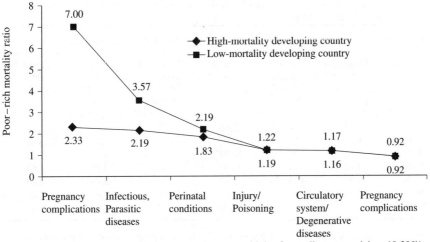

(Mortality among poorest 10-20% of population as a multiple of mortality among richest 10-20%)

Fig. 11.2 Poor–Rich differences in mortality from different causes in typical high- and low mortality developing countries

The principal findings are that:

- With the significant exception of the figures for neoplasms, all poor–rich ratios are above one—indicating that age-specific death rates for almost all causes, whether communicable or non-communicable, are higher for poor than for rich.

- The poor–rich ratios for the three largest categories of non-communicable diseases—circulatory system ailments, degenerative diseases, and neoplasms—are notably below the comparable ratios for complications of pregnancy and infectious/parasitic diseases. The poor–rich ratio with respect to infectious/parasitic diseases, for instance is two to three times as large as the poor–rich ratio for circulatory system and degenerative diseases (approximately 2.2 vs. 1.2 in the high-mortality society, around 3.6 vs. 1.2 in the low-mortality population). In other words, while the poor are at a disadvantage to the rich with respect to almost all causes, the disadvantage is particularly severe for maternal health and communicable diseases.

As was the case with respect to the age of death, discussed earlier, the findings from the global survey provide confirmation of intra-country findings like those just described. Data from this survey, which compares causes of death among people in poorest and richest 20% of the world's countries, appear in Table 11.6. As can be seen, the poor–rich ratio of death from non-communicable diseases

Table 11.6 Differences in mortality from different causes between the richest and poorest 20% of the world population

Age Group	Communicable diseases			Non-communicable diseases		
	Death rate in poorest 20% of global population	Death rate in richest 20% of global population	Poor–Rich ratio	Death rate in poorest 20% of global population	Death rate in richest 20% of global population	Poor–Rich ratio
0–4	35.16	2.78	**12.65**	1.92	1.11	**1.73**
5–14	1.91	0.03	**63.67**	0.78	0.16	**4.88**
15–29	1.52	0.07	**21.71**	0.61	0.26	**2.18**
30–44	3.12	0.17	**18.35**	1.48	0.99	**1.49**
45–59	3.49	0.23	**15.17**	8.37	5.13	**1.63**
60–69	7.03	0.57	**12.33**	26.80	16.07	**1.67**
70+	20.0	4.39	**4.56**	73.77	62.31	**1.18**

Source: Unpublished calculations by Michel Guillot, made in course of preparing Gwatkin and Guillot, 1999

is above one at every age level. But at every age level, the poor–rich ratio for death for non-communicable diseases is much smaller than that for communicable diseases. For example, in the age group 5–14, where the ratios peak for both non-communicable and communicable diseases, the poor die from non-communicable diseases five times as frequently as do the rich. But the comparable ratio for communicable diseases is more than 60:1—over ten times as large.

Given the obvious limitations of the data and techniques used, the results presented can be considered no more than crude approximations. However, they are no cruder or less reliable than the widely-used global burden-of-disease figures from which they are derived. And they gain in plausibility from their correspondence with what might be reasonably expected, given the well-established finding that communicable diseases tend to figure much more prominently in the disease profiles of poor population groups than of rich ones.

Changes over time

Very little information exists to indicate whether poor–rich differences are widening or narrowing over time. The information is equally unsatisfying with respect to inter-country and intra-country differences. About all that can be said with respect to the former is that application of common statistical measures of dispersion to standard international compilations of country data shows a modest to moderate narrowing of differences. For example, the standard deviation among all developing and transition countries fell from 9.6 to 9.3 years between 1970 and 1995, according to World Bank data. When developed countries are added in, the fall was larger: from 10.3 years in 1970 to 8.7 years in 1995 (Bacon, 1998, personal communication).

The only known information about trends in inter-group mortality within developing societies comes from a series of as-yet mostly unpublished manuscripts that covered six countries. The approaches and findings both varied widely. Martin Brockerhoff and Paul Hewett deal with ethnic differences in three African countries (Brockerhoff and Hewett, 2000). In the Côte d'Ivoire, differences in mortality under two years of age between the two groups studied remained approximately the same between the early 1970s and the early 1990s. In Kenya, over the same time period, the gap either remained unchanged, narrowed, or widened, depending upon the tribal groups concerned. In Senegal, the inter-group gap narrowed. Guy Stecklov and colleagues dealt with Uganda (Stecklov *et al.*, 1999). They found hints of a modest increase in the poor–rich differences with respect to infant mortality between the late 1980s and mid-1990s. Informal reports about initial findings from studies about Bangladesh and Chile suggest a significant narrowing of gender differences in the former, and an increase in mortality differences between poorly- and highly-educated people in the latter (Bhuiya, 1999).

Such varied findings are clearly insufficient to permit any generalization about intra-country trends. In the absence of more definitive data, the temptation to apply *a priori* reasoning—or, perhaps more accurately, to speculate—in an effort to produce a testable hypotheses becomes irresistible. Particularly tempting is the expectation that poor–rich gaps would widen at the early stages of the demographic–epidemiological transition, as the rich are the first to improve their nutrient intakes and take advantage of medical technology; then narrow, as the rich begin to push up against the natural limit of longevity and the poor catch up (see also chapter 6). This would imply that narrowing of gaps is likely in advanced developing countries, with some continued widening still possible in those less far along in the transition. However, one must note that a similar hypothesis about economic inequalities (the famous 'Kuznet's hypothesis') has not held up as well in the face of empirical investigation as some had anticipated. There is also the other, countervailing possibility that the financial resources available to the rich would permit them to take advantage of advanced medical technologies capable of raising the longevity limit among those fortunate few for whom the technologies' high cost does not represent a significant constraint.

In brief, neither data nor *a priori* considerations provide a firm basis for drawing any conclusion about trends in rich-poor health inequalities. The question of whether poor–rich health inequalities have generally been widening or narrowing remains unanswered.

Self-reported health status

Mortality rates are among the more objective indicators of health status of a population. Mortality is not a complete indicator, however, since it overlooks illnesses that cause great morbidity but are not in themselves fatal. Mortality is also difficult to measure accurately in sample surveys since it is a relatively rare event. For these and other reasons, household surveys have begun asking respondents how well or poorly they feel, or whether they have recently been ill. The responses provide an indication of self-perceived health status, whose relationship to health status as defined through external observation, based on measures like mortality or medical examinations, is not necessarily exact.

Most health professionals tend to consider self-perceived health status inferior to externally-observed conditions as a measure of a person's 'true' health situation. However, there are situations when self-perceived status is the more important for policy purposes. One such situation is in a market-oriented health system. There, consumer preferences are what count, and it is up to the patient to come forward (and pay) for the services; and the patient's, rather than the health professional's, view of the patient's health condition is what will determine whether or not the patient decides to consume and pay for services. Since most of the world seems to be in transition from governmentally-directed health systems toward mixed systems that incorporate a central role for private health services, the role of self-perceived health status is, for better or worse, growing as a matter of practical importance for health service planning.

As indicated earlier, there is not necessarily a one-to-one correspondence between self-perceived and externally observed health status; and there are suggestions that the two can often diverge in the developing world. As has been seen in the preceding section, the poor are clearly much worse off than the rich with respect to an externally-observed measure like mortality. But when one asks the poor and the rich how sick they have been, the result is mixed. Sometimes the poor say they have been sick more frequently than do the rich; but about equally often, it is the rich who say they have more often been sick. Table 11.7 shows that in seven of the nine country situations for which the relevant LSMS data are available, the richest 20% of the population, as measured by expenditures, reported more illness than the poorest 20%. This was the case in three of four rural areas (Ghana, Jamaica, Peru, but not Côte d'Ivoire) and in four of five urban areas (Ghana, Jamaica, Peru, Bolivia, but again not Côte d'Ivoire). In only four of the nine cases, however, was the increase or decrease in illness by income level monotonic.

The same was true for two (Kazakhstan, South Africa) of the five countries reporting results from an ongoing USAID-assisted international project. In the other three (Guatemala, Paraguay, Thailand), the poorest group reported more frequent illness (Rauch, personal communication).

This frequent finding that the rich feel sicker than the poor is a source of considerable consternation among researchers—especially since it seems contrary to

Table 11.7 Percentage of the population reporting illness or injury during the preceding four weeks

Country	Income group		Poorest 20% as a Multiple of richest 20%
	Poorest 20%	Richest 20%	
Rural			
Côte d'Ivoire	29	19	**1.5**
Ghana	25	45	**0.6**
Jamaica	14	18	**0.8**
Peru	36	45	**0.8**
Urban			
Bolivia	16	19	**0.8**
Côte d'Ivoire	20	18	**1.1**
Ghana	35	46	**0.8**
Jamaica	13	17	**0.8**
Peru	41	45	**0.9**
Unweighted Average	25	30	**0.8**

Source: Baker and van der Gaag, 1993

the finding of similar surveys in the developed countries, which tend to find a rather close correspondence between self-perceived and externally-observed health status (Idler and Benjamini, 1997). There are several possible reasons for the seeming paradox. One is that the questions are not being posed correctly and that properly-constructed survey instruments would produce the expected higher prevalence of illness among the poor. In developing countries surveys, respondents are typically asked how often they have been ill in the past few weeks. Developed country studies normally feature questions about how good or poor the respondent considers her or his health to be at the time of interview. Another is that the poor are not adequately well informed to recognize ill-health for what it is—it happens so frequently that they consider it a normal part of everyday existence. A third, of course, is that the rich are hypochondriac.

But hypochondriac or not, the prospect of so many rich people feeling so sick and thus wanting to use health services is disconcerting to those concerned with the health of the poor. For it raises the possibility that, in a market system, the rich will troop into the health facilities and crowd out the poor, whose physically-assessed health needs are considerably greater.

Differences in use of health services

Not surprisingly, the poor use health care services less frequently when they are sick than do the rich. The evidence on this point is fragmentary but consistent. In ten of eleven Sub-Saharan African countries in which DHS studies were

Table 11.8 Percentage of children from different socio-economic levels taken to medical centre or receiving no treatment for diarrhoea

Country	Taken to Medical Centre			Receiving No Treatment		
	Highest socio-economic level	Lowest socio-economic level	High–Low ratio	Highest socio-economic level	Lowest socio-economic level	High–Low ratio
Burkina Faso	30.0	14.9	**2.0**	19.5	32.2	**0.6**
Cameroon	22.2	16.3	**1.4**	24.9	30.0	**0.8**
Kenya	(49.7)	34.8	**1.4**	(31.2)	22.9	**1.4**
Madagascar	(47.6)	29.8	**1.6**	(13.5)	37.1	**0.4**
Namibia	68.4	66.9	**1.0**	25.2	23.6	**1.1**
Niger	26.0	9.0	**2.9**	26.9	48.5	**0.6**
Nigeria	30.9	16.7	**1.9**	56.2	66.3	**0.8**
Rwanda	(34.9)	20.3	**1.7**	(23.2)	34.8	**0.7**
Senegal	37.2	16.0	**2.3**	26.7	45.1	**0.6**
Tanzania	(43.0)	53.9	**0.8**	(44.8)	22.6	**2.0**
Zambia	62.6	46.1	**1.4**	12.1	26.1	**0.5**
Unweighted Average	41.1	29.5	**1.4**	27.7	35.4	**0.8**

Notes: The three economic classes were established on the basis of a simple, arbitrarily-constructed asset index. Information about the percentage of families belonging to each class is not available. Figures in parentheses are based on fewer than 50 (but more than 25) cases
Source: Gage *et al.*, 1996

undertaken during the period 1990–3, children from families in the highest (of three) socio-economic categories were more likely to be taken to a medical facility for treatment when ill from diarrhoea than were children in the lowest socio-economic category (see Table 11.8). In nine of the eleven countries, children in the highest category were correspondingly less likely to go untreated that were children belonging to families in the lowest class. On average, 41% of children from the high-class families were taken for treatment, compared with 30% in the lowest class; 27% in the highest class went untreated, compared with 35% in the lowest class.

Data on use by urban–rural status is available for a subset of the previously-cited LSMS data. As shown in Table 11.9, in all nine population groups (four rural, five urban) covered by the data, the richest 20% was more likely to receive care for reported illness or injury. Over one-half (55%) of the richest group received care on average, compared with about three-eighths (38%) of the poorest group. However, the poor–rich gradient was regular or monotonic across quintiles in only five of the nine groups.

In the 18 countries covered by DHS surveys in 1986–9, Table 11.10 shows women with secondary education were 20–40% more likely to take their children to a medical facility for treatment than were women with no education. For both fever and cough or difficult breathing, for instance, about 60% of mothers with

Table 11.9 Percentage of the ill population using treatment

Country	Income Group		Rich/Poor ratio
	Poorest 20%	Richest 20%	
Rural			
Côte d'Ivoire	23	44	**1.9**
Ghana	26	46	**1.8**
Jamaica	44	56	**1.3**
Peru	20	39	**2.0**
Urban			
Bolivia	61	69	**1.1**
Côte d'Ivoire	49	64	**1.3**
Ghana	40	59	**1.5**
Jamaica	43	60	**1.4**
Peru	35	57	**1.6**
Unweighted Average	38	55	**1.4**

Source: Baker and van der Gaag, 1993

Table 11.10 Percentage of uneducated and educated mothers who take ill children for medical treatment of common illnesses

Disease/ Symptom	Number of countries	Average for mothers with no education	Average for mothers with Secondary or Higher education	Educated– Uneducated ratio	Number of countries where Educated– Uneducated ratio is less than one
Diarrhoea	18	31.6	36.9	1.2	5
Fever	6	43.3	59.6	1.4	0
Respiratory	8	44.7	59.3	1.3	1

Notes: Figures presented are unweighted country averages. Particular care needs to be taken in interpreting maternal education in this case, since it almost certainly has an effect that is additional to and independent from its role as a proxy for economic status. Another complicating factor is that taking a child for medical treatment is not necessarily the preferable course of action for all diseases. Diarrhoea, for instance, can frequently be most efficiently treated by oral rehydration in the home, without recourse to medical treatment—and as a result, the lower use of medical facilities for diarrhoea on the part of highly educated women, found in five of the eighteen countries with available data, may be a reflection of the greater capability of educated women to handle the illness on their own rather than a reflection of inappropriate behaviour.
Source: Boerma et al., 1991

secondary or higher education took their children for medical attention, compared with around 45% of mothers with no education. For diarrhoea, fewer mothers of any educational level sought medical care; and the poor–rich differences were smaller. There were, however, several cases where uneducated women sought services more frequently than highly educated ones.

Differences in use of government health services

Public health service facilities are often thought to cater primarily to the poor, while the rich go to the private sector. Such evidence as is available, for nine countries, is summarized in Table 11.11. The evidence suggests that this common perception may well be right overall, in the sense that a higher percentage of the poor than the rich report using public sector facilities. However, the poor–rich differences are often modest. For example, public sector health care facilities are used by a somewhat higher proportion of the poorest group (usually the poorest quintile of the population measured in expenditure terms) than

Table 11.11   Percentage of total visits to public and private health facilities, poorest and richest 20% of the population

Country	Poorest 20% of Population			Richest 20% of Population		
	Public sector	Private sector	Public–Private ratio	Public sector	Private sector	Public–Private ratio
Ecuador	52.5	42.5	1.2	35.0	57.9	0.6
Ghana—Rural	39.2	58.5	0.7	47.9	48.6	1.0
Ghana—Urban	52.8	46.7	1.1	58.4	41.3	1.4
Guinea	35.0	65.0	0.5	25.4	74.6	0.3
India	15.5	84.6	0.2	0.0	100.0	0.0
Madagascar	73.0	27.0	2.7	60.0	40.0	1.5
Mongolia	100.0	0.0	Inf.	82.6	17.4	4.7
Pakistan	22.1	77.9	0.3	16.3	83.7	0.2
Tanzania	79.4	20.6	3.9	38.9	61.1	0.6
Trinidad and Tobago	56.5	43.5	1.3	39.1	60.9	0.6
Unweighted average	52.6	46.6	1.1	40.4	58.6	0.7

Notes:
1. All figures refer to population quintiles, measured in terms of income, expenditure, or assets, except for Ecuador and Tanzania. In Ecuador, the distinction is between people above and below the poverty line. In Tanzania, the population has been divided into high, medium, and low groups on the basis of an asset index. (No information is available concerning the percentage of the population belonging to each group.)
2. All figures refer to the percentage of people who seek medical care, and exclude those who treat themselves or go without care in the case of illness.
3. The private sector is defined as including the private commercial practitioners, mission or non-governmental organization facilities, traditional healers, and commercial pharmacies.
4. Public plus private percentage attendance figures do not always sum to 100% because of facilities whose nature could not be identified on the basis of available information.

Sources: Ecuador (World Bank, 1995a), Guinea (World Bank, 1997), Madagascar (World Bank, 1996a), Mongolia (World Bank, 1996b), Pakistan (World Bank, 1995b), and Trinidad and Tobago (World Bank, 1995c). For Ghana, the data are from a preliminary, unpublished draft of the 1997 core welfare indicators study. The data for India and Tanzania are from working papers of the International Health Policy Program: Ramesh Bhat, *Private health care in India: The private/public mix in health care in India*, pp 12–13; and Gaspar K. Munishi, *Private health care in Tanzania: Private health sector growth following liberalization in Tanzania*, p 13

of the richest group in eight of the nine countries (all except Ghana). On average, 53% of the poorest group used public sector facilities, compared with 40% of the richest group. Conversely, in eight of the nine countries (Ghana again being the exception), the situation is the reverse for the private health care sector: that is, such private facilities are patronized by a higher percentage of the rich than of the poor. Typically, 47% of total visits by the poorest group were to the private sector; while 59% of the richest group visited private sector facilities.

The figures of Table 11.11 tell only part of the story, however. One need not go far beyond them, in reading the studies from which they were drawn, to discover that the public and private health sectors are quite heterogeneous; and that there is considerable variation in the socio-economic profile of patients among different segments in each sector. For instance, within the public sector, tertiary institutions can have quite different utilization patterns than primary care facilities. Sometimes, as in Mongolia, the poor will predominate in the lower-level institutions and the rich in the higher-level facilities. Elsewhere, as in Madagascar, the situation is the reverse. While the poor may use the modern, commercial part of the private health care sector less than the rich, they can seek care in another part of the private sector—that is, the private traditional medical healer—much more than the rich. This is the case in Ghana and Madagascar. A look at the NGO component of the private sector produces a mixed picture. In Ghana, the situation is as one would expect: more—albeit only modestly more—of the rural poor (7%) than of the rural rich (6%) report visiting mission hospitals. But in Tanzania, the situation is the reverse: 38% of high-income people frequent voluntary agency facilities, compared with 7% of low-income people.

Also, it is quite possible for private facilities to be oriented primarily toward the rich, in the sense of serving more rich than poor, but still represent the principal source of the health services for the poor. A notable case is India, where one district study showed that a majority of the poor—84%—used private facilities. But an even larger percentage of the rich—100%, or virtually all—used those same private services, meaning that, overall, private sector providers saw more rich than poor patients. Other Indian studies produce similar results (Bhat, 1993).

In summary, the evidence points to enough complexity and country-to-country variation to argue against relying on any general rule of thumb derived from international experience. Informed judgement about the situation prevailing in any given country is likely to require a direct survey of conditions prevailing in that country.

Financial benefits received from government health services

The approach described in the previous section is not the only way to assess the use of public health service facilities by the poor and the rich. Another, often termed the 'benefit incidence' approach, can and in general does produce quite a different picture. Findings from this research tradition suggest that, subject to many important qualifications and exceptions, the government health service expenditures tend to provide greater benefits to the rich than they do to the poor.

The benefit incidence approach, which has been described more fully elsewhere (van de Walle, 1998; Castro-Leal *et al.*, 2000) measures the financial subsidies accruing to different socio-economic groups through the use of health services. It combines household data concerning the number of people using different kinds of government services when ill, with data on the unit cost of those services derived from government financial and service statistics. It does not necessarily produce the same results as information from household surveys alone, on which the preceding section was based; and it is quite possible for a benefit incidence study to show the majority of benefits accruing to the rich even when, say, only 20% of the rich compared to 40% of the poor use government facilities when they are ill. There are several reasons for this. One, noted above, is that the poor may consider themselves ill much less often than the rich. A second is that such use as the rich make of government health services may be concentrated in relatively expensive services, such as hospital care, while the poor use services that are much less costly.

The findings of benefit incidence studies undertaken in 23 countries are summarized in Table 11.12. Those findings suggest that in sub-Saharan Africa, which has been the site of the most systematic application of the benefit incidence approach, the rich clearly benefit financially more than the poor from government health services. This was the case in all seven of the countries covered by the principal systematic research effort thus far undertaken. The difference was particularly notable with respect to hospital services; but even primary care normally benefited the rich somewhat more than the poor. On average, the richest 20% of the population received well over twice as much financial benefit as the poorest 20% from overall government health service expenditures. In all but two of the seven countries, the richest 20% also gained more than the poorest 20% of the population from primary care expenditures.

In Asia, the situation appears quite mixed. On average, overall government health care expenditures in the five countries with available data appear to favour the rich slightly more than the poor. But this is an average of very dissimilar situations: three (Indonesia, Mongolia, Vietnam) in which the rich gain far more than the poor; two others (Malaysia, the Philippines) where the poor get larger financial benefits than the rich. It should be noted, however, that these findings may be less secure than for sub-Saharan Africa because the benefit incidence tradition is less well established in Asia than in Africa or Latin America. Also, no fully-published findings are available for the two largest countries, China and India; and the results for the five countries that are known to have been studied appear in differing formats that complicates direct comparison.

To judge from the two countries in central Europe for which data are available (Bulgaria, Romania), the situation appears similar to Africa. In each country, the rich gain more than the poor from primary as well as from hospital care. Overall, the financial benefit that government health services convey to the rich is nearly twice as large as that gained by the poor.

In Latin America, the situation appears somewhat different. There, information available for seven countries suggests that the poorest quintile gains more than the richest quintile in all but one (Brazil, where government health service coverage is highly regressive). On average, the poor in these countries receive twice as much benefit as the rich. However, these figures need to be viewed with caution, especially in comparison with those for Africa just cited, for two reasons. One is that government-delivered health services represent a much smaller percentage of total government health expenditures than elsewhere. Also important are the health benefits that flow through social security systems, on which Latin American governments tend to spend almost as much as on health services they provide directly. For example, according to one recent review, around 17% of Government health expenditures were through social security systems—compared with 16% for services provided directly by central governments, and 9% for local government services. Since such programmes focus on formal sector employees, they tend to be oriented toward the middle and upper classes; and when their benefit incidence is taken into account, the overall impact of government health care expenditures could well be regressive. A second consideration is technical: many of the Latin American studies appear to be based on the benefits accruing to households rather than to individuals. Since poorer families tend to be larger than rich ones, use of the household as the basis of analysis provides an impression of greater progressivity than do findings that refer to individuals (Lionel Demery, personal communication).

Such findings are quite instructive but deserve to be interpreted with care, since in addition to the specific considerations indicated with respect to Asia and Latin America, they are shaped by several general characteristics of the benefit incidence approach. Four are particularly worthy of note. First, in accordance with the tradition of the benefit incidence literature, the findings are presented in terms of absolute benefit (e.g. pesos per capita) rather than in terms of gain (i.e. percentage of per capita income). In relative terms, the poor are likely to benefit more than the rich because the incomes of the richest 20% are normally many times greater than those of the poorest 20%. Second, the conclusions are derived from estimates that cover only expenditures. These could differ quite significantly from conclusions that look at the revenue side as well, and measure only net benefits and incidence—that is, the amount a given income group gains from government health expenditures relative to the amount of taxes that the

Table 11.12 Percentage of financial subsidy from government health service accruing to poorest and richest 20% of the population: country data

Region/ Country	Year	Primary care		Hospital care						Total health care	
				Outpatient		Inpatient		Total			
		Poorest quintile	Richest quintile	Poorest quintile	Richest quintile	Poorest quintile	Richest quintile	Poorest quintile	Richest quintile	Poorest quintile	Richest quintile
Africa											
Côte d'Ivoire	1995	14	22	13	35	11	32	8	39	11	30
Ghana	1992	10	31							12	33
Guinea	1994	10	36					1	55	4	48
Kenya (Rural)	1993	22	14					13	26	14	24
Madagascar	1993	10	29					14	30	12	30
South Africa	1994	18	10					15	17	16	17
Tanzania	1993	18	21	11	37	20	36			17	29
Asia											
Bangladesh	1995	24	16					13	22	12	29
Indonesia	1990	18	16	7	41	5	41			29	11
Malaysia	1989									18	24
Mongolia	1995									26	11
Philippines	1988										
Vietnam	1993	20	10	9	39	13	24			12	29
E. Europe											
Bulgaria	1995	16	21					11	27	13	25
Romania	n.a.	16	22					12	30	12	29

	Year									
Latin America										
Argentina	1991								33	6
Brazil	1985								17	42
Chile	1982								22	11
Colombia	1992								27	13
Costa Rica	1986								28	11
Dominican R.	1980								41	9
Honduras	1997								23	5
Uruguay	1989								37	11
Africa		15 (7)	23 (7)	12 (2)	36 (2)	34 (2)	10 (5)	33 (5)	12 (7)	30 (7)
Asia		21 (2)	16 (2)	7 (1)	41 (1)	41 (1)	13 (1)	22 (1)	19 (5)	21 (5)
E. Europe		16 (2)	22 (2)	--	--	--	12 (2)	29 (2)	13 (2)	27 (2)
Latin America		--	--	--	--	--	--	--	29 (8)	14 (8)

Notes: The figures of Table 11.12 are summary statistics from a wide variety of studies undertaken using methodologies that often cannot be assessed on the basis of the information available and that may well vary in important respects. For this reason, the figures should be taken to represent no more than general orders of magnitude; and extreme care should be exercised in making inter-country comparisons, especially comparisons between countries in different regions.

Each figure in parentheses appearing in the regional average section indicates the number of countries included in the average that appears immediately to the parentheses' left.

Bangladesh figures for primary health care are unweighted averages of data for thana and union (lower-level) health centres.

Sources:

Bangladesh: Unpublished calculations by Abdo Yazbeck for the World Bank

Bulgaria, Argentina, Brazil, Chile, Colombia, Costa Rica, Dominican Republic, Malaysia, the Philippines, Uruguay: World Bank, 1996c

Côte d:Ivoire, Ghana, Guinea, Indonesia, Kenya, Madagascar, South Africa, Tanzania: Florencia Castro-Leal, Julia Dayton, Lionel Demery, and Kalpana Mehra, *Public Social Spending in Africa: Do the Poor Benefit?* (Draft, December 1977), pp. 6–7

Honduras: World Bank, 1977

Mongolia: World Bank, 1996d

Romania: K. Subbarao, presentation to the World Bank Workshop on Social Assistance and Poverty-Targeted Programs in the Africa Region, November 12, 1997

group pays for those services. The potential difference results from the fact that, while the poor may gain less from government health services, they may pay substantially lower taxes since they live outside the organized economy. Third, the distribution of financial benefits covered by the figures is not necessarily the same as the distribution of therapeutic benefit, which is arguably more relevant. The two would not correspond when, for example, the services that the poor receive consist principally of primary interventions that, although inexpensive, are quite effective in treating illness; while the expensive tertiary care received by the rich is of limited therapeutic value. Fourth, figures for the financial benefit accruing to any specific economic group provide no guidance on how well that benefit corresponds to need. For example, to say that the financial benefit accruing to the poor is twice that accruing to the rich sounds progressive; but it may not be if the poor need, say, four times as large a financial benefit as required by the rich in order to compensate for the greater degree of illness that the poor experience (Adam Wagstaff, personal communication, April 1999).

Conclusion

From what has been said in the preceding sections, it would clearly be unfair to say that nothing at all is known about the health of the poor in developing countries and about how it compares with that of the rich within the same countries. However, the knowledge that has been cited is often unsatisfying, for several reasons.

First, while it sometimes provides fresh insights, it tends more often simply to confirm the intuitively obvious. For instance, it is perhaps unexpected to find that the financial benefits of even primary care in Africa often flow more to the than to the poor than to the rich, and that the poor do not always consider themselves sicker than the rich. But many other findings are in line with anticipation. For example, although it is useful to document the magnitude of poor–rich differences in health status that exist, few readers are likely to have been surprised by the findings that the poor are generally much less healthy than the better-off when health is measured in terms of some externally-observable, objective standard. Nor is it particularly startling to find that the poor generally tend to use health services less frequently than the rich.

Second, the existing knowledge about many important issues is quite inconclusive. An example is the question of whether the poor tend primarily to use government health services, while the rich look more to the private health sector. Another is the related issue of whether the financial subsidies provided through government health services in different parts of the world benefit the poor more or less than they do the rich. In each case, there appears to be a great deal of variation from country to country, for reasons that remain to be determined. As a result, it is very difficult to draw generalizations of value for the guidance of health policies.

Third, there are glaring gaps and imbalances. A particularly obvious gap concerns the almost total lack of information about recent time trends in health inequalities, whether within or among countries. This makes it impossible to determine whether poor–rich health differences have been increasing, declining, or remaining about the same. Arguably even more important is the nearly complete absence of information about how to reduce the health inequalities that have been uncovered. The benefit incidence material presented earlier, for all its important limitations, raises clear doubts about the effectiveness of government health service expenditures—often seen as one of the principal tools available for correcting poor–rich inequalities. But practically no attention has been paid to research into alternative interventions that might work better.

Fourth, several methodological issues limit the degree of confidence that can be placed on those results that are available. An illustration is the finding that the poor often consider themselves sicker than do the rich. This could in fact be the case. But it is also possible that this finding is simply an artefact of the way in which the survey instrument concerned was constructed; and that there exists an alternative, more intuitively appealing construction that would produce the opposite result. Another instance is the finding that the financial benefits of government health programmes appear to accrue primarily to the rich in Africa, whereas in Latin America, the poor are the primary beneficiaries. Is this difference real, or does it result simply from the difference between the practice of focusing on individuals in African studies, and on households in the Latin American investigations? And to the extent that this difference in practice is in fact the source of differences in the findings, what basis is there for preferring one practice over the other?

Shortcomings like this are obviously important. However, their existence does not justify despair. As noted at the outset, the incomplete and imperfect findings reported appears likely to be superseded by the results of a new generation of studies that are currently under way. These promise to provide new information that is far less subject to the methodological limitations of the findings that are currently available. What remains less clear is whether the new generation of research will provide the information that policy makers most clearly need in order to move ahead. While opinions about policy makers' needs in this regard will no doubt vary, a plausible argument can be made for giving priority to two types of information.

The first type consists of reliable estimates of time trends in health status and service use among different population groups, defined in terms of some socio-economic or other indicator (such as gender or ethnic affiliation) of a dimension of inequality whose continuation can plausibly be considered inequitable. Information of this sort is a prerequisite for the effective introduction of health policies and programmes oriented toward the achievement of goals relevant for the disadvantaged and the reduction of differences between them and other groups in society. The information currently available concerning country-wide averages with respect to health status and service use is suitable for tracking progress toward health goals that pertain to overall societal conditions. But, as was argued earlier, such goals are of limited relevance for the reduction of inequalities or for improvements in conditions prevailing among the disadvantaged. What matters from this perspective is progress toward goals expressed in terms of the inequality reduction or amount of improvement among the disadvantaged that is to be achieved. Yet such goals, while of at least some heuristic and hortatory value in themselves, will be able to realize only a small portion of their full potential in the absence of information that can reliably track the pace of progress toward them.

The second type of necessary information features identification of measures that can effectively reduce inequalities and improve conditions among the poor. To identify and measure inequalities, through the type of research that has thus far dominated work on that topic, is obviously an important initial step. But identification of a problem does not necessarily in itself lead to effective action to deal with that problem. Now that inequalities are being much better documented and are being widely recognized as unjust, it is time to begin taking the next steps and working to reduce those inequalities. In this, there will be an important role for types of research that have thus far received little attention. One such type is research into the determinants or causes of inequalities, in anticipation that a better understanding of causes will provide clues about how to counter their impact. Another type is intervention research—such as field trials or the evaluation of large-scale operational programmes—directed toward determining what works and what does not work in terms not simply of improving overall conditions, but also of reaching the disadvantaged and lessening inequalities.

In brief, the principal challenge before researchers concerned with health inequalities and the health interventions is to move beyond diagnosis toward effective action. This will require not simply more and better research; but also, and even more importantly, types of research that are different from those undertaken thus far.

REFERENCES

Baker JL, van der Gaag J. Equity in health care and health care financing: evidence from five developing countries. In: van Doorslaer E, Wagstaff A, Rutten F (eds) *Equity in the finance and delivery of health care: an international perspective*. Oxford: Oxford University Press, 1993, p 382

Bhat R. The private/public mix in health care in India. *Health Policy and Planning*, 1993; **8**:43–56

Bhuiya A, Vega J. *World Bank consultation on current activities and future directions in health equity*. Presentations on Bangladesh at Rockefeller Foundation, Alexandria, Virginia, 24 June 1999

Bicego G, Ahmad OB. *Infant and child mortality: demographic and health surveys comparative studies No. 20*. Calverton, Maryland: Macro International, 1996

Boerma JT, Sommerfelt AE, Rutstein SO. *Childhood morbidity and treatment patterns: demographic and health surveys comparative studies no. 4.* Columbia, Maryland: Institute for Resource Development/Macro International, 1991, pp 20, 26, 31

Brockerhoff M, Hewett P. Inequality of child mortality among ethnic groups in sub-Saharan Africa. *Bulletin of the World Health Organization*, 2000; **78**:30–41

Bulatao R. Mortality by cause, 1970 to 2015. In: Gribble JN, Preston SH (eds) *The epidemiological transition: policy and planning implications for developing countries.* Washington, DC: National Academy Press, 1993, pp 42–68

Carr D, Gwatkin DR, Fragueiro D, Pande R. *A guide to country-level information about equity, poverty, and health available from multi-country research programs.* Washington: World Bank Health, Nutrition, and Population Department, November 1998

Castro-Leal F, Dayton J, Demery L, Mehra K. Public spending on health care in Africa: do the poor benefit? *Bulletin of the World Health Organization*, 2000; **78**:66–74

Demographic and Health Survey. http://www.measuredhs.com, 15 August, 2000

Gage AJ, Sommerfelt AE, Piani AL. *Household structure, socioeconomic level, and child health in Sub-Saharan Africa, demographic and health surveys analytical reports no. 1.* Calverton, Maryland: Macro International, 1996, p 38

Gwatkin DR. Distributional implications of alternative strategic responses to the demographic–epidemiological transition—an initial inquiry. In: Gribble JN, Preston SH (eds) *The epidemiological transition: policy and planning implications for developing countries.* Washington, DC: National Academy Press, 1993, pp 197–228

Gwatkin DR, Guillot M. *The burden of disease among the world's poor: current situation, future trends, and implications for policy.* Washington, DC: World Bank and Global Forum for Health Research, 1999

Gwatkin DR, Guillot M, Heuveline P. The burden of disease among the global poor. *Lancet*, 1999; **354**:586–9

Hakulinen T, Hansluwka H, Lopez AD, Nakada T. Global and regional mortality patterns by cause of death in 1980. *International Journal of Epidemiology*, 1986; **15**:226–33

Idler EL, Benjamini Y. Self-rated health and mortality: a review of twenty-seven community studies. *Journal of Health and Social Behavior*, 1997; **38**:21–37

Murray CJ, Lopez AD (eds). *The global burden of disease: a comprehensive assessment of mortality from diseases, injuries and risk factors in 1990 and projected to 2020.* Cambridge, MA: Harvard University Press, 1996

Organization for Economic Cooperation and Development, Development Assistance Committee. *Shaping the twenty-first century: the contribution of development co-operation.* Paris: Organization for Economic Cooperation and Development, 1996

Preston SH. *Mortality patterns in national populations.* New York: Academic Press, 1976

Stecklov G, Bommier A, Boerma T. *Trends in equity in child survival in developing countries: an illustrative analysis using Ugandan data.* Paper presented at the 1999 meeting of the Population Association of America, March 1999

van de Walle D. Assessing the welfare impacts of public spending. *World Development*, 1998; **26**:365–79

Wagstaff A. Socioeconomic inequalities in child mortality: comparisons across nine developing countries. *Bulletin of the World Health Organization*, 2000; **78**:19–29

World Bank. *Honduras: improving access, efficiency, and quality of care in the health sector*. Report No. 17008-HO. Washington DC: World Bank, 1977, p 6

World Bank. *World Development Report 1980*. New York: Oxford University Press, 1980

World Bank. *Ecuador—poverty assessment*. Sector report: 14533-EC. Washington DC: World Bank, 1995*a*

World Bank. *Pakistan—poverty assessment*. Sector report: 14397-PAK. Washington DC: World Bank, 1995*b*

World Bank. *Trinidad and Tobago—poverty assessment*. Sector report: 14382-TR. Washington DC: World Bank, 1995*c*

World Bank. *Madagascar—poverty assessment*. Sector report: 14044-MAG. Washington DC: World Bank, 1996*a*

World Bank. *Mongolia—poverty assessment*. Sector report: 15723-MOG. Washington DC: World Bank, 1996*b*

World Bank. *Poverty reduction and the World Bank: progress and challenges in the 1990s*. Washington DC: World Bank, 1996*c*

World Bank. *Mongolia poverty assessment in a transition economy*. Report No. 15723-MO. Washington DC: World Bank, 1996*d*, p 69

World Bank. *Guinea—poverty assessment*. Sector report: 16465-GUI. Washington DC: World Bank, 1997

World Bank. *1998 World Development Indicators*. Washington: World Bank, 1998

World Bank. Living standards measurement survey of the World Bank. http://www/worldbank.org/lsms, 13 December 1999

World Health Organization. *Primary health care: report of the International Conference on Primary Health Care, Alma-Ata, USSR, 6–12 September 1978*. Geneva: World Health Organization, 1978

World Health Organization. *World Health Report 1999: making a difference*. Geneva: World Health Organization, 1999

12 Poverty, inequality, and mental health in developing countries

Vikram Patel

The relationship between poverty and mental health is a topic which, at best, inspires cautious scepticism, and at worst, dismissal from public health practitioners in developing countries. Mental health has always been the Cinderella of health concerns in developing countries, even though health policy and international consensus defined health in its broadest context of physical, mental, and social components nearly 30 years ago. More recently, attempts to place mental health on the global public health agenda compete for attention with old and new infectious scourges ravaging the low-income world, and the threat of non-communicable disorders such as heart disease and diabetes becoming a reality. Amidst all these health priorities and concerns about economic inequality and poverty, where does mental health fit in? Can we really afford to be mentally well when our bodies are sick and our stomachs empty? Can cash-strapped health services divert any resources to mental illness, with its vague, fuzzy boundaries and its connotations of asylums, shock therapy, and madness? Is mental illness not largely due to consumerism and materialism? These are just some of the clichés and challenges faced in a discourse on impoverishment and mental health in developing countries. This chapter presents evidence to demonstrate that, far from being a luxury or peripheral item, mental health is in fact a central component of health problems arising out of inequality and, indeed, contributes to the perpetuation of inequality in developing countries. The chapter will tackle this complex and still little-understood issue in three parts. First, it will present evidence to justify that mental illness is a serious public health issue in developing countries; second, it will present evidence to demonstrate that there is a relationship between impoverishment and mental health; and third, it will consider various hypotheses on the potential explanations for this relationship and discuss their public health implications.

Mental illness: its relevance to public health in developing countries

Mental illnesses, like physical disorders, constitute a wide range of specific disorders. Thus, the very diverse conditions of infantile autism and hyperactivity, depression and schizophrenia, alcohol and drug abuse, Alzheimer's disease and learning disabilities all fall under the broad umbrella of mental health. Even though mental illnesses are such a varied group of health problems, in most developing countries they are typically regarded as being composed of a rather narrower group of psychotic disorders, such as schizophrenia. It is this group of disorders which are the predominant conditions in psychiatric hospitals in developing countries. However, from a public health context, the major mental health priorities which this chapter will focus on are depression and anxiety disorders (also referred to as 'Common Mental Disorders') and alcohol abuse, which are common but rarely seen in psychiatric clinics. The vast majority of patients with these conditions consult general practitioners, primary health care professionals or alternative medical practitioners (Goldberg and Huxley, 1992; World Health Organization, 1992; Patel *et al.*, 1997*a*).

Common Mental Disorders (CMD) are characterized by a mixture of medically unexplained somatic symptoms such as tiredness, weakness, and aches and pains; behavioural symptoms such as sleep and appetite disturbances; and psychological symptoms such as loss of interest and suicidal feelings. Evidence that there is an enormous burden of unmet needs among millions with CMD in developing countries has been accumulating over the past 20 years. Studies showing high prevalence have been conducted in a range of settings in low-income countries, from rural Lesotho and Uganda to primary health clinics in Chile and India (Orley and Wing, 1979; Hollifield *et al.*, 1990; Araya *et al.*, 1994; Patel *et al.*, 1998*b*). These studies reveal prevalence figures approaching 30% of women in the community and up to 40% of adult primary care populations. CMD often run a chronic course, with up to 40% of patients in treatment settings remaining ill for 12 months or more (Weich *et al.*, 1997; Patel *et al.*, 1998*b*). Patients frequently consult health practitioners, but, due to stigma and other factors, tend to present with somatic complaints rather than psychological complaints; indeed, this is one of the key problems in using terms such as 'depression'. Most health workers in developing countries will simply not encounter patients who state their complaint as 'feeling depressed.' However, even the simplest questions about mood and cognition often reveal the classic, 'hallmark' features of depression (Patel *et al.*, 1998*c*).

Alcohol abuse is another mental health problem that has assumed considerable public health significance in many developing countries. There is mounting evidence that alcohol abuse, apart from being the commonest addiction in developing countries, can have a major impact on the drinker's physical and mental health and is a major cause of impoverishment among already poor families. It is also related to the high rates of domestic violence and road traffic accidents in developing countries (World Health Organization, 1992; Zwi, 1993; Patel, 1998). Yet the vast majority of persons with drinking problems receive treatment only for the injuries or ailments resulting from the alcohol abuse, with no specific help for the addiction itself. In a study from Harare, not one of the nearly 20% of 500 consecutive primary care attenders with hazardous alcohol consumption was even asked about their drinking history and, unsurprisingly, not one diagnosis of substance abuse was recorded (Chinyadza *et al.*, 1993).

A popular belief is that mental illnesses are of lower priority because they are not associated with disability or mortality. However, the evidence suggests quite the opposite. The recent Global Burden of Disease study (Murray and Lopez, 1996) listed the most important causes of disability (as measured by Disability Adjusted Life Years, a measure of the number of years of life lost by disability due to a specific illness). To the surprise of many public health experts, five of the top ten causes of disability were mental disorders, of which depression and alcohol abuse were the most important (Table 12.1). Depression was the single most disabling disorder, accounting for more than one in ten years of life lived with disability. There is also evidence that mental illness can lead to increased mortality. In particular, the risk of death by suicide in persons with depression or substance abuse is well described (Gelder *et al.*, 1989). Further, there is growing concern of the rising rates of suicide in many developing countries, particularly amongst adolescents and young adults, in whom suicide is one of the three leading causes of death (Ramsay, 1996). In India, for example, the suicide rate increased by 6.2% per annum between 1980 and 1990; the highest growth in suicide rates was for young adults (Shah, 1996). Deliberate self-harm (i.e. self-harm which does not lead to death) is far commoner than completed suicide and is fast becoming the commonest reason for emergency medical treatment in some developing countries such as Sri Lanka (Eddleston *et al.*, 1998). Even after excluding suicide, a recent cohort study from the UK demonstrated a higher

Table 12.1   The leading causes of disability in the world, 1990

All Causes	Total DALYs (millions)	Percent of total
Unipolar major depression	50.8	10.7
Iron deficiency anaemia	22	4.7
Falls	22	4.6
Alcohol use	15.8	3.3
Chronic obstructive pulmonary disease	14.7	3.1
Bipolar disorder	14.1	3
Congenital anomalies	13.5	2.9
Osteoarthritis	13.3	2.8
Schizophrenia	12.1	2.6
Obsessive–compulsive disorder	10.2	2.2

Source: adapted from Murray and Lopez, 1996

mortality rate in patients with CMD (Lloyd *et al.*, 1996). The association of alcohol abuse with higher mortality through suicide, injuries, accidents, and gastrointestinal disease is well demonstrated (Gelder *et al.*, 1989).

Another myth is the notion of mental illnesses being 'untreatable'. This myth ignores the considerable progress made in pharmacological and psycho-therapeutic treatments for a variety of mental disorders. Psychopharmacological innovations have included effective treatments for schizophrenia, bipolar affective disorder, and depression. More recently, efforts are under way to develop new approaches to the management of disorders such as substance abuse and dementias. Psychotherapeutic interventions have been demonstrated to be effective in a variety of mental disorders, ranging from psychoses and substance abuse to depression and childhood psychiatric disorders. Recent consensus papers review the treatment evidence and lay down practice guidelines for the management of schizophrenia and CMD (Paykel and Priest, 1992; Kane and McGlashan, 1995). Though there are effective, and relatively cheap, treatments for most mental illnesses, the majority of patients in developing countries do not have access to these, and are instead given sleeping pills and other symptomatic medications and subjected to numerous investigations and tests (Patel *et al.*, 1998*a*; Linden *et al.*, 1999). The difficulties in providing mental health services in low-income countries and settings where health services are poorly developed have been described by many authors (e.g. Srinivasa Murthy, 1998; Somasundaram *et al.*, 1999). However, even in middle-income countries, such as some Arab nations, which enjoy high per capita income, mental health services are inadequately developed (Okasha and Karam, 1998). It would appear that for many non-EuroAmerican societies, mental health is simply not a relevant issue for public health policy or programming.

Thus, mental illnesses are common and disabling causes of ill-health which are associated with higher mortality. There is little doubt then that mental illnesses cannot be regarded as transient, unimportant, trivial, or irrelevant health issues in developing countries, notwithstanding the other pressing health concerns already plaguing these societies.

Impoverishment and mental health: is there a relationship?

Two examples from Indian society in the past few years demonstrate vividly the relationship between impoverishment and mental health. This experience is likely to be reflected in other countries too. First is the case of droughts, crop failure, debts, and suicide amongst farmers in several states of India. Since the mid-1990s, the seasonal monsoon has consistently failed in some central regions of India, leading to low harvests and, subsequently, lower incomes for farmers. Those who have suffered the most have been the poorest subsistence farmers, those who were not credit-worthy enough to get bank loans and had to borrow money at exorbitant rates of interest to tide themselves over the financial crisis. With their crops failing, the farmers were faced with the stark choice of selling whatever few assets they still had or becoming bonded labourers to the money-lender until the debt was repaid. These events have been extensively chronicled in the Indian press.[1] An analysis of the patterns of suicides also revealed another source of inequality in Indian society. In the state of Maharashtra, 82% of those who killed themselves belonged to the socially and economically disadvantaged Dalit community, who constituted just 12% of the state's population.[2] Stressful life events have been associated with a variety of health outcomes, particularly depression (Brown and Harris, 1978). Stresses unique to farming and their relationship to high suicide rates in this occupational group have been described in developed countries as well (e.g. Malmberg *et al.*, 1999). Examples of these stresses include unpredictable weather conditions, unexpected market fluctuations, and social isolation. In addition to these stressful life events, experienced by farmers all over the world, farmers in India also had to cope with life events which threaten the very existence of the individual or his family, viz., the stress and fear presented by the money-lender in a system where there is limited access to organized banking and state-funded social welfare. It is not surprising, then, that these circumstances are likely to be associated with suicide

Consider a second example. Alcohol abuse is associated with serious health, social, and economic consequences in developing countries. Domestic violence and an exacerbation of poverty have made alcohol abuse the single most important problem for women in India. A recent study in Goa showed that poor women attending primary care clinics were likely to cite a drinking relative as a key problem in their homes, to have problems with making ends meet, and to suffer from a depressive or anxiety disorder (Patel *et al.*, 1998a). Another study in an alcohol treatment setting found that the monthly cost of alcohol dependence was more than half of the monthly wage of the individual (Leela *et al.*, 1996). Thus, alcohol is killing men, is impoverishing families, and is associated with psychological illness in women. Non-governmental organizations have successfully mobilized millions of women and struck a sensitive chord in identifying alcoholism in their families as being a potentially preventable cause of poverty and abuse. Alcohol abuse has become such an enormous problem that it is now the main issue on which elections are being fought and won, with policies to promote prohibition a major vote-winner in many states. For example, the Telegu Desam party in Andhra Pradesh won a landslide victory on its single-plank policy of prohibition in 1995, as did the Haryana Vikas Party in the state of Haryana in 1996. Has prohibition worked? In both states (Andhra Pradesh and Haryana), the government had to abandon the policy, admitting that it had been a complete failure for many reasons: there was an increase in criminal activity linked to smuggling alcohol, and a series of deaths associated with drinking improperly distilled alcohol. Most importantly, from an economic perspective, prohibition led to reduced government revenues and increasing unemployment.[3] In Andhra Pradesh, alcohol breweries, a lucrative industry, were shut with the loss of hundreds of jobs, virtually bankrupting the state. The government attempted to counter the budgetary deficit by raising taxes, and amazingly, the cost of subsidized rice, the staple food of local people. Despite this, the deficit continued to spiral out of control, reaching a third of the annual budget outlay. Finally, the Reserve Bank of India threatened to withdraw the overdraft facility to the state, leading the state government to reverse the policy, replacing complete prohibition with a more regulated alcohol retailing system. Despite the considerable grassroot and NGO activity and political manoeuvring on the issue of alcohol and prohibition it is striking that there has been almost no discussion of the public health dimension of the issue of alcohol abuse or of the need to develop public health initiatives to tackle alcohol abuse.

The above two examples are powerful, real-life narratives which demonstrate vividly the relationship between impoverishment and mental health. But there is also epidemiological evidence which demonstrates this relationship. Five cross-sectional surveys of treatment seekers and community samples from Brazil, Zimbabwe, India, and Chile were collated to examine the gender and economic risk factors for CMD. In all five studies there was a consistent, and significant, relationship between low income and vulnerability to suffer a CMD (Table 12.2). There was also a relationship between proxy indicators of impoverishment and CMD; for example those who had experienced hunger recently were more likely to suffer CMD (OR 3.2, 95% CI 1.9–5.2 in Goa, India; OR 2.1, 1.3–3.2 in Harare, Zimbabwe) as were those who had been in debt (OR 2.8, 1.7–4.6 in Goa, India). In addition, all five studies, like most other studies from developing countries, showed that women were two to three times more likely to suffer from such disorders; low education as estimated by the number of years of schooling was also strongly associated with CMD (Patel et al., 1999). A population-based study from Indonesia found strong associations between

Table 12.2 Association of income (categorized in tertiles) with common mental disorders

	HARARE (Zimbabwe)	OLINDA (Brazil)	PELOTAS (Brazil)	SANTIAGO (Chile)
Income	(personal)	(household per capita)	(household per capita)	(household total)
Tertile 1	1	1	1	1
Tertile 2	0.59 (0.3, 1.1)	0.66 (0.4, 1.1)	0.75 (0.5, 1)	0.7 (0.6, 0.9)
Tertile 3	0.46 (0.2, 0.9)	0.47 (0.3, 0.8)	0.54 (0.4, 0.8)	0.5 (0.4, 0.7)
Chi square tests for trend	5.6, $p = 0.05$	11.4, $p = 0.003$	15.8, $p<0.001$	60.2, $p<0.001$

Notes: All Odds Ratios adjusted for age and sex with 95% confidence intervals. Tertile 1 is the lowest income tertile and is the reference value
Source: Patel et al., 1999

CMD and education and household amenities such as electricity, and ownership of a television (Bahar *et al.*, 1992). In this study, the rates of disorder were strongly associated with the degree of economic development of the villages, with a rate of 28% in the least developed as compared to 13% in the most developed ($p < 0.05$). Similar findings have been replicated by several other cross-sectional studies in developing countries (Mumford *et al.*, 1997; Amin *et al.*, 1998).

There is also evidence, from prospective longitudinal studies, that economic deprivation is associated with persistence and incidence of CMD. A study from Zimbabwe showed that economic variables such as being in debt and having cash savings were associated with the incidence of CMD. Thus, the incidence rate amongst those who had experienced hunger due to the lack of money to buy food in the previous month was 30%, compared with 12% in those who had not (OR 3.1, 1.2–7.8, $p = 0.01$), while the incidence rate amongst those without any current cash savings was 24%, compared with 11% amongst those who had savings (OR 2.6, 1–6.4, $p = 0.03$) (Todd *et al.*, 1999). Impoverishment was also associated with the persistence of morbidity; thus, in a cohort of subjects with CMD, those who had experienced an economic stressor at recruitment but were no longer experiencing it at 12 months had a lower case rate than those who had new economic problems. For example, the proportion of cases in the former group for the variables of indebtedness and hunger was 31% and 32% respectively, the comparable figures in the second group were 56% and 65% (Patel *et al.*, 1998*b*). It is worth noting that there is also substantial evidence of an association between socio-economic deprivation, as represented by unemployment (Bartley, 1994; Gunnell *et al.*, 1995; Lewis and Sloggett, 1998), low income (Weich *et al.*, 1997), standard of living (Lewis *et al.*, 1998), and lower social class (Brown and Harris, 1978), and suicide rates and psychological disorder in developed countries. While these findings may not have a direct bearing on developing countries, they do indicate that the association of economic inequality with mental distress is a universal human experience. We can therefore conclude that there is considerable epidemiological and real-life evidence which supports a substantive and consistent linkage between impoverishment and mental illness.

Impoverishment and mental illness: what is the relationship?

The bulk of evidence linking impoverishment and mental illness comes from cross-sectional studies. It is therefore not possible to be definitive about causal associations between them. How far is the association between impoverishment and mental illness due to mental illness 'causing' impoverishment as opposed to impoverishment 'causing' mental illness? It is obvious that poverty in itself does not cause mental illness, in the same way that poverty *per se* does not cause any physical illness. However, we would agree that the poor are more likely to suffer from tuberculosis, an obviously infectious disease with a clearly defined causal agent, because of the associations of poverty with overcrowding and limited access to adequate health care. In much the same way, we can search for reasons to explain why the poor are more likely to suffer depression and anxiety because of the proxy associations of stress-related behaviour such as alcohol abuse. We do not need to look very far to understand this relationship. Poverty in developing countries is associated with many stressors. It is relevant to note that both absolute impoverishment and also relative impoverishment (and inequality) can lead to mental health consequences.

The rapid pace of urbanization is posing great strains on traditional social support systems across the developing world (Harpham, 1994). The lack of social support and the breakdown of kinship structures is probably the key stressor for the millions of migrant labourers flooding the urban centres of Asia, Africa and South America. This migration leaves in its wake vulnerable persons in the rural areas whose only hope of survival are the remittances that their relatives will send from distant cities. This phenomenon is an inherent component of our current models of development; rural areas of many countries are witnessing a withering and slow death, with the disintegration of communities and loss of social and personal identity typical of agrarian societies. Such a major upheaval, which has happened in less than a generation for most people, is likely to be a major source of stress and mental illness. Brown and Harris (1978), in their seminal work on the social origins of depression, identified factors such as having no one to confide in as one of the vulnerability factors for depression. It is not difficult to deduce that young women who are married far from their parental homes, and live for most of the year without their husbands, may become depressed. Then there are the obvious material stresses which accompany poverty. The daily worries about paying essential bills and being able to afford food under inflationary conditions could be expected to preoccupy even the strongest minds. The living conditions of the poor, characterized by over-crowding, lack of safe drinking water or sanitation, noise, pollution, and crime, can hardly be conducive to good mental health.

Next, there is the obvious association between poverty and lack of opportunity. One of the strongest and most consistent predictors of mental disorder is lack of education, and it is obvious that the poor are more likely not to have adequate education (Patel *et al.*, 1999). The lack of opportunity in a society where there is huge income inequality, high unemployment and under-employment, and no social welfare provision can be expected to lead to feelings of hopelessness, anger, and despair. Then, there is the well-recognized association between poverty and a higher burden of physical ill-health, particularly infectious diseases, along with inadequate access to good, cheap health care. This may mean that many poor persons with mental health problems go untreated, or are treated inappropriately and suffer for long periods.

The potential stresses imposed by absolute poverty may differ considerably from those of relative poverty. It is suggested that the psychological impact of 'relative' poverty is the result of both the indirect effects (e.g. increased exposure to behavioural risk factors due to psycho-social stress) and the direct effects (e.g. physiological effects of chronic mental and emotional stress) of psycho-social circumstances associated with social position. One proposed mechanism is that of 'cognitive comparison', whereby people are made aware of the vast difference in socio-economic status that prevails, and the knowledge of how the richer 'other half' live affects psycho-social well-being and, thus, overall health status (Wilkinson, 1997). This mechanism may be the most important factor in explaining the association between impoverishment and mental disorder in developed societies where absolute poverty is relatively uncommon, but economic inequality is also rising. Whether the existing hierarchical structures in developing societies, such as the caste system in India, act as buffers to the negative effects of such cognitive comparison, as a result of the greater acceptance of the relative inequality, is unclear.

Can mental illness lead to impoverishment? There is strong reason to support this possibility, with evidence for two major mechanisms. First, the evidence that mental disorders lead to disability, which has been described earlier. A range of studies have demonstrated that CMD are profoundly disabling, leading to a range of social and occupational disabilities (Ormel et al., 1993; 1994). For example, studies of primary care attenders in India and Zimbabwe showed that subjects with CMD spent more than twice the number of days in the previous month in bed or being unable to do their daily activities as compared to others (Patel et al., 1997b; 1998c). Thus, patients are often incapable of being economically productive to their full potential. The impact of severe mental disorders is likely to be even more catastrophic, not only because of the considerable occupational and social disability caused by these disorders, but also due to the stigma attached to them, which makes persons much less likely to find a job (Westermeyer, 1984). Second, there is evidence that persons with mental illnesses spend more on health care and, because this is often inappropriate, remain unwell for longer. In many health systems, both in developing and developed countries, depressed persons are typically subjected to numerous costly investigations and polypharmacy and consult many health practitioners in an attempt to gain relief from their illness (Ustun and Sartorius, 1995). Rarely are any structured counselling therapies or antidepressants used; in most developing countries the latter are not even on the essential drugs list and thus remain unavailable to patients in public health care settings. The precise costs incurred due to multiple consultations, multiple investigations and drugs, chronicity, and other poor health outcomes related to misdiagnosis and inappropriate treatments can only be guessed, since there are no reliable economic estimates from developing countries. However, there is substantial evidence of the enormous economic burden of CMD in developed countries (Croft-Jefferys and Wilkinson, 1989). In addition to these mechanisms, alcohol dependence can lead to impoverishment through the obvious route of income being spent on purchasing alcohol and, over time, the high costs of sustaining the dependence.

Thus, the nature of the relationship between impoverishment and mental illness is complex, bi-directional, and dynamic, leading to a vicious cycle of impoverishment and mental illness (Fig. 12.1). An example of such a vicious cycle could be as follows: while material stressors and domestic violence may be stressors which trigger depression in a woman already facing other deprivation-related problems, depression in turn robs the woman of the necessary coping skills and energy to overcome her problems and leads her to spend money and time seeking relief from various health practitioners, often without any benefit.

Implications for public health policy

The earlier discussion has pointed out that factors related to both absolute and relative poverty are linked to mental illness. People in the lowest income groups of any society are more vulnerable to depression, irrespective of the overall state of development of the society they live in (Lewis *et al.*, 1998; Patel *et al.*, 1999). Thus, while development policies which succeed in raising absolute income levels would potentially reduce the burden of mental illness, if these policies led to greater income inequality, these benefits could be negated or even reversed. Unfortunately, the economic reforms being implemented throughout the low-income world have only increased the inequalities in the distribution of income and access to education and other basic needs. For example, in Brazil the proportion of the GNP consumed by the poorest 50% of the population dropped from 17.4% to 12.6% from 1960 to 1989, while the equivalent figures for the richest 10% rose from 39.6% to 51.3% (Pereira, 1988). In Zimbabwe, a 1995 poverty

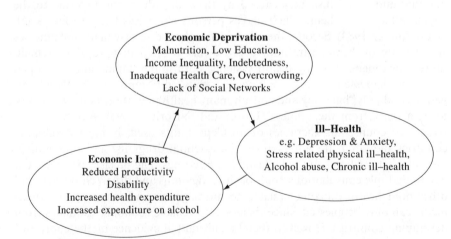

Fig. 12.1 The vicious cycle of impoverishment and mental disorder

assessment survey found that 45% of households were living below the food poverty line and 61% below the total consumption line (Government of Zimbabwe, 1996). Thus, economic inequality is being enhanced, which in turn may lead to higher levels of depression and suicide amongst low income groups. Arguably, the main implication of this association is that economic development policies must aim not only to elevate average incomes and thus abolish absolute poverty (as many developed countries have done), but to ensure in doing so that income inequality is also reduced (a goal which many developed countries are also struggling to achieve).

Prevention

There is potential for both primary and secondary preventive strategies. In terms of *primary prevention,* a strong risk factor which may have a considerable impact on mental disorders is education. It is perhaps important to recognize that the key factor may not be whether 100% of children are in primary school, but rather the proportion of children who fail to complete the minimum years needed to obtain a secondary school certificate (10–12 years in most countries). This is a far more significant landmark in society for, without it, the number of years of schooling is irrelevant to prospective higher educational institutions or employers. Thus, even though there are impressive gains in increasing school enrolment, there may need to be further emphasis on reducing school drop-out rates; in many developing countries, less than half the children who are in primary school go on to complete their ten years of secondary education. One of the reasons for this high dropout rate is the need to earn money very early in life (Haq and Haq, 1998). Education reflects the socio-economic circumstances of the family in early life and is an important cause of perpetuating inequalities, given its role in sorting individuals into occupations (Rutter and Madge, 1976; Sinha, 1997). Education permits greater choices in life decisions, and influences aspirations, self-image, and opportunities to acquire knowledge, which may motivate attitudes and behaviour toward lifestyle and health status (BMA, 1987). It can be argued that rising unemployment, particularly amongst the edu- cated, makes the very prospect of education less attractive to young people. Thus, there is an equal need for generating new employment opportunities to motivate those in schools to stay and complete their education.

In many developing countries, indebtedness to loan-sharks is a consistent source of stress and worry. This was best demonstrated by the anecdote on farmers earlier. Indeed, it is not uncommon for the children of a family to spend their lives toiling to repay the interest on relatively small loans taken out by their parents. It is clear that here lies another potential preventive strategy, in that local banks could step in and review their process of assessing credit-worthiness for persons who belong to the poorest sectors of society. Radical community banks and loan facilities, such as those run by SEWA in various parts of India and the Grameen Bank in Bangladesh, could be involved in setting up such loan facilities in areas where they do not exist (see also Chapter 16, this volume). A potential research theme would be evaluating mental disorder and suicidal behaviour in populations who have access to such facilities and comparing them to populations with similar economic and social circumstances but without loan facility access. It is likely that many other protective factors which have yet to be identified may be amenable to primary preventive strategies; identification of these factors must therefore be an important objective for public health and psychiatric research in developing countries.

The key to secondary prevention is placing mental illness, in particular CMD and alcohol abuse, onto the priority agenda for primary health care by local policy makers. There is need to move these mental illnesses from their current home within the isolated and marginalized realm of psychiatry into the broader, community-oriented public health arena. There needs to be much greater co-operation and collaboration between mental health and public health workers. There would need to be greater emphasis and time on training general health workers on common mental health problems. Individual clinicians need training to recognize and treat depression and alcohol problems effectively. The message is clear: depression and other mental health problems are already in the primary health clinic; they are amongst the commonest of all health problems; they are profoundly disabling and prone to chronicity; and there are cheap and effective pharmacological and psycho-social remedies for them. Just as clinicians must treat tuberculosis, even if they cannot get rid of the overcrowding, so too must we persuade otherwise the clinicians who argue that if their patients are poor, and therefore are depressed, there is little they can do about it. The best argument is that the majority of the poor do not get depressed, they are only at greater risk than the rich.

Outstanding questions

Despite the compelling evidence of an association between mental illnesses, in particular CMD, and economic deprivation, it is important to recognize that the majority of people living even in squalid poverty remain well, cope with the daily grind of existence, and do not succumb to the stressors they face in their lives. Indeed, this is the real challenge for public health researchers: to identify the protective and nurturing qualities in those who do not become depressed when faced with awful economic circumstances—for therein lies a potential to help and prevent mental health problems (see chapter 7, this volume). Could informal local community social networks protect some from depression? Could religious or spiritual involvement limit alcohol abuse in some men, and help prevent suicide in women and teenagers? Could micro-credit schemes, which are challenging existing notions about who knows how to handle money properly, help prevent some from succumbing to despair? Could being close to one's family provide the necessary support? Could a caring local councillor's efforts to clean up a slum help reduce the suicide rate? These are the practical research questions arising from the relationship between poverty and mental illness. In societies where mental health services are poorly developed (when compared to the developed world), it may be argued that preventive strategies aimed at strengthening protective factors in local communities may be a more sensible investment of scarce resources than duplicating the extensive mental health care systems of the developed world (whose existence has not led to any significant reduction in the prevalence of mental disorders).

Conclusion

The social factors known to be linked to depression and other mental illnesses are on the increase throughout the developing world, as the formula for economic development adopted by many countries is leading to a reduction in public health expenditure; a rising inequality between the rich and poor; and increased migration to urban areas, with its attendant rise in urban squalor and rapid culture change as the great urban centres take on a cosmopolitan flavour. There is convincing evidence that depression and other mental illnesses are associated with profound disability independent of any co-existing physical illness. Thus, those who are already vulnerable due to their economic circumstances risk becoming ill with a disorder which will further disable them and render them less able to cope with the adverse circumstances that they already face. Despite the above evidence, most individuals with mental illnesses remain undiagnosed and untreated. There are several strategies which may be employed to deal with the public health implications of mental disorders and their association with impoverishment; arguably, the single most important strategy will be to convince public health experts and policy makers in developing countries of the importance of giving priority status to mental health problems, particularly Common Mental Disorders and alcohol abuse, in the public health agenda of their countries.

Acknowledgements

I am grateful to Glyn Lewis and David Leon for their helpful comments on an earlier draft of this chapter.

Notes

1. For example, *India Today*, April 27, 1998 (pp 31–3).
2. See editorial by Gail Omvedt ('Dalit suicides'), *The Hindu newspaper*, 24 April 1999.
3. Discussions on the political and economic impact of prohibition can be found in a number of Indian newspapers and magazines; for example *The Hindustan Times* (19 January 1997); *Indian Express* (21 March 1997/9 February 1997); *Outlook newsmagazine* (8 January, 1997).

REFERENCES

Amin G, Shah S, Vankar GK. The prevalence and recognition of depression in primary care. *Indian Journal of Psychiatry*, 1998; **40**:364–69

Araya R, Wynn R, Leonard R, Lewis G. Psychiatric morbidity in primary health care in Santiago, Chile. Preliminary findings. *British Journal of Psychiatry*, 1994; **165**:530–3

Bahar E, Henderson AS, Mackinnon A J. An epidemiological study of mental health and socioeconomic conditions in Sumatra, Indonesia. *Acta Psychiatrica Scandinavica*, 1992; **85**:257–63

Bartley M. Unemployment and ill health: understanding the relationship. *Journal of Epidemiology and Community Health*, 1994; **48**:333–7

British Medical Association. *Deprivation and ill-health*. London: British Medical Association, 1987

Brown GW, Harris T. *Social origins of depression: a study of psychiatric disorder in women*. London: Tavistock, 1978

Chinyadza E, Moyo IM, Katsumbe TM *et al.*. Alcohol problems among patients attending 5 primary health care clinics in Harare city. *Central African Journal of Medicine*, 1993; **39**:26–32

Croft-Jefferys C, Wilkinson G. Estimated costs of neurotic disorder in UK general practice 1995. *Psychological Medicine*, 1989; **19**:549–58

Eddleston M, Rezvi Sheriff MH, Hawton K. Deliberate self-harm in Sri Lanka: an overlooked tragedy in the developing world. *British Medical Journal*, 1998; **317**:133–5

Gelder M, Gath D, Mayou R. *The Oxford textbook of psychiatry*, (2nd edn). Oxford: Oxford University Press, 1989

Goldberg D, Huxley P. *Common mental disorders: a biosocial model*. London: Tavistock/Routledge, 1992

Government of Zimbabwe. *Poverty assessment study survey 1995*. Harare: Ministry of Public Service, Labour and Social Welfare, 1996

Gunnell DJ, Peters TJ, Kammerling RM, Brooks J. Relation between parasuicide, suicide, psychiatric admissions, and socioeconomic deprivation. *British Medical Journal*, 1995; **311**:226–30

Harpham T. Urbanization and mental health in developing countries: a research role for social scientists, public health professionals and social psychiatrists. *Social Science and Medicine*, 1994; **39**:233–45

Haq M, Haq K. *Human development in South Asia: the education challenge*. Karachi: Oxford University Press, 1998

Hollifield M, Katon W, Spain D, Pule L. Anxiety and depression in a village in Lesotho, Africa: a comparison with the United States. *British Journal of Psychiatry*, 1990; **156**:343–50

Kane JM, McGlashan TH. Treatment of schizophrenia. *Lancet*, 1995; **346**:820–5

Leela S, Balaji W, Bengal V, Jain S, Chandrasekhar CR. The cost of alcoholism. *Indian Journal of Psychiatry*, 1996; **38(suppl 2)**:35

Lewis G, Sloggett A. Suicide, deprivation and unemployment: record linkage study. *British Medical Journal*, 1998; **317**:1283–6

Lewis G, Bebbington P, Brugha T. Socioeconomic status, standard of living and neurotic disorder. *Lancet*, 1998; **352**:605–9

Linden M, Lecrubier Y, Bellantuono C, Benkert O, Kisely S, Simon G. The prescribing of psychotropic drugs by primary care physicians: an international collaborative study. *Journal of Clinical Psychopharmacology*; 1999; **19**:132–40

Lloyd KR, Jenkins R, Mann A. Long term outcome of patients with neurotic illness in general practice. *British Medical Journal*, 1996; **313**:26–8

Malmberg A, Simkin S, Hawton K. Suicide in farmers. *British Journal of Psychiatry*, 1999; **175**:103–5

Mumford DB, Saeed K, Ahmad I, Latif S, Mubbashar MH. Stress and psychiatric disorder in rural Punjab. A community survey. *British Journal of Psychiatry*, 1997; **170**:473–8

Murray CL, Lopez AD (eds). *The global burden of disease*. Boston: Harvard School of Public Health, 1996

Okasha A, Karam E. Mental health services and research in the Arab world. *Acta Psychiatrica Scandinavica*, 1998; **98**:406–13

Orley J, Wing JK. Psychiatric disorder in two African villages. *Archives of General Psychiatry*, 1979; **36**:513–20

Ormel J, Von Korff M, Van Den Brink W, Katon W, Brilman E, Oldehinkel T. Depression, anxiety, and social disability show synchrony of change in primary care patients. *American Journal of Public Health*, 1993; **83**:385–90

Ormel J, Von Korff M, Ustun TB, Pini S, Korten A, Oldehinkel T. Common mental disorders and disability across cultures. Results from the WHO collaborative study on psychological problems in general health care. *Journal of the American Medical Association*, 1994; **272**:1741–8

Patel V. The politics of alcoholism in India. *British Medical Journal*, 1998; **316**:1394–5

Patel V, Simunyu E, Gwanzura F. The pathways to primary mental health care in Harare. *Social Psychiatry and Psychiatric Epidemiology*, 1997a; **32**:97–103

Patel V, Todd C, Winston M *et al.*. Common Mental Disorders in primary care in Harare, Zimbabwe: associations and risk factors. *British Journal of Psychiatry*, 1997b; **171**:60–4

Patel V, Pereira J, Coutinho L, Fernandes R, Fernandes J, Mann A. Poverty, psychological disorder and disability in primary care attenders in Goa, India. *British Journal of Psychiatry*, 1998a; **171**:533–6

Patel V, Todd C, Winston M *et al.* The outcome of common mental disorders in Harare, Zimbabwe. *British Journal of Psychiatry*, 1998b; **172**:53–7

Patel V, Pereira J, Mann A. Somatic and psychological models of common mental disorders in primary care in India. *Psychological Medicine*, 1998c; **28**:135–43

Patel V, Araya R, Lima M, Ludermir A, Todd C. Women, poverty and common mental disorders in four restructuring societies. *Social Science and Medicine*, 1999; **49**:1461–71

Paykel ES, Priest RG. Recognition and management of depression in general practice: consensus statement. *British Medical Journal*, 1992; **305**:1198–202

Pereira LT. *Economia Brasileira*. Sao Paulo: Editiora Brasiliense SA, 1988

Ramsay RF. Suicide prevention strategies within a United Nations context. In: Ramsay RF, Tanney BL (eds) *Global trends in suicide prevention: toward the development of national strategies for suicide prevention*. Mumbai: Tata Institute of Social Sciences, 1996, pp 1–24

Rutter M, Madge N. *Cycles of disadvantage: a review of research*. London: Heinemann, 1976

Shah G. Suicide prevention in India. In: Ramsay RF, Tanney BL (eds) *Global trends in suicide prevention: toward the development of national strategies for suicide prevention*. Mumbai: Tata Institute of Social Sciences, 1996, pp 233–52

Sinha D. Psychological concomitants of poverty and their implications for education. In: Atal Y (ed) *Perspectives on educating the poor*. New Delhi: Abhinav Publications, 1997, pp 57–118

Somasundaram DJ, van de Put W, Eisenbruch M, De Jong J. Starting mental health services in Cambodia. *Social Science and Medicine*, 1999; **48**:1029–46

Srinivasa Murthy R. Rural psychiatry in developing countries. *Psychiatric Services*, 1998; **49**:967–9

Todd C, Patel V, Simunyu E *et al.* . The onset of common mental disorders in primary care attenders in Harare, Zimbabwe. *Psychological Medicine*, 1999; **29**:97–104

Ustun TB, Sartorius N. *Mental illness in general health care: an international study*. Chichester: John Wiley and Sons, 1995

Weich S, Churchill R, Lewis G, Mann A. Do socio-economic risk factors predict the incidence and maintenance of psychiatric disorder in primary care? *Psychological Medicine*, 1997; **27**:73–80

Westermeyer J. Economic losses associated with chronic mental disorder in a developing country. *British Journal of Psychiatry*, 1984; **144**:475–81

Wilkinson RG. Socioeconomic determinants of health. Health inequalities: relative or absolute material standards? *British Medical Journal*, 1997; **314**:591–95

World Health Organization. *Project on identification and management of alcohol-related problems*. Geneva: World Health Organization, 1992

Zwi A. Injury control in developing countries. *Health Policy and Planning*, 1993; **8**:173–9

13 Injuries, inequalities, and health: from policy vacuum to policy action

Anthony Zwi

Injuries account for a significant burden of mortality, morbidity, disability, and health care costs. Injuries differentially affect age and sex groups, but, more impressively, demonstrate massive inequalities in occurrence at global, national, and sub-national levels. Within countries, it is the poorest who suffer most and who have least access to the mechanisms for altering their exposure to risk. Addressing inequalities in injury occurrence and their effects would play a valuable role in reducing the differential burden of ill-health between rich and poor. Despite these features, and despite the fact that there is evidence for many effective injury-related interventions, limited attention has been focused upon addressing injuries as a public health priority, with few exceptions. This chapter seeks to highlight these issues and to question why attention has been limited to date. It suggests policy action necessary to support the issue being addressed as a mainstream concern for national and international health policy-makers, necessitating the mobilization and commitment of funds and resources.

The chapter considers the public health burden of injuries and violence; illustrates the range of inequalities that characterize the occurrence of injuries and violence; highlights the scope for public health action and considers the extent to which policies that reduce the overall burden of injuries may also reduce inequalities in their occurrence; and examines why there has been a limited policy response to date, suggesting ways of advancing the agenda.

Public health burden of injuries

Injuries are a heterogeneous group of conditions, often categorized by cause as being either intentional (homicide, suicide, other forms of interpersonal physical and sexual violence, and war-related) or unintentional (road traffic injuries, falls, burns and scalds, drowning, poisoning, and occupation-related). There may be considerable imprecision in how particular injuries are classified and recorded: even the key issue of intentionality may be difficult to ascertain in cases of, for example, traffic crashes, drowning, or poisoning. Other types of injuries, such as various forms of interpersonal violence and war-related deaths, may be intensely political, and hence subject to manipulation and widely different interpretations.

Injuries account for a significant proportion of disability adjusted life years lost (DALYs) in all regions and age groups, and are responsible for what the World Health Organization and World Bank term 'an accelerating epidemic' (Jamison, 1996). Table 13.1 reflects estimated levels of the global burden of injuries in 1990 and 2020, over which time injuries are projected to increase from 15% of DALYs lost globally to 20% (Jamison, 1996). Road traffic injuries are projected to increase in rank from the ninth most important to the sixth most important cause of death by 2020, and suicide from twelfth to tenth. Road traffic injuries accounted for almost as many DALYs lost as tuberculosis, widely recognized as a 'global health emergency'.

Projections generated by the Global Burden of Disease study (Jamison, 1996) indicate that the global burden of injuries could equal that due to non-communicable diseases by 2020, and in several developing regions, including China, Latin America, and the Caribbean, may exceed communicable diseases by that time. Trends in accelerating globalization, urbanization, motorization, and industrialization, at the same time as increasing poverty and a widening of the gap between rich and poor between and within some countries, are likely to increase the future injury burden. Earlier studies have shown a complex link between traffic injuries and per capita income. Using data on GNP per capita and traffic injury fatalities for 1990 (or the closest year) one study revealed an increasing risk of traffic-related fatalities as per capita GNP increased for countries with a per capita GNP of $5000 or less (Soderlund and Zwi, 1995). This trend was reversed among wealthier countries, suggesting that, despite having more cars, richer countries learn to adopt better mechanisms for protecting

Table 13.1 Proportion of DALYs lost world-wide as a result of injuries

Injury types	% of global burden of disease	
	1990	2020
All unintentional	11.0	13.0
Road-traffic related	2.5	5.1
Other unintentional	8.5	7.9
All intentional	4.1	7.1
Self-inflicted	1.4	1.9
Violence	1.3	2.3
War-related	1.5	3.0
Total injuries	15.1	20.1

Source: World Health Organization, 1998

against traffic-related injuries and deaths. This observation is reinforced by examining individual countries such as New Zealand, Australia, or the UK, in which traffic-related fatalities have fallen dramatically in recent decades. In the US, highway safety has improved tremendously; the death rate has declined from 15.6 deaths per 100 million vehicle miles in 1930, to 5.1 in 1960 and 2.1 in 1990 (US Department of Health and Human Services, 1992). A key challenge to lower income countries, as they develop, is to learn lessons from elsewhere and to avoid experiencing massive increases in road traffic and other injury fatalities before directing resources at reducing the burden (Zwi *et al.*, 1996).

Inter-personal violence is projected to increase across the globe over the next few decades, from 1.3% of DALYs lost in 1990 to 2.3% projected for 2020. In some regions, particularly Latin America and the Caribbean, violence is one of the leading public health problems, exacerbated by the ready availability of firearms. DALYs lost from war are also predicted to increase, although the assumptions upon which this is based are uncertain. Some areas which appeared to be relatively stable during the Cold War, such as most of Central and Eastern Europe and the former Soviet Union, have in recent years succumbed to significant political conflict, with substantial loss of life and population displacement. The acceleration of globalization has placed many economies under strain and in some cases has widened inequalities (UNDP, 1999), thus increasing the risk of more widespread interpersonal and collective violence. Since the 1990 Global Burden of Disease assessments, crises have erupted or been exacerbated in virtually every region of the globe, with immense public health and human rights impact in Rwanda, Bosnia, Kosovo, Chechnya, Afghanistan, Angola, Congo, Sierra Leone, and East Timor, to mention but a few.

The costs of injuries, both in human and financial terms, to individuals, their families, and society more generally, have been poorly documented and assessed; this remains a significant gap if an enhanced policy response is to be promoted (see Table 13.2). A study in the US estimated that injuries cost the country around $180 billion in 1988 (US Department of Health and Human Services, 1992). Injury deaths typically occur at younger ages than cancer or cardiovascular deaths, and are therefore responsible for substantially greater productivity losses per death than results from these other conditions ($334,851 per injury death versus $88,000 for cancer and $51,000 for cardiovascular (Rice *et al.*, 1989)). In most low- and middle-income countries, it has been estimated that 1–2% of GDP is lost as a result of injuries and traffic crashes and collisions. In Thailand in 1987, the economic losses associated with injuries were calculated as being in the region of 1.5 billion dollars. It is especially children and young adults who bear the brunt of injury fatalities, and hence contribute substantially to the associated social and economic costs. The WHO has noted that, because injuries are concentrated in those between the ages of one and 45 years:

> they tend to affect productivity severely, particularly among the lowest income groups whose exposure to risk is greatest and whose earning capacity is most likely to rely on physical activity (Jamison, 1996, p. 68).

Table 13.2 Identifying injury research needs and gaps

	Epidemiology and social sciences	Economics and social sciences	Policy research
Descriptive	Who is affected? By what types of injuries? How large is the problem? When and how do these injuries occur? What are the trends in injury occurrence? Do injuries occur more frequently in particular countries, and, within countries, in specific age, gender, or social class groups? How do people perceive particular injuries and the extent to which they can be prevented? Are there social class differences in the distribution of injuries, and/or in the availability of interventions to respond to them? Are the trends in injury occurrence the same for people of different social class? How are indigenous people affected?	What are the direct and indirect costs of injuries? What are the costs of resultant disabilities/lost production and loss of life? Who incurs these costs? What do people or might people pay to avoid and or/to treat these injuries? How does society value these losses? Are different social classes affected by injuries in the same way? Are those with injuries willing and able to pay for services? Do resultant disabilities affect the rich and poor similarly?	To what extent has the state identified injuries as an important health and social problem? What are the objectives for any interventions? To what extent is reducing the difference in occurrence of injuries among rich and poor, and improving access to services, an explicit or implicit objective? Who are the main other groups with a concern for injuries? What are their interests, priorities, and commitments? What is the context within which interventions need to be considered?

Analytic	What are the key risk factors for the occurrence of different types of injuries? Do particular risk situations predispose to high rates of injuries in particular groups? Which structural factors contribute most to injury occurrence in marginalized and poorer sections of society? Do interventions exist for these problems? How effective and efficacious are they in general, and in these risk situations in particular? To what extent can interventions developed elsewhere be adopted in the setting in question?	What is the cost-effectiveness of available interventions? What priority has been and should be given to primary, secondary, and tertiary interventions? What are the opportunity costs of introducing interventions? Who benefits most from different types of interventions? Which interventions contribute most to reducing inequalities in injury occurrence and in access to quality treatment and rehabilitation services?	What resources should be allocated to injury control? How do these rank relative to other conditions? To what extent is reducing inequalities considered to be a desirable policy objective? What is the role of the state and private sector in terms of provision and financing of services? Who should monitor quality? What are the equity implications of interventions? What is the role of civil society organizations?
Interventions	Towards evidence-based policies: which policies are known to be most effective in reducing inequalities in injury occurrence and in access to appropriate care? In what sorts of contexts are these interventions applicable? How feasible are these policies in the setting in question? How can the likelihood of effective implementation be increased? What incentives can be offered to the range of stakeholders to increase their support for desirable interventions? What are the equity implications of the proposed policies? How sustainable are they? To what extent do bureaucrats, policy makers, international donors, and civil society organizations support the proposed interventions? What is the information base upon which needs have been defined and interventions promoted? To what extent have policies to reduce injuries been prioritized to ensure that those that reduce injury inequalities gain greatest attention and resources?		

Young adults have received substantial societal investment in the form of schooling and employment training, and often carry substantial responsibilities in both the work and home environments. The burden on health services in the form of primary care, out-patient care, surgery, and rehabilitation needs are substantial, given that injuries often require health care interventions and the more serious injuries, such as those affecting the abdominal cavity, chest, head, and spinal cord, are associated with significant disabilities and long hospital stays.

Inequalities, injuries, and violence

Inequalities in the occurrence of injuries and violence are consistently apparent in relation to age and sex. In addition to these dimensions are inequalities between countries, and within countries between regions, between social classes, and in relation to other determinants of health.

Differences in injury morbidity, mortality, and disability reflect biological as well as socially mediated variations. Differences by age group may reflect the developmental stage in an individual's life (young children aged one to four years may be at greatest risk of unintentional poisoning, burns and scalds, and drowning); differential exposure to risk within the home or workplace (and between the two, where traffic injuries often occur); and gender differences resulting from how societies bring up their boys and girls, thus influencing what they do, the risks to which they are exposed, and their relationships with one another (gender-based violence is a significant problem wherever it has been studied). Aside from differences in the occurrence of injuries, there may be substantial differences in access to, and the quality of health and rehabilitation care available between groups. Socio-economic and political transitions may place some groups, particularly those dependant on societal social safety nets, at greatly increased risk, as reflected in massive increases in homicides, suicides, and other external causes of death in Russia in recent years (Leon *et al.*, 1997; Leon and Shkolnikov, 1998; Notzon *et al.*, 1998).

Recent data from numerous countries reflect the differences. Figures 13.1 and 13.2 demonstrate variations in mortality from injuries of children of different social classes in the UK. Not only are inequalities present, but the gap between rich and poor appears to be widening over time, partly reflecting reductions in mortality in those better off, and a lack of reduction or, in the case of intentional injuries, a worsening, of mortality over time.

Studies from Europe, North America, and Australia demonstrate that injury rates differ by socio-economic group, with a relatively consistent pattern of higher rates being found among those of lower socio-economic status. Data from the Australian National Injury Surveillance Unit database were analysed, linking injury rates for each postcode with measures of disadvantage derived from the census data. There was a consistent pattern of significant associations (Pearson correlation coefficients generally 0.30–0.60) between measures of disadvantage and injury rate at the postcode level of aggregation. This association

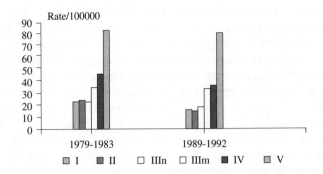

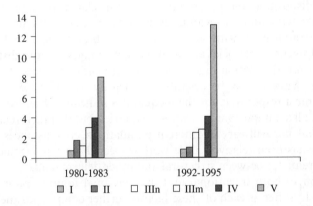

Fig. 13.1 Unintentional injury deaths/100,000 children (0–15 years), England and Wales, by social class
Source: Roberts *et al.*, 1998a

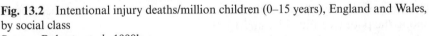

Fig. 13.2 Intentional injury deaths/million children (0–15 years), England and Wales, by social class
Source: Roberts *et al.*, 1998b

was present across cities, age groups, and type of injury, and for those hospitalized as well as those treated as outpatients. It was concluded that residence in a low income area was a significant predictor of child injury in Australia (Jolly *et al.*, 1993). Particular groups within countries may be exposed to high risk situations and have raised levels of injury deaths. Native Americans in the US had much higher unintentional injury death rates (77/100,000) compared with White Americans (41/100,000) in 1980–6, while death rates from homicide were even more unequally distributed (32/100,000 in American Blacks, 14/100,000 in Native Americans, and 6/100,000 in White Americans) (Baker *et al.*, 1992).

There are fewer data linking poverty and injuries and their effects in low income countries. A study of children and adolescents in four cities in Brazil, Chile, Cuba, and Venezuela found that children of parents with a low educational level (primary or less) in Brazil experienced a 2.9-fold increase in the risk of injury in the home environment (Bangdiwala and Anzola-Perez, 1990). The same study, however, indicated that these same children were at less risk of motor vehicle injuries, highlighting the importance of considering exposure factors when comparing injury occurrence. A study of intra-urban differentials in mortality in São Paulo revealed that homicides in men aged 15–44 years were three times higher in deprived areas compared to the most privileged areas (Stephens *et al.*, 1994). The process of development may differentially affect the distribution of risk and exposure among different groups and areas: poor rural children, for example, may have very limited exposure to motor vehicles in many low-income countries, while their urban counterparts may be increasingly exposed to traffic and violence-related hazards.

As with all health problems, there is obvious patterning by social class, the result of a range of influences. LaFlamme (1998) summarizes the range of possible explanations put forward for inequalities in health generally as reflecting genetic predisposition and programming, health-related social mobility, differences in lifestyles and behaviour, differences in exposures to risks, socio-economic stratification with accumulation of disadvantage in lower social strata, reinforcement of social and health disadvantages, relative distribution of income and social cohesion in society, and inequalities in access to and use of health care. While it may be desirable to identify which one or combination of these is most responsible for the inequalities in health observed, it could be argued that all are important in relation to injuries, but that their relative importance and balance will vary in different populations, circumstances, and injury type. There has been relatively little work, especially in low-income countries, which differentiates between structural and other determinants.

In relation to both intentional and unintentional injuries, poor people are more likely to suffer as each of these factors further compounds the other with a heaping of disadvantage in relation to many of the factors mentioned above, among the poor (see Figs 13.1 and 13.2)

Aside from inequalities between social classes within countries, there are also important differences between countries within different regions. A study examining injury mortality in children across Europe (ECOHOST, 1998), observed dramatic age, sex, and geographic variations, reflecting differences in the determinants of injuries reinforced by socio-economic, cultural, environmental and political features. The massive differences in mortality intensify from West to East and from North to South across Europe and the former Soviet Union (Fig. 13.3). The rates are eight to ten times higher in the Southern Newly Independent States than in the Nordic countries. Although the study does not examine the social stratification of injuries within the countries of Eastern Europe and the Newly Independent States, there is no reason to anticipate a departure from general social stratification, which indicates that the poor suffer most.

Unexpected causes of death, such as drowning and poisoning, account for a major proportion of the difference in deaths between East and West (ECOHOST, 1998). Mortality from all external causes among children aged 1–14 years was,

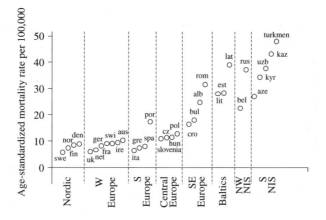

Fig. 13.3   ECOHOST data, showing geographic inequalities in childhood injury mortality across Europe
Source: WHO *Health for all*

on average, 4.5 times greater in the Newly Independent States than in the European Union in 1996, while in central and eastern Europe it was 2.4 times higher. This pattern is apparent across all ages and sex groups, although the differences are less in older children (Table 13.3).

Reducing mortality from injuries in Eastern Europe to the same levels as those in Western Europe would avoid approximately 31% of the deaths among those aged 1–19 years (ECOHOST, 1998). Furthermore, as these injury-related deaths contribute to a substantial proportion of the difference in mortality between East and West, it is apparent that these differences could be substantially reduced or even eradicated by controlling injuries (Table 13.4). The latter is hypothetical, however, in that competing causes of death would undoubtedly contribute to raising mortality even if injury-related deaths could be avoided.

This section has sought to illustrate some of the inequalities present in injury mortality between geographic and social class groups. The examples given echo those that are apparent wherever they have been examined in relation to both mortality and morbidity. Poor people are more likely to suffer from occupational injuries, pedestrian fatalities, and burn fatalities than those better off (Jamison, 1996). Similar patterns are present in relation to intentional injuries. In the US, deaths from intentional injuries are twice as high in low-income areas as in high-income areas (Jamison, 1996); a classic study from the US showed dramatically that Black men in Harlem had a 14 times greater risk of death from homicide than American whites in 1979–81, and that Black men from Harlem had lower life expectancy than men in Bangladesh (McCord and Freeman, 1990).

Addressing inequalities in injury mortality and morbidity would clearly contribute to reducing inequalities in health (Table 13.4). Can this be done?

Table 13.3 Ratio of external-cause mortality rates in the countries of Central and Eastern Europe (CEE) and the Newly Independent States (NIS) to the European Union (EU) average, 1992/93

| | Age group | | | | | | | |
| | Region 1–4 years | | 5–9 years | | 10–14 years | | 15–19 years | |
	M	F	M	F	M	F	M	F
EU*	1.0	1.0	1.0	1.0	1.0	1.0	1.0	1.0
CEE	2.5	2.5	2.5	2.4	2.1	1.6	1.2	1.1
NIS	5.0	5.2	5.1	4.5	4.0	3.0	2.5	2.5

* Reference group
Source: ECOHOST, 1998, based upon WHO Mortality data

Table 13.4 Percentage reduction in the total mortality gap between the West and each transition sub-region that would occur *if* external cause mortality rates were reduced to those in the West, 1992–3

| Sub-region | 1–4 years | | 5–9 years | | 10–14 years | | 15–19 years | |
	M	F	M	F	M	F	M	F
Southern NIS	20	18	50	40	53	33	45	22
North/West NIS	49	45	73	61	80	59	84	68
Baltics	74	56	80	64	87	77	95	70
South/Eastern Europe	26	23	56	43	65	40	41	25
Central Europe	53	49	82	74	>100	54	>100	44

Note: Mortality rates for the 'West' used to construct this table were the average rates for the three 'West' sub-regions: Western Europe, Southern Europe, Scandinavia.
Source: ECOHOST, 1998

Evidence of effective interventions

It is apparent that injuries are an important global (and local) public health problem, and that there are vast disparities and inequalities in how these deaths and the other ill-effects of injuries are distributed. The public health response has been muted at best, for reasons discussed below. It is important, however, to question whether we can do much about injuries before arguing that the response has been inadequate to date.

A variety of simple approaches to injury control have been developed. Haddon (1980) provided key pegs around which to develop interventions. One simple observation was the value of identifying the pre-event, event-related, and post-event factors that influence mortality and morbidity outcomes. A second key insight was to consider those factors which were amenable to interventions in relation to the person affected, the agent of injury, and the environment

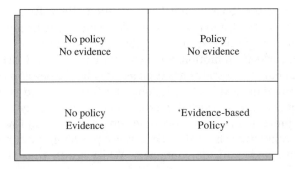

No policy No evidence	Policy No evidence
No policy Evidence	'Evidence-based Policy'

Fig. 13.4   Evidence–policy matrix

(physical and social) in which the injury occurs. Considering both these dimensions allows the establishment of a matrix which can help to guide policy action, which furthermore needs to be adapted to the socio-economic and cultural context.

In considering the feasibility of policy interventions, it is also valuable to consider engineering, environmental, educational, and enforcement mechanisms for enhancing safety. Other useful factors are primary, secondary, and tertiary preventive actions: primary prevention seeks to ensure that injurious events do not occur (e.g. through the use of traffic calming measures in built-up environments); secondary prevention is aimed at minimizing health damage should an injurious event occur (e.g. wearing a helmet will reduce the severity but not the occurrence of motorcycle injuries); and tertiary prevention is geared to ensuring that, even if injuries occur, their most severe manifestations are mitigated (e.g. through improving pre-hospital, hospital, and rehabilitation services to reduce the long-term side-effects of the injury). Measures can be directed at high-risk individuals and/or at the population at large.

People in poverty typically have lower educational attainment, may be more stressed, and have less scope for providing adequate supervision of, for example, children's play. Or they may be exposed to less well-maintained equipment and vehicles, and live in poorer physical and social conditions, in which the health service response to injuries is inadequate. Experiences of earthquake-related property damage and deaths in Turkey in 1999 highlighted the failure of civic authorities to ensure adherence to building requirements, necessary for sustaining an earthquake. The poor suffered most—it was they who were exploited by profit-hungry contractors and surveyors, whereas the better off were able to protect their property and assert their interests.

Data to demonstrate the inequitable occurrence of these risks and of the policy response may assist in targeting action (Fig. 13.4). There is evidence of the effectiveness of many injury interventions (National Committee for Injury Prevention and Control, 1989; Baker *et al.*, 1992; Nuffield Institute for Health and NHS Centre for Reviews and Dissemination, 1996; Rivara *et al.*, 1997*a*; 1997*b*; Barss *et al.*, 1998; and many more). These include reducing traffic injuries through the use of speed controls, safety belts, control of drunk driving, safety belt and child car seat promotion, and helmet use for motorcyclists and cyclists. Avoiding fatal burns and scalds has been assisted by the development of smoke alarms, fire-retardant textiles for clothing and furniture, and control over the maximum temperature to which domestic water supplies can be heated. Drowning has been prevented by improving protection placed around swimming pools and covering other water hazards such as wells; poisoning by introducing child-proof medicine and pesticide containers. While health education may be of value in helping prevent many of these injuries, it is erroneous to assume that education is the most effective means of bringing about behaviour change.

There is evidence, then, that many injury prevention strategies work, although data on their cost-effectiveness, feasibility in different types of settings, acceptability, and adaptability to different contexts has been relatively untested. This may be part of the reason, but not the main reason, for the lack of policy action to date.

Understanding the limited international policy response to injuries

Why has there been a poor response to injuries in so many settings? One important reason is that the poor suffer most, but also have least influence over policy decisions. As a result, there is limited public concern: it affects 'them, not us', and therefore does not attract attention. Furthermore, the poor in most settings have limited political influence and may have more difficulty engaging local policy-makers with their concerns.

The response to injuries to date can be characterized by *ambivalence* and *neglect*. Ambivalence, because injuries and the response to them are often seen as the focus of sectors other than public health—traffic injuries pertain to transport departments; monitoring and responding to homicide and interpersonal violence is construed as a job for the police; intervening in relation to violence against women is seen as a private matter with which the family must deal. The complexity of mounting multi-sectoral responses is considerable. There is little experience, expertise, and documentation of how best to address this, leading to poor co-ordination between health and other sectors. In addition, it is conceivable that the middle classes focus more on behavioural changes which affect injury exposure, and devote less attention to making the environment safer for others. Wearing a seat belt, or purchasing a car with airbags, may be seen as appropriate action for car owners and users, but such measures are of little benefit to the poor, who will not sit in that car, but are still at risk of being hit by it.

Neglect is reflected in the limited international financial and scientific effort expended to identify and respond to injuries. WHO has acknowledged that 'health researchers have devoted scarcely any attention or resources to these problems' (Jamison, 1996, p 68). On average between 1990 and 1992 the amount spent on injury-related research was between $24 million and $33 million a year, a tiny fraction of the $56 billion for health research per year (Jamison, 1996). Further, there is virtually no support for research on injuries in low- and middle-income countries (Jamison, 1996). Only a small number of extremely wealthy countries, such as the US, Sweden, the Netherlands, Canada, the UK, New Zealand, and Australia, have in recent decades begun to acknowledge the public health burden of injuries and to direct resources at research and interventions. In the US, the National Institutes of Health spent nearly $200 million on injury-related research in 1996. However, this amount was still about two-thirds of the resources devoted to diabetes, despite injuries contributing substantially more hospital days, mortality, years of life lost, and estimated DALYs (Gross *et al.*, 1999).

The response to date also reflects limited awareness of what can be done, and of what works and in what contexts. While the evidence base for effective responses is undoubtedly building up, many policy-makers and members of the public remain uncertain as to how to respond. The term 'accidents' is a manifestation of this: injury events were often seen as an 'act of God', unpredictable and unpreventable, although this perspective is increasingly challenged in today's 'risk society' (Green, 1999)—at least in well-resourced and educated populations. Key data for making decisions are often lacking. Most notable is the paucity of information on the costs and consequences of injuries and of the cost-effectiveness of different preventive and treatment strategies. Even in wealthy countries, the situation is not much better. Relatively little is known about the economic costs to individuals and health services of injuries, and the associated medical care and rehabilitation needs. Even less is known about the attitudes, perceptions, and concerns of community members regarding risks, injuries, violence, and their predictability and preventability. Furthermore, there is little documentation of the evaluation of high profile initiatives such as the Healthy Cities and Safe Communities programmes, and there is considerable difficulty in carefully evaluating and costing multi-sectoral and multi-dimensional interventions.

Some of the data required for attracting international attention is 'hidden'. International efforts have prioritized the infectious diseases of children under five, maternal health in women of reproductive ages, and chronic diseases and cancers in older adults. Ill-health associated with alcohol and tobacco have similarly attracted recent attention. Although injury deaths clearly occur in all these groups (children under five are at great risk of death from falls, poisoning, drowning and burns; young women are exposed to various forms of violence and abuse; older adults are at risk of falls, and traffic and work-related injuries), the age groups at greatest risk of injury mortality are children, adolescents, and young adults. The latter two have received very limited attention.

Vested interests may constrain interest in some forms of injury control. The firearms lobby, represented by the National Rifle Association (NRA) in the US (Davidson, 1993), has opposed measures directed at gun control, despite good evidence of the effectiveness of such measures in reducing both externally and self-directed violence. Firearm deaths are a highly significant proportion of deaths in adolescents and young adults, and comprise a considerable proportion of the excess deaths in poor and minority communities. The NRA is so powerful that it has imposed constraints, through the US Congress, on the ability of the Centers for Disease Control to advocate public health-based policies around gun control.

Civil society organizations and the public health community have not developed links to channel concern or outrage that may be key to developing the political momentum and resource base necessary for effective injury control. Countries with a history of centralized and/or repressive government, in which independent civil society structures are seen as a threat, have been slow to develop initiatives around injuries. Efforts to control excessive childhood injuries in Eastern Europe and the Newly Independent States appear to be way behind equivalent efforts in Western Europe (see McKee *et al.*, in press), where non-governmental organizations, the trade union movement, and the media have been instrumental in demanding attention to safety and injury control issues.

The above section stresses the inadequacy of policy responses to date. The picture is not all bleak, however. There are some impressive exceptions in both wealthy and poor countries: examples include the attention given by the US Centers for Disease Control to establishing injury control and research programmes; efforts by the Malaysian and Zimbabwean ministries of health and transport to develop injury control activities; South African initiatives to address interpersonal violence, safety and security; and the identification in the UK of reductions in injury mortality and morbidity as an important public health target. At international level, there is some evidence of increased appetite for responding to injuries. The Melbourne Declaration on Injury Prevention and Control (Australian Institute of Health and Welfare, 1996) demanded attention to this neglected issue. The WHO (Jamison, 1996) has identified the lack of injury-related research as an 'immediate priority'. The World Health Assembly in 1997 approved a policy directed at developing a public health response and enhancing WHO's role in relation to violence (WHO, 1997). A current WHO initiative will see the publication of a World Report on Violence within the next couple of years. International injury control meetings have been held in Atlanta, Melbourne, Amsterdam, and Delhi, India. At least one new journal, *Injury Prevention*, has recently been established; another, *Injury Policy and Control*, is due. A number of non-governmental organizations have been established to tackle particular forms of injury in different countries, and new networks have been established to take forward public health advocacy and research. The World Bank established the Global Road Safety initiative in 1998 and sought to bring together leading players in this field to define and develop the agenda. The

Global Forum on Health Research recently invited the submission of a traffic safety related research initiative. In 1999, the European Ministerial Conference on the environment identified injuries as a major problem deserving attention, and called on member states to develop a systematic response to them.

Advancing the agenda: addressing the public health burden of injuries and stimulating an effective policy response

How can the renewed interest in injuries be further developed and consolidated? It is helpful to look at different stages of the policy process, to identify what might be accomplished, how to develop capacity in low-income countries, and the role donors can play.

Get key issues onto the agenda

Evidence of magnitude, trends, severity, costs, and an assessment of the current policy response help build the necessary attention to stimulate action. Data demonstrating the differential impact of injuries on different social classes, or between better and worse off regions of a country, may provide powerful evidence of the need for action. Trends in the decline or exacerbation of injury mortality, and their relationship to social class, may provide additional background data. Such information may be complemented, or overtaken, by unique events which immediately attract public, and therefore policy-maker, attention. In Zimbabwe, a bus crash in which over 90 schoolchildren died led to hasty policy responses to control speeds of long-haul public transport vehicles. Unfortunately, this response was short-lived, due to opposition from stakeholders. More focused policy attention and action followed firearm-related massacres of children in Dunblane, Scotland, and in Port Arthur, Tasmania.

Research needs to be available at crucial moments, and helps to garner support for policy action (Kingdon, 1984). In the absence of such data, policy makers have to (and are more free to) interpret events and potential action without evidence. Reich (1995) draws attention to the importance of symbolism in propelling policy action (photographs of injured children, media using language such as 'injuries' over 'accidents'): civil society organizations and the media have an important role to play in highlighting and responding to inequalities in injury occurrence. Public attention and media interest increase the desire of politicians to seek solutions. Organizations such as Mothers Against Drunk Driving in the US have effectively mobilized such attention and demanded policy action. The absence of evidence or public views enable government to get on with its business without responding to the needs of often marginalized and disenfranchised segments of society.

Policy formulation

Acknowledgement of the extent of the injury burden needs to be complemented by evidence of effective interventions and key data. However, such data need to be supplemented by considerations of population concern, local ownership, sustainability, equity, cost, and feasibility in a given context. Moving towards evidence-based policy requires a panoply of evidence (Table 13.2) beyond that traditionally associated with the evidence-based medicine movement.

Formulating appropriate policy, which is evidence-based, sustainable, and likely to be implemented, requires the participation of a wide range of stakeholders in the policy debate. Public and private sectors need to be engaged, as do service providers, researchers, community members, and civil society organisations. Unlikely partners may come forward to participate in such initiatives: representatives of the alcohol industry in Zimbabwe supported efforts to control drunk driving, arguing that the latter gave drinking a 'bad name'. The military in a number of countries have supported the International Campaign to Ban Landmines, because it has become a technology that is too destructive to the general population, is easily used by those outside military control, and has attracted immense media and celebrity support.

A key shift away from the public health community's concerns with 'injuries' and their control, to acknowledging the much broader societal concerns with safety and security, may well be instrumental in facilitating greater involvement in policy debate and change. Safety and security are already high on public agendas everywhere—working within this agenda rather than creating a new one may encourage more radical and sustainable action. Highlighting 'safety and security' fits well with renewed efforts to recognize and kindle social capital whereas 'injuries' may be seen as a technical issue in which communities can participate little.

Promote policy implementation: build on the evidence base

Despite knowledge of what can be done, policy formulation and implementation are often inadequate. Researchers and practitioners may be surprised at the extent to which 'the wheel has to be reinvented', and at the inadequacy of lessons transferred from one setting to another. The lack of uptake of the results of scientific enquiry and research reflects numerous barriers between researchers and policy-makers: conflicts over priorities, values, and funds; attitudes to time invested in research and time to disseminating policy-relevant findings; methods of making decisions; weight of scientific relative to other types of data; degree of precision of findings; differences in the use of language, jargon and style of presentation; the balance between research and action; and key differences in the extent to which scientific and technical data should influence policy making (see Walt, 1994).

Innovative responses to these problems are possible and require explicit attention which recognizes the gap between knowledge and practice, that appropriate 'messages' need to be conveyed by credible 'messengers', that processes and not just the content of change needs to be considered, that this necessitates the engagement of key stakeholders, and that contextual understanding is crucial. Identifying likely impediments to change and the positions of different groups, and seeking to support those who advocate change while removing the concerns of those opposing it, is central to developing strategies to overcome barriers and lever change.

Policy implementation thus depends on ensuring that key stakeholders are 'on board' and support the initiative; facilitating their role in the process of policy formulation and implementation; developing commitment from civil society, government and private sector; ensuring that appropriate systems and institutions are in place; and ensuring that resources are made available for effective implementation. Setting public targets which are challenging and publicly monitored can contribute to keeping the issue on the agenda and in maintaining the pressure for implementation. Documenting innovative means of reaching the targets through effective policy development and implementation is of value to those in other settings. Good-practice interventions to reduce inequalities in injury occurrence and care may be transferable and adaptable to many other settings. Linking policy initiatives concerning injuries to other, broader social policy issues will broaden debate and participation by relevant groups.

Strengthen within-country resources

Within affected countries, undertaking situation analyses will assist in identifying the most significant injury problems, in terms of health losses, service loads, and economic costs. Situation analyses contribute to identifying lead agencies and their roles, responsibilities, strengths, and limitations. Promoting equity, through addressing inequalities in injury occurrence, in the distribution of determinants of injuries, and in injury care, presupposes focusing on the countries, regions, and communities which have a disproportionate injury burden. Added to these assessments are identification of those that have the willingness and commitment to respond. Wherever possible, linkages between injury control and other community- and service-based initiatives should be promoted. Local capacity for research, policy formulation, and intervention invariably requires support; facilitating innovative public–private partnerships may provide one important means of promoting this, especially given global moves around corporate governance and social responsibility among industry leaders. Multinational corporations operating in car manufacture, construction, fuels, technology transfer, life insurance, and alcohol, all have reason to support pro-equity and pro-safety activities and should be challenged to do so.

Donor community role

Lastly, donors, because of their economic power and policy influence, can play a significant role in getting injuries and safety on the agenda, and in addressing inequities in injury distribution as the major target. The UK Department for International Development has recently published its white paper on development assistance and also on its health strategy: both highlight the importance of addressing poverty if better health is to be promoted. Injuries are experienced more acutely by the poor, and contribute to the poor becoming more poor due to health service costs, rehabilitation needs, and employment and education foregone. Supportive donors may assist in developing regional initiatives and in providing support to the development of national capacity to monitor and respond to injuries and their control. New initiatives, such as funding road construction, should assure a concomitant safety audit; the World Bank already assures this in relation to roads construction. New developments, such as enhancing injury surveillance and control activities, are difficult to promote in a period of resource constraints, especially as the benefits may be seen to accrue to other sectors. It should be noted, however, that the health sector itself stands to gain substantially through improved injury control efforts: notably through a reduction in service loads. Donors can play a key role in bringing together key actors within a region: the Open Society Institute and Schweitzer Seminars have facilitated such activity in Kyrgyzstan, with a view to potentially rolling this out to a broader range of countries in the region. UNICEF has funded activities to increase the recognition of injuries as a significant cause of death and in inequalities between East and West Europe (ECOHOST, 1998).

Conclusion

This chapter has sought to identify the importance of injuries as a global and local health problem, which is important both in its own right and in the contribution it makes to inequalities in health. The chapter provides some evidence of the burden and the relationship with inequalities, and highlights the relative lack of attention to injury control to date. Reference to existing evidence of effective interventions is presented, and suggestions made as to why there has been little attention to date. The final section proposed key issues to be considered in taking injury control forward.

Injuries reflect the 'fine-grained' inequalities which are present for many health conditions. There are effective interventions available, and emerging evidence of how to stimulate appropriate policy action. Improving our understanding of the present knowledge of injuries, and feeding this into a process which is sensitive to contextual and process-related factors, and which builds around current actors, institutions, systems, and resources, can play a significant part in kick-starting injury control efforts. The public and private sector, academic organizations, donors, and most importantly, civil society, have key roles to play in emerging from the policy vacuum around injuries to promoting the policy action that will contribute to reducing inequity in health and health care.

REFERENCES

Australian Institute of Health and Welfare. Melbourne declaration on injury prevention and control. Melbourne: Australian Institute of Health and Welfare, 1996

Baker SP, O'Neill B, Ginsburg MJ, Li G. *The injury fact book* Second edition. Oxford: Oxford University Press, 1992

Bangdiwala SI, Anzola-Perez E. The incidence of injuries in young people: II. Loglinear multivariable models for risk factors in a collaborative study in Brazil, Chile, Cuba and Venezuela. *International Journal of Epidemiology*, 1990; **19**:125–32

Barss P, Smith G, Baker S, Mohan D. *Injury prevention: an international perspective. Epidemiology, surveillance and policy.* Oxford: Oxford University Press, 1998

Davidson, OG. *Under fire: the NRA and the battle of gun control.* New York: Henry Holt and Company, 1993

European Centre on Health of Societies in Transition (ECOHOST). *Childhood injuries. A priority area for the transition countries of Central and Eastern Europe and the Newly Independent States. Final Report.* London: London School of Hygiene & Tropical Medicine, 1998

Gilson L. In defence and pursuit of equity. *Social Science and Medicine*, 1998; **47**:1891–6

Green J. From accidents to risk: public health and preventable injury. *Health, Risk and Society*, 1999; **1**:25–39

Gross CP, Anderson GF, Powe NR. The relation between funding by the National Institutes of Health and the burden of disease. *New England Journal of Medicine*, 1999; **340**:1881–7

Haddon W. Advances in the epidemiology of injuries as a basis for public policy. *Public Health Reports*, 1980; **95**:411–21

Irwig L, Zwarenstein M, Zwi A, Chalmers I. A flow diagram to help select interventions and research for health care. *Bulletin of the World Health Organization*, 1998; **76**:17–24

Jamison DT. *Investing in health research and development.* Report of the Ad Hoc Committee on World Health Organization Health Research Relating to Future Intervention Options. Geneva: WHO, 1996

Jolly DL, Moller JN, Volkmer RE. The socio-economic context of child injury in Australia. *Journal of Paediatrics and Child-Health*, 1993; **29**:438–44

Kingdon J. *Agendas, alternatives and public policies.* Boston: Little Brown and Co., 1984

La Flamme L. Social inequality in injury risks—knowledge accumulated and plans for the future. Stockholm: Sweden National Institute of Public Health, 1998

Leon DA, Shkolnikov VM. Social stress and the Russian mortality crisis. *Journal of the American Medical Association*, 1998; **279**:790–1

Leon DA, Chenet L, Shkolnikov *et al.* Huge variations in Russian mortality rates 1984–94; artefact, alcohol or what? *Lancet*, 1997; **350**:383–8

McCord C, Freeman HP. Excess mortality in Harlem. *New England Journal of Medicine*, 1990; **332**:173–7

McKee M, Zwi A, Koupilova I, Sethi D, Leon D. Injury in Eastern Europe: role of civil society organisations. *Health Policy and Planning* (in press)

National Committee for Injury Prevention and Control. Injury prevention, meeting the challenge. *American Journal of Preventive Medicine*, 1989; **5(suppl 3)**

Notzon FC, Komarov YM, Ermakov SP, Sempos CT, Marks JS, Semos EV. Causes of declining life expectancy in Russia. *Journal of the American Medical Association*, 1998; **279**:793–800

NHS Centre for Reviews and Dissemination. Unintentional injuries in young people. *Effective Health Care Bulletin*, 1996; **1**:1–16

Reich M. The politics of agenda setting in international health: child health versus adult health in developing countries. *Journal of International Development*, 1995; **7**:489–502

Rice DP, Mackenzie EJ *et al*. Cost of injury in the United States. A report to Congress. San Francisco: Institute for Health and Ageing, University of California and Injury Prevention Center, Johns Hopkins University, 1989

Rivara FP, Grossman DC, Cummings P. Injury prevention: first of two parts. *New England Journal of Medicine*, 1997*a*; **337**:543–8

Rivara FP, Grossman DC, Cummings P. Injury prevention: second of two parts. *New England Journal of Medicine*, 1997*b*; **337**:613–8

Roberts I, *et al*. Childhood injuries: extent of the problem, epidemiological trends, and costs. *Injury Prevention*, 1998*a*; **4 Supp**:56–70

Roberts I, Li L, Barker M. Trends in intentional injury deaths in children and teenagers. *Journal of Public Health Medicine*, 1998*b*; **20**:463–6

Soderlund N, Zwi AB. Traffic-related mortality in industrialized and less developed countries. *Bulletin of the World Health Organization*, 1995; **73**:175–82

Stephens C, Timaeus I, Akerman M, *et al*. Environment and health in developing countries: An analysis of intra-urban differentials using existing data. London School of Hygiene & Tropical Medicine, 1992

UK Department for International Development Eliminating World Poverty—a challenge for the 21st century. London: HMSO, 1997

United Nations Development Programme (UNDP). *Human Development Report 1999*. New York: Oxford·University Press, 1999

US Dept of Health and Human Services. Position papers from The Third National Injury Control Conference. Setting the national agenda for injury control in the 1990s. Atlanta 1992

Walt G. How far does research influence policy? *European Journal of Public Health*, 1994; **4**:233–5

Whitehead M, Dahlgren G. What can be done about inequalities in health? *Lancet*, 1991; **338**:1959–63

World Health Organization. Investing in health research and development. Report of the Ad Hoc Committee on Health Research Relating to Future Intervention Options. Geneva: World Health Organization, 1996

World Health Organization. *World Health Report 1998*. Geneva: World Health Organization, 1998

Zwi AB, Forjuoh S, Murugasampillay S, Odero W, Watts C. Injuries in developing countries: policy response needed now. *Transactions of the Royal Society of Tropical Medicine & Hygiene*, 1996; **90**:593–595

14 Inequalities in health: is research gender blind?

Sally Macintyre

In this chapter, I want to argue that much research on the relationship between socio-economic status and health has been gender blind, and that this gender blindness may hinder attempts to understand the causal mechanisms which create and maintain social patterning in health. Examining differences and similarities between men and women in the relationship between socio-economic status and mortality or morbidity may direct attention both to potential explanations for socio-economic gradients in health, and to potential explanations for gender differences in health, and may advance our understanding of the relationship between social and biological processes and outcomes.

Ruiz and Verbrugge have suggested that there are two types of gender bias in health research. The first is the assumed equality of men and women. They note that:

> the many clinical trials that have been conducted only among men carry the assumption that results can automatically be applied to women, as if women had been studied too (Ruiz and Verbrugge, 1997).

Secondly, they note that for diseases which are common in both sexes but perceived to be more prevalent in men (the classic example would be heart disease), the knowledge on which diagnosis, prognosis, and risk factor assessments are made may be obtained only from studies of men (one may note that the reverse may happen for conditions stereotyped as being female, such as anorexia nervosa). Thirdly, it is common in epidemiological studies for sex to be controlled for in multivariate analysis as if it is 'noise' and there is some pure, ungendered, relationship between risk factor and disease which one wishes to uncover.

The second assumption is that men and women are fundamentally different. The basis of these differences is often unquestioned and this assumption may be expressed in different outcome measures (e.g. safe units of alcohol per week, or cut off points of body mass index for obesity), or in a lack of any systematic comparisons. For example some symptoms experienced in midlife may be assumed to be menopausal and therefore only females asked about them, so we do not know the prevalence of similar symptoms in the same age groups in men; and although we know something about the prevalence of post natal depression in mothers, we know little about the prevalence of depression in new fathers.

In the field of socio-economic inequalities in health there are similar gender biases. The first, related to Ruiz and Verbrugge's first gender bias, is gender blindness. Many of the key studies examine socio-economic gradients in men only. Examples are the analysis of the relationship between median household income in the zip code in the US MRFIT study (Davey Smith et al., 1996); the Whitehall I Study (Marmot et al., 1984); international comparisons of mortality by social class (Kunst and Mackenbach, 1994); and the British Regional Heart Study (Shaper et al., 1981). For each study there may be a good reason for only using men (e.g. because the original intention was to examine heart disease, or because occupational distributions are harder to compare for women than for men). The net effect however has tended to be that socio-economic gradients observed in these studies have been seen as being the gold standard, and as generalizable to all people in these contexts.

A second type of gender blindness in the field of socio-economic inequalities in health is that some studies simply combine both sexes and look at age-adjusted mortality for men and women combined. Some have done this without mention of or control for sex (Kennedy et al., 1996; van Doorslaer et al., 1997; Lynch et al., 1998), while others control for sex but do not examine interactions with sex (Dahl, 1994; Benzeval et al., 1996; Daly et al., 1998). Finally there are some which probably only include men but which do not mention the gender of subjects in the design and methods section (Abramson et al., 1982).

A third type of gender bias is that alternative forms of social classification are frequently developed for women (for example incorporating marital and parenting roles) but not for men. Thus we know little about the effect, if any, on men's socio-economic gradients in health of including information about their wives' occupation, education, or income.

In previous work Kate Hunt and I have argued that gender differences in health may not be as constant over time, cultural context, and health measure as is often assumed (Macintyre et al., 1996; Macintyre and Hunt, 1997). We have also suggested that, with the exception of cardiovascular disease, social inequalities in health tend to be less steep for women than for men (Macintyre and Hunt, 1997; Hunt and Macintyre, in press). What I want to do in this chapter is to present further evidence of the shallower socio-economic gradients among women than men in a range of health measures, using a variety of socio-economic measures, as a way of illustrating how this raises questions about the mechanisms producing socio-economic gradients in health.

Note that all the data I present here comes from industrialized countries. This is because not only are there few published data on socio-economic inequalities in health in developing countries (as Davidson Gwatkin points out in his chapter in this volume (see chapter 11)), but even fewer reports present these data separately by gender.

Data from the US on age-adjusted death rates among adults of working age show that, whether measured by education or income, the difference between the top and bottom socio-economic groups is greater for men than for women among the white population. Among the black population this was true of income but not of education, where the difference between the top and bottom groups was similar for men and women (Pappas *et al.*, 1993) (see Table 14.1). This then raises two questions: why should there be a bigger difference for men than women, and why does this differ between whites and blacks? What is it that income and education are measuring, and what are the pathways linking these to death among men and women?

Changing country, socio-economic measure, and outcome measure, we see a similar picture for life expectancy by deprivation level (measured by Jarman scores based on 1991 census variables) of Health Authority districts in England (Raleigh and Kiri, 1997) (see Table 14.2).

As expected, females have longer life expectancy than men, but they also have a less steep gradient in life expectancy by deprivation of district than do men—2.4 years difference between the top and bottom compared to 4 years for men,

Table 14.1   Rate ratios: (bottom to top SES group) for age-adjusted death rates in 1986 among persons 25–64 by education and income groups, sex and race, USA

	White		Black	
	Men	Women	Men	Women
Education	2.71	1.88	2.83	2.81
Income	6.66	4.06	5.42	3.30

Source: Pappas *et al.*, 1993

Table 14.2   Life expectancy at birth by sex in 1992–4 by deprivation level of district, in England

Deprivation level	Males	Females	F/M differences (yrs)
(least) 1	75.2	80.2	4.9
2	75.0	80.1	5.1
3	74.8	80.0	5.3
4	73.2	79.1	5.5
5	73.0	78.7	5.6
6	72.9	78.9	6.0
(most) 7	71.2	77.8	6.6
Difference	4 years	2.4 years	
% p.a. increase 1984–6 — 1992–4	0.35%	0.25%	

Source: Raleigh and Kiri, 1997

an even smaller relative difference given women's greater longevity. One of the consequences is that the gender gap differs by deprivation of district, ranging from 4.9 years in the least deprived to 6.6 years in the most deprived districts. While one might think that education and income might be distributed differently, or mean something different, among women as compared with men, the notion that average deprivation score in the district of residence is more strongly associated with life expectancy among men than women, tends to raise issues about different exposure or vulnerability to area level deprivation among men as compared with women. Note too that, between 1984–6 and 1992–4, the percentage annual increase in life expectancy was greater for men, at 0.35%, than for women, at 0.25%.

Similar data for Scotland around the time of the 1991–3 census show the same picture. Usually all-cause mortality by deprivation of postcode sector of residence has been presented for males and females separately. We re-analysed the data separately for men and women and found steeper gradients for men than for women (see Fig. 14.1). Similarly, when we grouped postcode sectors into quintiles of average household income in the area, there was a stronger relationship with mortality for men than for women (see Fig. 14.2).

Before moving on to cause-specific mortality and other health measures, I want to raise the issue of national differences, and also differences in the way socio-economic status is operationalized. In a recent study, Ossi Rahkonen, Sara Arber, and colleagues looked at the relationship between self-perceived poor health and both individual and household income and for men and women in Finland and Britain. For gross individual income there was a linear relationship with self-perceived poor health among Finnish women (most of whom are employed) but no relationship among British women (fewer of

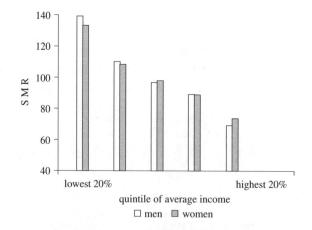

Fig. 14.1   Standardized mortality ratios (SMRs) (ages 0–64) by quintiles of average household income in postcode sectors, Scotland, 1991–3

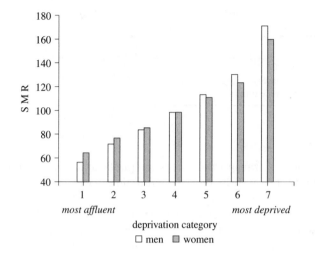

Fig. 14.2 Standardized mortality ratios (SMRs) (ages 0–64) for men and women in each Carstairs deprivation category, Scotland, 1991–3

whom are in employment). Among British women in the quintile of lowest personal income, rates of poor self-perceived health are quite low; this group probably includes non-employed or part-time employed women married to men in a higher income bracket. The picture changes with household income, there being steep gradients in poor self-perceived health among British women as well as Finnish. The difference between the top and bottom quintiles of income in poor health was greater for men than women in both Britain and Finland. Thus, there were differences between countries, sexes, and ways of representing income, in the steepness of the gradient of health by income (Rahkonen *et al.*, 2000).

However, as noted earlier, it is not only by income and social class that women's socio-economic gradients are less steep; deprivation of local area (whether at postcode sector level in Scotland or district health authority level in England) is more strongly associated with men's than women's mortality. In a study in the West of Scotland we have found that limiting long-standing illness is similarly more closely associated with three measures of material assets—housing tenure, household car access, and household income adjusted by household size—among men than among women. Among women in this study—which was designed to explore the reasons for associations between housing tenure, car access and health—household car access was not significantly related to health among women, and indeed in some age groups women in households with cars had poorer health than those in households without cars (see Table 14.3). This raises questions about what household car access is measuring: is it a marker of wealth, or of prestige, or of the availability of a

Table 14.3 Odds* of reporting limiting longstanding illness by tenure, car access, and income quintile by sex, West of Scotland

	Men	Women
Social renters v. owners	2.03	1.63
No car access v. car access	2.24	1.05 (ns)
Lowest v. highest income quintile	4.91	2.11

* Age-adjusted

convenient form of transport for accessing public and private services? Are cars used differently by, and do they have different social meanings for, men and women?

Gender differences in socio-economic inequalities are also observable for health outcomes commonly assumed to be strongly socially patterned. In Britain, for example, major accidents are more common among men than women at younger ages, but what is less often noted is that they only show a strong socio-economic gradient among men (and only at younger ages, i.e. below 50) and not among women (Prescott-Clarke and Primatesta, 1998). Similarly with drug dependence: in Britain, both alcohol and drug dependence show steep social class gradients among men but not among women (Meltzer et al., 1995).

If we look more closely at specific causes of death or types of health measure, we can see differences in the male/female socio-economic differences. Data on mortality by educational level in Russia in 1989 show the common pattern of greater socio-economic differences (here measured by comparing the lower with the higher education groups) for men than for women for all-cause mortality, the male/female ratio in socio-economic group differences being 1.12 (see Table 14.4). This was most marked for infective and parasitic diseases, respiratory cancers, and suicides. In Russia accidents and violence and digestive diseases showed little difference between men and women in socio-economic gradients; circulatory diseases and, perhaps more surprisingly, deaths related to alcohol showed steeper gradients for women than for men (Shkolnikov et al., 1998).

The observation of steeper socio-economic gradients among women for cardiovascular disease is a common one. Data for England and Wales among adults of pre-retirement age show a bigger social class difference among women than among men for coronary heart disease, the ratio of death rates in social class IV and V to social class I and II being 2.69 for women compared to 1.66 among men (Harding et al., 1997).

Perhaps related to this steeper socio-economic gradient for women for cardiovascular disease, we have also found steeper socio-economic gradients among women for anthropometric measures which may predict CVD. We have found steeper gradients for women than for men by household income in pulse rate, weight, body mass index, and waist:hip ratio (Der et al., in press).

Table 14.4 Rate ratios (lower v. higher education groups) of specific-cause mortality in Russia 1989, aged 20–69

	Men	Women	M/F ratio
All causes	1.71	1.45	1.12
Infections, parasitic	4.53	2.35	1.93
Respiratory	3.39	2.24	1.51
Neoplasm	1.57	1.08	1.45
Suicide	2.72	1.77	1.28
Accidents and violence	2.32	2.12	1.09
Digestive	1.56	1.49	1.04
Circulatory	1.41	1.56	0.90
Related to alcohol	3.45	4.63	0.75

Source: Shkolnikov *et al.*, 1998

To summarize so far: there appear to be steeper socio-economic gradients in many measures of morbidity and mortality for men than for women. These steeper gradients are observable using a range of indicators of material and social resources, at the individual, household, and area level. The main exceptions are cardiovascular disease and body shape measures.

The question this observation raises is why this should be so. Kate Hunt and I have previously suggested three possible explanations: artefact, exposure, and vulnerability (Hunt and Macintyre, in press). The first reaction of many researchers in the field to our observation of less steep socio-economic gradients among men compared to women is that this must be an artefact of the way socio-economic status is measured. In particular it is argued that occupational social class schema have been developed around male occupations and do not adequately capture differentiation among women's occupations, and that personal, individual income means something different for men and women.

However, the observation seems to remain generally true whether one measures socio-economic status by education, household income, asset-based measures such as housing tenure or access to a car, or area-based deprivation measures.

Further, we feel that what are often dismissed as being artefacts of measurement may more accurately be described as differences in exposure or vulnerability. One example is that men's occupations span a range from highly dangerous blue collar jobs (mining, fishing, fire fighting, infantry men etc.) to highly privileged and supported white collar jobs (top rank civil servants, barristers, doctors etc.) in a way that women's occupations do not in most industrialized societies. (The lowest status, least skilled female jobs are not concentrated in dangerous sectors, and being a top rank civil servant, barrister, doctor etc. may be more stressful than a routine white collar occupation for women.) (Hunt and Macintyre, in press.) The domestic roles of men and women within employment settings may also vary in potentially health-relevant ways; for example we have found in three white collar organizations (a bank, a university, and the civil service) that women in senior positions are much less likely than their male counterparts to be married or have children (Emslie *et al.*, 1998). The point is that rather than thinking of these occupational differences as artefacts, it might be more productive to think of them as real, causal differences in exposures or vulnerability that might help explain both socio-economic and gender differences in health.

There has been very little research on the possibly different vulnerability (whether social or biological) of men and women to the physical and social environment—a lack I always found astonishing given the seven-year or so life expectancy gap between men and women and the fact that males are more likely to die at every age (including *in utero*) than females. There are other hints that males may be more biologically vulnerable to the environment; for example, they are more likely to experience growth retardation in adverse childhood circumstances. A fascinating but unresearched observation is that changes in mortality rates over time may be faster among men than women in industrialized countries. For example, there have been faster increases in socio-economic inequalities, and faster increases in life expectancy, among men than among women over the last few decades, and the life expectancy of men in Russia decreased much faster than that of women in the recent troubled times. In this context, it would be interesting to see whether mortality in under-five-year-olds in developing countries is higher among boys than girls, more sharply socially-patterned among boys than girls, and changing faster among boys than girls.

The idea that men and women may be differentially exposed, or vulnerable, to features of the physical and social environment, suggests that we need to examine, and to be more precise about, specific pathways and mechanisms, and specific health outcomes.

The fact that many people dismiss the observation of steeper male gradients as artefactual can stem from an often unconscious further set of gender biases. These are based on two rather essentialist assumptions; firstly that there are some real (and possibly constant) socio-economic gradients in health, and that the issue is how best to tap into these gradients. This assumption is frequently manifest in the rather circular idea that the 'best' measure of socio-economic status is the one that produces steepest gradients in health (Berkman and Macintyre, 1997). The second assumption is that there are real and enduring gender differences in health, and that the issue is of how best to measure these differences by controlling out extraneous factors (such as reproductive related mortality among women in industrialized countries in the nineteenth century, or female infant neglect in some developing countries). Both these assumptions can lead to the view that less steep socio-economic gradients or smaller gender differences than some notional gold standard (in the socio-economic case usually based on early studies of men), are artefacts rather than interesting observations that can trigger thinking about mechanisms.

My view is that both socio-economic and gender differences in health are produced and maintained by social, economic, and cultural processes, which will vary by:

- historical period;
- political system;
- stage of economic development;
- cultural and subcultural context;
- measure of material well-being or social position; and
- measure of health and well-being.

Given men and women's different biology, and their different situations in these different historical and socio-economic and cultural settings, it should not surprise us that there might be differences between men and women in socio-economic gradients and that these might vary over time. I do not believe these should be treated as artefacts, but as clues to aetiological and inequality-producing processes.

Acknowledgements

I am employed by the UK Medical Research Council.
I would like to thank the following for help in drafting this paper: Kate Hunt for her collaboration on work on gender and health over many years, and Rosemary Hiscock, Philip McLoone and Ossi Rahkonen for providing unpublished data. The data on housing tenure and car access are from a study funded by the Economic and Social Research Council under the Health Variations Programme (grant ref. L128 25 1017).

REFERENCES

Abramson JH, Gofin R, Habib J, Pridan H, Gofin J. Indicators of social class. A comparative appraisal of measures for use in epidemiological studies. *Social Science and Medicine*, 1982; **16**:1739–46

Benzeval M, Judge K, Shouls S. Household income and self reported health. *Journal of Epidemiology and Community Health*, 1996, **50**:594–5

Berkman L, Macintyre S. The measurement of social class in health studies; old measures and new formulations. In: Kogevinas M, Pearce N, Susser M, and Boffetta P (eds) *Social inequalities and cancer*. Lyons: International Agency for Research in Cancer, 1997, pp 51–64

Dahl E. Social inequalities in ill-health: the significance of occupational status, education and income-results from a Norwegian survey. *Sociology of Health and Illness*, 1994; **16**:644–67

Daly MC, Duncan GJ, Kaplan GA, Lynch JW. Macro-to-micro links in the relation between income inequality and mortality. *The Milbank Quarterly*, 1998; **76**:315–39

Davey Smith G, Neaton JD, Wentworth D, Stamler R, Stamler J. Socioeconomic differentials in mortality risk among men screened for the multiple risk factor intervention trial. 1: white men. *American Journal of Public Health*, 1996; **86**:486–96

Der G, Macintyre S, Ford G, Hunt K,West P. The relationship of household income to a range of health measures in three age cohorts from the West of Scotland. *European Journal of Public Health* (in press)

Emslie C, Hunt K, Fuhrer R, Stansfeld S, Macintyre S. Gender differences in minor morbidity amongst bank employees, civil servants, and university employees. Abstracts from the Society of Social Medicine Conference 1998. *Journal of Epidemiology and Community Health*, 1998; **52**:699

Harding S, Bethune A, Maxwell R, Brown J. Mortality trends using the longitudinal study. In: Drevor F, Whitehead M (eds) *Health inequalities: decennial supplement.* DS Series No. 15. London: The Stationery Office, 1997

Hunt K, Macintyre S. Sexe et inegalités sociales en santé. In: Grandjean H, Kaminski M, Leclerc A, Fassin D, Lang T (eds) *Inegalités et Disparités Sociales en Santé.* Paris: Editions La Decouverte (in press)

Kennedy BP, Kawachi I, Prothrow-Stith D. Income distribution and mortality: cross sectional ecological study of the Robin Hood index in the United States. *British Medical Journal*, 1996; **312**:1004–7

Kunst AE, Mackenbach JP. International variations in the size of mortality differences associated with occupational status. *International Journal of Epidemiology*, 1994; **23**:742–50

Lynch JW, Kaplan GA, Pamuk ER *et al.* Income inequality and mortality in metropolitan areas of the United States. *American Journal of Public Health*, 1998; **88**:1074–80

Macintyre S, Hunt K. Socio-economic position, gender and health; how do they interact? *Journal of Health Psychology*, 1997; **2**:315–34

Macintyre S, Hunt K, Sweeting H. Gender differences in health; are things as simple as they seem? *Social Science and Medicine*, 1996; **42**:617–24

Marmot MG, Shipley MJ, Rose G. Inequalities in death; specific explanations of a general pattern. *Lancet*, 1984; **i**:1003–6

Meltzer H, Gill B, Petticrew M, Hinds K. The prevalence of psychiatric morbidity among adults living in private households. London: HMSO, 1995

Pappas G, Queen S, Hadden W, Fisher G. The increased disparity in mortality between socioeconomic groups in the United States 1960 and 1986. *New England Journal of Medicine*, 1993; **329**:103–9

Prescott-Clarke P, Primatesta P. *Health Survey for England '96.* London: The Stationery Office, 1998

Rahkonen O, Arber S, Lahelma E, Martikainen P, Silventoinen K. *Understanding income inequalities in health among men and women in Britain and Finland. International Journal of Health Services*, 2000; **30**:27–47

Raleigh S, Kiri V. Life expectancy in England: variation and trends by gender, health authority, and level of deprivation. *Journal of Epidemiology and Community Health*, 1997; **51**: 649–58

Ruiz MT, Verbrugge LM. A two way view of gender bias in medicine. *Journal of Epidemiology and Community Health*, 1997; **51**:106–9

Shaper AG, Pocock SJ, Walker M *et al.* British Regional Heart Study: cardiovascular risk factors in middle-aged men in 24 towns. *British Medical Journal*, 1981; **283**:179–86

Shkolnikov VM, Leon DA, Adamets S, Andreev E, Deev A. Educational level and adult mortality in Russia: an analysis of routine data 1979 to 1994. *Social Science and Medicine*, 1998; **47**:357–69

van Doorslaer E, Wagstaff A, Bleichrodt H *et al*. Income-related inequalities in health: some international comparisons. *Journal of Health Economics*, 1997; **16**: 93–112

15 From science to policy: options for reducing health inequalities

Hilary Graham

Tackling health inequalities is moving up the public health agenda, at both international and national level. In the international arena, the Declaration of the 1998 World Health Assembly confirmed that a reduction in socio-economic inequalities in health is a priority for all countries. In Europe, the EU Action Programme on Public Health is giving priority to improving the health of disadvantaged groups. Alongside this, the WHO has launched its new health strategy for Europe, *Health 21*. Improving health and promoting equity are again the organising principles around which the health strategy is built (WHO, 1998). Underlying this two-track strategy is the recognition that reducing health inequalities is an essential pre-requisite for wider gains in public health. In other words, improved health turns on greater equity in health.

This two-track strategy is evident, too, in national public health policies. As one recent example, the UK government has launched new public health strategies in England, Northern Ireland, Scotland, and Wales built around the twin goals of reducing health inequalities and improving population health. As in the UK, governments elsewhere are recognising that achieving these goals requires a broader and more radical vision of public health policy. It is one that not only targets individuals and their risk behaviours, but also tackles the inequalities in life chances and living standards which shape people's lifestyles. Tackling health inequalities requires a comprehensive strategy which, in the words of the New Zealand report on health inequalities, 'addresses the fundamental socio-economic determinants of health' (New Zealand National Advisory Committee on Health and Disability, 1998). Or as the Public Health Strategy for England put it, 'tackling inequalities generally is the best way of tackling health inequalities in particular' (Great Britain Department of Health, 1998).

Tackling inequalities generally is clearly an ambitious policy objective, particularly at a time of rapid social and economic change. People's working and domestic lives are being transformed by the growth of the global economy, by increasing job insecurity and unemployment, and by a shift away from lifelong marriage. These changes are fuelling a wider process of social polarization in many societies, marked by a widening gap in living standards between work-rich, two-earner households and work-poor, no-earner households. This process of polarization is being played out on the international stage, with rich economies based on capital-intensive industries gaining at the expense of poor countries dependent on labour-intensive industries (UNDP, 1996).

Social change and social polarization provide the backdrop against which the international community and national governments are seeking to reduce inequalities in health. And they are turning to the scientific community for advice on how to do so. Governments are looking, in the words of the WHO's strategy for Europe, for 'a scientific framework for decision makers' and 'a science-based guide to better health development' (WHO, 1998). Research programmes and evidence-based reviews are being launched to furnish these science-based guides: in the Netherlands, Finland, Sweden, New Zealand, and elsewhere (Mackenbach et al., 1994; Kunst, 1997; Arve-Pares, 1998; New Zealand National Advisory Committee on Health and Disability, 1998). The Independent Inquiry into Inequalities in Health, established by the UK government, is the latest example of this international trend. The Inquiry's terms of reference were to review the scientific evidence on health inequalities in order to identify policies with the potential to reduce them: in other words, to bring the science of health inequalities to bear on the process of policy development (Great Britain Independent Inquiry into Inequalities in Health, 1998).

But what is the science of health inequalities? It clearly includes epidemiological studies which, since the nineteenth century, have mapped the persistent association between individual socio-economic status and individual health. It includes, too, the more recent and smaller seam of experimental research which has sought to evaluate the effectiveness of interventions designed to narrow socio-economic differentials in health. I will discuss these fields of research briefly below.

But the science of health inequalities potentially covers a much larger canvas: one which moves beyond description and evaluation to explanation. This broader science is concerned with how inequalities in health result from inequalities in socio-economic status and how inequalities in socio-economic status are produced and maintained. It is a science concerned with what the socio-economic structure is doing to individual socio-economic circumstances as well as what individual socio-economic circumstances are doing to health. This dual scientific focus, structural and individual, upstream and downstream, is particularly important at times of social transformation, when the occupational structure is changing and income inequalities are widening. The central sections of the chapter broaden the base of health inequalities research to include these processes of change, moving beyond the disciplines of social epidemiology and public health to the social science disciplines of sociology, social policy, and welfare economics.

The science of health inequalities: describing health inequalities

At the core of health inequalities research is the long tradition of collecting data on the health and socio-economic status of individuals. In the nineteenth century, it was these data which brought the fact and scale of health inequalities to the attention of policy makers, prompting major investment in environmental health and sanitation. It is this descriptive science which revealed how socio-economic inequalities in childhood health had all but disappeared in Sweden by the 1960s (Whitehead and Diderichsen, 1997). And it is this descriptive science which is pointing to widening inequalities in mortality in a number of countries, including the UK (Drever and Whitehead, 1997). Recording and publicising these trends has been an important catalyst in the policy process, ensuring that health inequalities remain on and move up the political agenda (Haines and Smith, 1997).

These descriptive studies also convey a simple, and compelling, policy message. Health inequalities are dynamic: their scale, and the causes of ill-health which underlie them, vary over time and between countries. The fact that health inequalities are not fixed and immutable provides evidence that they can be reduced.

The science of health inequalities: intervention studies

The evaluative studies are concerned with identifying interventions with the potential to reduce health inequalities. They represent, as is widely acknowledged, a small and underdeveloped field, and one where the research designs of the randomized control trial are ill-suited to assessing the impact of macro-trends and policies. As a result, evaluative research on health inequalities is disproportionately weighted towards the evaluation of interventions targeted at individuals rather than at the circumstances in which they live. Systematic reviews have found a predominance of interventions designed to reduce risk-related behaviours, like cigarette smoking, through providing individuals with information and support (NHSCRD, 1995; Gepkins and Gunning-Schepers, 1996). There is little evidence that these behavioural interventions have either a positive effect on those in lower socio-economic groups or one that is differentially beneficial for these groups. As the Scottish public health green paper puts it (Scottish Office, 1998; italics and emphasis in original):

> Simply addressing disease and lifestyle cannot deliver what is needed. *The first part* of a cohesive strategy for a healthier, more equitable, Scotland must be to counter the *life circumstances* which can give rise to poor health, and foster those which generate good health. These include a job, a home, a good education and an attractive environment.

There are few evaluated interventions designed to counter adverse life circumstances. The few, however, point to the potential impact that interventions targeted at life circumstances could have on health inequalities.

One example is of an intervention designed to achieve health gain by increasing financial resources to low-income families. In a randomized control trial conducted in the early 1970s in Indiana, USA, the intervention group of low-income mothers received an expanded income support plan which guaranteed them a minimum income. Mothers at high risk of adverse pregnancy outcome who were in the intervention group had heavier babies than control-group mothers (Kehrer and Wolin, 1979). Another example is the introduction of measures to reduce traffic accidents, a major cause of injury and death to children which displays a sharp socio-economic gradient. The introduction of 20 mph zones is associated with, on average, a 60% drop in pedestrian casualties and a 70% reduction in child pedestrian and cycling casualties (GB DETR, 1997).

A third, and more developed, field of intervention is the provision of out-of-home day care to improve the current and future life circumstances of disadvantaged children. Evidence from randomized control trials indicates that such interventions have positive effects on children's well-being and, through its impact on cognitive development and school performance, on future socio-economic status (Zoritch et al., 1998).

While providing a guide to policy, the range of intervention studies is currently too limited to provide the evidence base on which a comprehensive strategy to reduce health inequalities could be built. In its place, scientists and policy makers are looking to a third area of health inequalities research, where evidence is derived from the analysis of causal pathways and not the effectiveness of interventions. As the New Zealand report on health inequalities puts it (NZ National Advisory Committee on Health and Disability, 1998):

> Even if there is no specific evidence on the health outcomes of interventions, if there is
>
> • evidence for a strong and consistent association between a particular socio-economic factor and health **and**
>
> • there is good evidence that the association is causal **then** specific initiatives, including policies that show a positive effect on that factor, are highly likely to lead to improved health.

The science of health inequalities: explanatory studies

This third area, concerned with consistent associations and causal pathways, has been traditionally resourced by social epidemiology. The dominant epidemiological model tracks the socio-economic patterning of individual health back through a series of intermediate factors to individual socio-economic status (Fig. 15.1). As the figure indicates, the causal chain is short and links up a range of individual-level influences on health. Some epidemiological models lengthen the causal chain to include the social structure as the upstream, independent variable (e.g. International Centre for Health and Society, 1998; Diderichsen, 1998). However, the social structure features as an unanalysed variable: placed within, but not incorporated into, these extended models.

We need to look beyond social epidemiology to other disciplines, and to sociology and social policy in particular, for analyses which track macro-level influences on individual socio-economic status. And the evidence from these disciplines suggests that the socio-economic structure of many societies is undergoing a process of rapid change, and fracturing in ways which are widening inequalities in living standards and life chances. This suggests that the science of health inequalities needs, to coin a well-used UK phrase, to be a 'joined up' one. It should include both epidemiological research on individual health and sociological research on social inequality. Although these fields of research have developed separately, there is considerable potential for synergy. As one example, longitudinal studies of the socio-economic patterning of health over the life course could be integrated into sociological analyses of social polarization. Such an integration highlights a set of interlocking links in the chains which run from the social structure to individual health. Together, these two seams of research are uncovering how health is fashioned by:

- risk exposures across the life course...
- within pathways of disadvantage, shaped by...
- broader changes in the socio-economic structure.

As a case study—and I would emphasise that it is only one example—the sections below look in more detail at this joined-up science of health inequalities and at the policy framework it provides.

An example of a joined-up science of health inequalities

(i) Culminative exposure to disadvantage

As Fig. 15.1 indicates, social epidemiology has identified a cluster of individual-level factors which link individuals' socio-economic circumstances and their health. These include material factors, like poor housing and poor living standards, and psycho-social factors, like life events and chronic difficulties and the social networks and relationships which support people through them. These

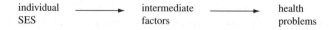

Fig. 15.1 An individual-level model of health inequalities
Source: Mackenbach, 1998, Fig. 1

intermediate factors also include behavioural influences, like cigarette smoking and a diet with a limited nutrient base.

An important seam of research has described how these proximate influences cluster together. They have demonstrated that an individual exposed to material disadvantage is more likely to be disadvantaged with respect to their psycho-social environment and their health behaviour, while an individual protected from material hazards is more likely to have a protective psycho-social environment and to engage in health-promoting behaviours (Marmot and Davey Smith, 1997). These factors can also interact. For example, low levels of social support have been found to have a more negative effect on the psychological health of those living in poverty, and poverty has its most substantial effects on the psychological well-being of those who had limited access to social support (Whelan, 1993).

However, longitudinal studies are now tracking how these risks and resources not only cluster together but accumulate over the life course (Power *et al.*, 1996; van de Mheen, 1998). The British 1958 birth cohort study provides a powerful and chilling insight into this process of culminative disadvantage. It has followed children born in one week in 1958 through their childhood up to the age of 33 (Power and Matthews, 1997). And it is revealing how girls and boys born into families at the bottom of the class hierarchy (based on father's occupation) are much more likely to be exposed to material, psycho-social, and behavioural risks in the process of growing up than those in higher social classes. For example, they are more likely to live in overcrowded homes, to experience such life events as the divorce of their parents, and to be exposed to parental smoking.

(ii) Pathways of disadvantage

Longitudinal studies are not only uncovering the socio-economic patterning of health risks—material, psycho-social, and behavioural—across the life course. They are also uncovering the socio-economic trajectories of which these exposures are part. In other words, they are beginning to move beyond individual socio-economic status to the social structure, identifying the pathways through which the occupational structure shapes the lives and life chances of individuals (Fig. 15.2). Again, the 1958 National Child Development Survey provides an instructive example. Analyses of the 1958 cohort to the age of 33 indicate that those born and brought up on the lower rungs of the class ladder are more likely than their more advantaged peers to follow disadvantaged pathways across their adult lives. Their employment pathways are more likely to be characterized by

(changes in) ⟶ socio-economic ⟶ individual ⟶ culminative ⟶ health
social structure   pathways   SES   risk exposures   outcomes

Fig. 15.2 A society-level model of health inequalities

low educational qualifications, unemployment, redundancy, and receipt of means-tested benefits.

Figure 15.3 maps the employment trajectories of young adults by their social class at birth (Power and Matthews, 1997). The proportion of young people entering the labour market without educational qualifications, facing redundancy, and being in receipt of means-tested social security benefits increases in line with declining social class—with working-class men particularly exposed to the risk of redundancy. Ethnicity mediates the employment pathways young people follow into and through the labour market. UK studies point to an 'ethnic penalty' paid by young people from minority ethnic groups in which they do less well with respect to employment and job level than similarly qualified whites. African-Caribbean and Bangladeshi/ Pakistani groups, in particular, face higher rates of unemployment and of employment in low-skilled jobs than their white peers (Modood, 1997).

Socio-economic status also structures young people's domestic pathways, with low SES linked to pathways which run through early parenthood, and for

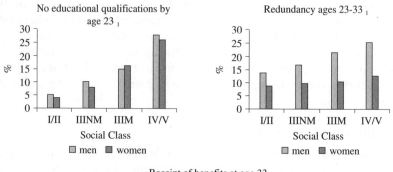

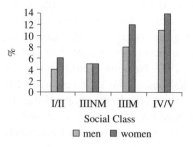

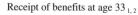

Notes

1. p < 0.001
2. includes income support, supplementary unemployment benefit, participant or partner

Fig. 15.3   Socio-economic pathways by social class at birth, National Child Development Study
Source: Power and Matthews, 1997

women, lone parenthood (Fig. 15.4). As Fig. 15.4 indicates, there is a sharp socio-economic gradient in the proportion of young people becoming parents by their early twenties. Among men in the highest social class at the age of 23, less than 1 in 10 are fathers by that age; among women in the lowest social class, more than 6 in 10 are mothers. Single parenthood shows even more pronounced gender and class differences. Few men are lone fathers by the age of 33 and it is not patterned by their socio-economic status. The chances are significantly higher for women and are closely related to occupational circumstances in early adulthood. The domestic pathways which run through early and lone parenthood bring additional layers of disadvantage, restricting opportunities to gain the skills and work experience necessary to move out of unemployment and low-paid work and into the better-paid and more secure sectors of the labour market. The result is a high level of dependency on means-tested social security benefits, with living standards significantly below those taken for granted by the majority of the population (Bradshaw, 1993; Burstrom *et al.*, 1999).

As Figs 15.3 and 15.4 suggest, longitudinal studies are broadening the scientific framework of health inequalities research, introducing a temporal as well as a spatial dimension to socio-economic status. It is not simply where an individual is in the socio-economic hierarchy which matters, it is how this position shapes exposure to health-damaging influences across their lives which is crucial.

The life-course perspectives provided by longitudinal studies have moved the science of health inequalities closer to the social structure, enabling it to measure the effects of disadvantage on the paths which individuals follow across their lives. But their individual-level focus means that the structural-level forces which shape these pathways remain hidden from view. Leaving out structural-level

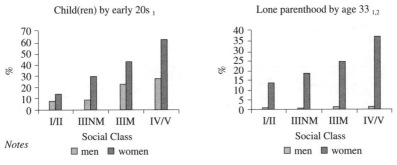

Notes

1. p < 0.001
2. ever been a lone parent (greater than 1 month)

Fig. 15.4 Domestic pathways by social class at age 23, National Child Development Study
Source: Unpublished data, Sharon Matthews, Institute of Child Health

processes is particularly problematic during periods in which the social structure is undergoing rapid change. These are periods when the size and composition of the occupational categories which underpin the class structure are changing, and with them the socio-economic trajectories that individuals can expect to follow across their lives.

(iii) Changes in the socio-economic structure

The science of health inequalities needs to include society-level as well as individual-level analyses, because the pathways that people track through their lives are framed by the wider socio-economic structure: by how life chances and living standards are distributed through the labour market, and by the tax and welfare system. The international pattern, repeated across Europe, the US, and in the emergent economies of Africa, Asia, and South America, is of rising unemployment linked to a collapse in demand for low-skilled manual workers. However, the effect of these labour market changes on the distribution of income, and on the class structure more broadly, varies between countries. The UK provides an instructive example of a society in which the process of social polarization is well advanced.

From the mid 1970s to the mid 1990s, inequalities in living standards in the UK increased at a pace and to a scale unmatched in Europe (Goodman *et al.*, 1997). While better-off households enjoyed rising living standards, the proportion of the population living in poverty rose sharply. Figure 15.5 plots the proportion of the UK population living in households below the EC poverty line, represented by a household income below half of national average income. As

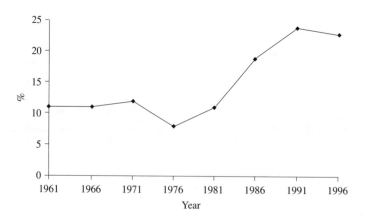

Fig. 15.5 Proportion of the population below 50% of average income (after housing costs) 1961–96, UK
Source: Goodman and Webb, 1994; Great Britain Department of Social Security, 1998

it indicates, 7% were in poverty in the mid 1970s; by the mid 1990s, nearly a quarter (24%) of the population were living in households with incomes less than half the national average (after housing costs) (Endean, 1998).

Rising unemployment and widening income inequalities have been associated with a wider process of social polarization. Underlying this process have been changes in the structure of the labour market, and, in particular, a rapid decline in manual and low-skilled work. As a result, unemployment rates for those in unskilled manual socio-economic groups have doubled, reaching 30% among white men and over 60% among African Caribbean men by the early 1990s (ONS, 1998). Rising unemployment at the bottom of the class hierarchy has been matched by rising earnings among high-paid workers.

As elsewhere in Europe and in the US, changes in the structure of the labour market and in the dispersal of earnings have been associated with a more far-reaching change. They have fuelled a redistribution of employment between households. Across the last two decades, there has been a rapid shift away from households containing a mix of employed and non-employed adults and a corresponding increase in two-earner and no-earner households (Gregg and Wadsworth, 1996). The proportion of no-earner households has doubled since the late 1970s, from less than 1 in 10 households in 1979 to more than 1 in 5 in 1995.

Changes in household composition, and in particular the growth in single-parent households and childless single-adult households, explains some of the growth in no-earner households. To take account of this demographic trend, Fig. 15.6 is restricted to the dominant household form. It focuses on two-adult households, which represent about 60% of all households in Britain. As the figure indicates, male-earner households have given way to two-earner and no-earner households. The upward trend in no-earner households reflects the toll of

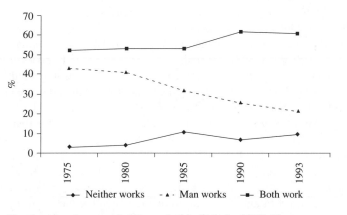

Fig. 15.6 Employment in two-adult households, Britain, 1975–93
Source: Gregg and Wadsworth, 1996

increasing unemployment. However, new jobs have disproportionately been taken by those living in households where another member is already in work (Gregg and Wadsworth, 1996).

With the changing household distribution of work, the clumping of households on middle incomes has begun to break up. In its place, a new income distribution has emerged, characterized by high and rising real incomes for working households and low and stagnant incomes for non-working households (Jenkins, 1996; Cowell et al., 1997; Hills, 1998). For no-earner households dependent on means-tested benefits, real incomes have not even been stagnant: they have declined.

These trends suggest that the UK class structure no longer consists of a hierarchy of unequal but relatively stable positions. Increasingly, it is a structure composed of unequal and diverging socio-economic trajectories. Those in secure and well-paid jobs can expect to increase their command over the material, psycho-social, and behavioural resources associated with good health: enjoying, for example, high living standards, high control at work, and high nutrient intake. Those in disadvantaged positions face the prospect of downward socio-economic trajectories. Low and declining living standards are likely to restrict opportunities to avoid the health risks which come with a poor material and psycho-social environment or to break health-damaging patterns of behaviour.

In examining the effects of macro socio-economic change on individual socio-economic trajectories, it is instructive to compare the UK with countries where labour market changes have been associated with less pronounced changes in the distribution of living standards and life chances. Finland provides an illuminating example. There the rapid economic growth which marked out the 1970s and 1980s gave way to deep recession at the beginning of the 1990s. The economic reversal was rapid and profound: unemployment climbed from less than 4% in 1990 to over 18% in 1993 (Fig. 15.7).

As in the UK, earnings differentials between higher-paid white collar workers and lower-paid blue collar workers widened and, with them, income inequalities increased. But the widening of income inequalities has been relatively small in comparison with the UK (Keskimaki et al., 1999). This is because fiscal and welfare policies have moderated the effects of rising unemployment. Tax rate increases have contained the rise in real incomes of those in better-paid jobs while, despite cuts, the social security system has protected the living standards of the increasing proportion of the population dependent on them for their economic survival. As a result, the cost of recession has been redistributed and shared. By 1996, real incomes for most income groups were below their pre-recession level. Only the higher-income decile have seen a rise in real incomes. As Keskimaki et al. (1999) note, the Finnish fiscal and welfare systems have been relatively successful in maintaining an equitable distribution of income in the face of forces which, in the UK, resulted in a rapid widening of income inequalities.

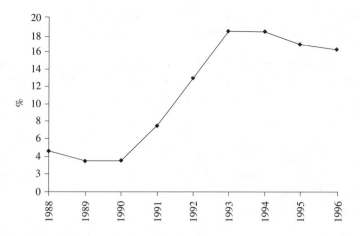

Fig. 15.7 Unemployment rate in Finland 1988–96
Source: Keskimaki *et al.*, 1999

Policy options for reducing health inequalities

In the sections above, I have drawn selectively on health inequalities research. I have drawn particularly on epidemiological research on life-course influences and sociological research on socio-economic inequality to illustrate how, in the words of the WHO *Health 21* strategy, research can yield 'a scientific framework for decision makers'. The framework highlights a set of interlocking processes in the production of the socio-economic gradient in health, and in particular: *cumulative exposure to risks along disadvantaged pathways* framed by *wider structures of inequality*. In so doing, it reveals multiple points where policy leverage can be exerted, as scientific and policy reviews have made clear (Great Britain Independent Inquiry into Inequalities in Health, 1998; NZ National Advisory Committee on Health and Disability, 1998). Two are highlighted below.

Pathways of disadvantage

The evidence that exposure to health risks—material, psycho-social, and behavioural—is patterned by the socio-economic pathways individuals follow across their lives has a clear policy message. It argues for policies which intervene in the disadvantaged pathways which increase exposure to health risks.

One policy option is to target points and periods in the life course when individuals are making changes likely to have long-term effects on their future socio-economic status. These critical life transitions include entering pre-school care and education, moving from primary and secondary school, (early) school leaving and entering the labour market, becoming redundant, becoming a (lone) parent and, particularly for women, moving through separation and divorce. Recognizing these critical life transitions, and especially those relating to childhood and adolescence, offers a number of advantages.

Firstly, governments are already involved in helping and directing individuals through the key transitions which mark out childhood and adulthood: for example, entry into pre-school and compulsory education, into and off means-tested benefits, through pregnancy and into parenthood are all life events which are closely regulated by state agencies. Secondly, targeting these transitions goes with the grain of welfare policy. It is a principle and practice already integrated into welfare programmes and expenditure plans. There are many examples of programmes which aim to improve the educational levels and outcomes for children from disadvantaged communities and to promote education and training for low-skilled young people.

Informed by evaluations of established programmes, particularly those in the US, early childhood programmes are being developed in the UK, New Zealand, and elsewhere with the aim of lifting disadvantaged children onto more advantaged socio-economic trajectories. The Sure Start programme in England is a targeted programme providing child care and primary health care services in 250 areas, reaching about 5% of the national population of 0–3 year olds. While a programme from which important research and policy messages will flow, its targeted focus means that its broader population impact will be limited.

Like the early childhood programmes, New Deal and Welfare-to-Work programmes are designed to break into disadvantaged socio-economic pathways by providing targeted groups with a springboard onto more advantaged trajectories. In the US and the UK, these programmes are part of a wider set of policies aimed to help move key claimant groups off social security benefits and into paid work, by offering access to training and education and to subsidised jobs. In the UK, the largest recipient group for the Welfare-to-Work Programme are young adults aged 18 to 24 who have been claiming unemployment benefits (job seekers allowance) for 6 months or more.

Enhancing the skills of unemployed people is what economists call a supply side approach to tackling unemployment and reducing poverty. The aim is to increase the skills and employment chances of unemployed people, who are considerably less skilled than those in paid work. However, evaluated New Deal schemes have produced disappointing results. Employment rates among those recruited to the schemes are only fractionally above rates among welfare recipients excluded from them (Solow, 1998). This suggests that the schemes require parallel demand-side initiatives to improve the availability of the low-skilled jobs sought by unemployed people. Further, providing gateways out of unemployment for some groups offers little to those who remain on means-tested benefits (Graham et al., 1999). To address these structural dimensions of disadvantage requires policies which generate low-skilled jobs and which improve the living standards of those unable to earn their living.

Structures of inequality

In the UK, life chances and living standards polarized across two decades in which inequality was off the political agenda. From 1979 to 1997, the country was led by a Conservative government which adopted a free market approach to economic, social, and fiscal policy. As a result, inequalities resulting from labour market restructuring and the emergence of new patterns of family life were magnified rather than moderated.

As the example of the UK suggests, national state policies play an important part in mediating the effects of social and socio-economic change. Change—whether at the level of the transitional corporation and the global labour market or in our patterns of cohabitation and parenthood—is not inevitably linked to widening inequalities in health and opportunity. Whether and how far social and economic change results in widening inequalities depends on national state policies: social, economic, and fiscal (Bradshaw, 1996; Breen and Rothman, 1998; Black *et al.*, 1999).

The role of social policy in tempering social inequality is underlined in a recent analysis by Richard Breen and David Rothman (1998). They analysed the occupational structure and extent of class inequality and mobility in countries occupying core positions in the global labour market (Australia, Belgium, France, Italy, Japan, the US, Germany, Norway, and Sweden) and peripheral locations (Philippines and Malaysia). They concluded that national policies shape class structures and buffer the effects of low social class on life chances and living standards:

> Welfare and other state policies enacted and implemented in diverse ways at the level of the national state shape class structures and the consequences of class membership. The specifics of such policies are important vehicles linking class position and life chances. As a result, national states that occupy a similar niche within the world (economic) system present us with diverse class structures, degrees of openness (as manifest in social mobility) and degree of class inequality.

As their analysis indicates, national state policies form an integral part of a public health strategy to reduce health inequalities. Attention has been drawn, in particular, to employment, income, and the provision of services like public housing, health care, and transport as mechanisms through which to temper inequalities in the labour market and improve the living standards of those groups whose earning power is low (for example, Great Britain Independent Inquiry into Inequalities in Health, 1998; NZ National Advisory Committee on Health and Disability, 1998; Black *et al.*, 1999). In these policy domains, governments exercise a high degree of direct control, providing considerable opportunity for leverage and impact.

Participation in paid employment is the major determinant of living standards, with poverty concentrated among households outside the labour market. The sharp socio-economic differentials in the opportunities for paid work are widely recognised by governments, with Welfare-to-Work programmes seeking to reduce unemployment among low-skilled workers. However, analyses suggest that the demand for low-skilled labour in an increasing number of societies is falling short of the supply, even when the quality of that supply is enhanced through welfare-to-work programmes. Increasing the availability of low-skilled jobs in the public sector is one—and an important—policy option (Solow, 1998).

A second option is to act directly on the distribution of income. The tax and social security systems are redistributive systems through which governments can influence the scale of income inequality and can protect the living standards of the poorest groups. As evidence from Finland and Sweden indicates, progressive tax structures narrow differentials in (post-tax) incomes while the introduction of a more regressive tax structure in the UK widened inequalities in income (Hills, 1998; Burstrom and Diderichsen, 1999; Keskimaki et al., 1999). The simplest way of protecting the living standards of households dependent on social security benefits is to peg benefit levels to average earnings. This maintains their relative value and avoids the downward drift in living standards experienced by welfare recipients in the UK (Hills, 1998).

A third potential lever on inequalities is provided by publicly-funded welfare state services. These include health care and education, subsidised housing, personal social services (social work and social care), subsidised public transport, and local amenities (parks, playgrounds, leisure centres) open to and free for the whole community. Evidence from the UK suggests that poorer households derive significantly greater benefit than richer households from these services (Sefton, 1998). As a result, universally-provided welfare services are an important mechanism for raising the living standards of the poor, for moderating the impact of income inequalities, and for redistributing wealth. Services which are targeted at, and disproportionately used by, those in need, like subsidised rented housing, personal social services, and subsidised bus networks, have the most pronounced redistributive effects. Investment in these elements of the welfare state therefore offers an effective strategy for targeting groups and areas in which disadvantage is concentrated.

Conclusion

My review of the science/policy interface has been necessarily selective. I have looked briefly at descriptive and evaluative studies and, in more depth, at the scientific contribution of longitudinal studies of individuals and of time-series analyses of societies. In this narrow focus, key areas have been omitted. I have not, for example, discussed how areas and communities exert their own and independent effects on the class gradient in health and how gender and ethnicity mediate the effects of class disadvantage. Nonetheless, I hope my selective approach has uncovered the long interface that runs between science and policy.

I have highlighted how socio-economic inequalities are—at least in part—the outcome of risks accumulated along disadvantaged life-course pathways which, in turn, are fashioned by wider structures of inequality. I have pointed to how science can inform and intersect with policy, underlying the importance of policies which intervene in disadvantaged pathways and temper socio-economic inequality.

My selective focus also has a broader policy message. Because health inequalities are multi-determined, policies need to exert leverage at multiple points. As the Acheson report concludes, a broad-front approach is required. I give my final word to the report (Great Britain Independent Inquiry into Inequalities in Health, 1998):

> A broad front approach reflects scientific evidence that health inequalities are the outcome of causal chains which run back into and from the basic structure of society. Such an approach is necessary because many of the factors are inter-related. It is likely to be less effective to focus solely on one point if complementary action is not in place which influences a linked factor in another policy area.

Acknowledgements

I would like to thank Sharon Matthews, Institute of Child Health, for unpublished data from the National Child Development Study, and Tanya Richardson for help with typing the chapter.

REFERENCES

Arve-Pares B (ed). *Promoting research on inequality in health.* Stockholm: Swedish Council for Social Research, 1998

Black D, Morris JN, Smith C, Townsend P. Better benefits for health: plan to implement the central recommendation of the Acheson report. *British Medical Journal,* 1999; **318**:724–7

Bradshaw J. *Household budgets and living standards.* York: Joseph Rowntree Foundation, 1993

Bradshaw J. *The employment of lone parents: a comparison of policy in 20 countries.* London: Family Policy Studies Centre, 1996

Breen R, Rottman DB. Is the national state the appropriate geographical unit for class analysis? *Sociology,* 1998; **32**:1–22

Burstrom B, Diderichsen F. Income related policies in Sweden, 1990–8. In: Mackenbach JP, Droomers M (eds) *Interventions and policies to reduce socio-economic inequalities in health.* Rotterdam: Erasmus University Rotterdam, 1999

Burstrom B, Diderichsen F, Shouls S, Whitehead M. Lone mothers in Sweden: trends in health and socio-economic circumstances, 1979–1995. *Journal of Epidemiology and Community Health,* 1999; **53**:750–6

Cowell FA, Jenkins SP, Litchfield JA. The changing shape of the UK income distribution: kernal density estimates. In: Hills J (ed) *New inequalities: the changing distribution of income and wealth in the United Kingdom.* Cambridge: Cambridge University Press, 1997

Diderichsen F. Understanding health equity in populations—some theoretical and methodological considerations. In: Arve-Pares B (ed) *Promoting research on inequality in health*. Stockholm: Swedish Council for Social Research, 1998

Drever F, Whitehead M (eds). *Health inequalities: decennial supplement*. London: The Stationery Office, 1997

Endean R (ed). *Households below average income, 1979 to 1996/97*. Leeds: Department of Social Security, 1998

Gepkins A, Gunning-Schepers LJ. Interventions to reduce socio-economic health differences. *European Journal of Public Health*, 1996; **6**:218–26

Goodman A and Webb S. *For richer, for poorer: the changing distribution of income in the United Kingdom*. London: Institute for Fiscal Studies, 1994

Goodman A, Johnson P, Webb S. *Inequality in the UK*. Oxford: Oxford University Press, 1997

Graham H, Benzeval M, Whitehead M. Social and economic policies in the UK with a potential impact on health inequalities. In: Mackenbach JP, Droomers M (eds) *Interventions and policies to reduce socio-economic inequalities in health*. Rotterdam: Erasmus University Rotterdam, 1999

Great Britain Department of Environment, Transport and the Regions. *Road safety: current problems and future solutions*. London: DETR, 1997

Great Britain Department of Health. *Our healthier nation*. London: The Stationery Office, 1998

Great Britain Department of Social Security. *Social security statistics 1997*. London: The Stationery Office, 1998

Great Britain Independent Inquiry into Inequalities in Health. *Report of the Independent Inquiry into Inequalities in Health: Report*. London: The Stationery Office, 1998

Gregg P, Wadsworth J. More work in fewer households. In: Hills J (ed) *New inequalities: the changing distribution of income and wealth in the United Kingdom*. Cambridge: Cambridge University Press, 1996

Haines A, Smith R. Working together to reduce poverty's damage, (Editorial). *British Medical Journal*, 1997; **314**:529–30

Hills J. *Income and wealth: the latest evidence*. York: Joseph Rowntree Foundation, 1998

International Centre for Health and Society. Socio-economic circumstances and health outcomes. In: Great Britain Independent Inquiry into Inequalities in Health (1998). *Report of the Independent Inquiry into Inequalities in Health*. London: The Stationery Office, 1998, Figure 2

Jenkins S. Recent trends in the UK income distribution: what happened and why? *Oxford Review of Economic Policy*, 1996; **12**:29–46

Kehrer B, Wolin V. Impact of income maintenance or low birth weight, evidence from the Gary experiment. *Journal of Human Resources*, 1979; **14**:434–62

Keskimaki I, Lahelma E, Koskinen S, Valkonen T. Policy changes related to income distribution and income differences in health in Finland in the 1990s. In: Mackenbach JP, Droomers M (eds) *Interventions and policies to reduce socio-economic inequalities in health*. Rotterdam: Erasmus University Rotterdam, 1999

Kunst AE. *Cross-national comparisons of socio-economic differences in mortality*. Rotterdam: Erasmus University, 1997

Mackenbach JP. The Dutch experience with promoting research on inequality in health. In: Arve-Pares B (ed) *Promoting research on inequality in health*. Stockholm: Swedish Council for Social Research, 1998

Mackenbach JP, Kunst AE, Cavelaars AE, Groenhof F, Geurts JJ. Socio-economic inequalities in morbidity and mortality in Western Europe. *Lancet*, 1994; **349**:1655–9

Marmot MG, Davey-Smith G. Socio-economic differentials in health. *Journal of Health Psychology*, 1997; **2**: 283–96

Modood J. Employment. In: Modood J, Berthoud R (eds) *Ethnic minorities in Britain: diversity and disadvantage*. London: Policy Studies Institute, 1997

New Zealand National Advisory Committee on Health and Disability. *The social, cultural and economic determinants of health in New Zealand: action to improve health*. Wellington: National Health Committee, 1998

NHS Centre for Reviews and Dissemination. *Review of the research on the effectiveness of Health Service interventions to reduce variations in health*. York: NHS Centre for Reviews and Dissemination, University of York, 1995

Office for National Statistics. *Living in Britain: results from the 1996 General Household Survey*. London: The Stationery Office, 1998

Power C, Matthews S. Origins of health inequalities in a national population sample. *Lancet*, 1997; **350**:1584–5

Power C, Bartley M, Davey-Smith G, Blane D. Transmission of social and biological risk across the life course. In: Blane D, Brunner E, Wilkinson R (eds) *Health and social organisation*. London: Routledge, 1996, pp 188–203

Scottish Office. *Working together for a healthier Scotland*. Edinburgh: The Stationery Office, 1998

Sefton T. *The changing distribution of the social wage*. London: STICERD, London School of Economics, 1998

Solow RM. *Work and welfare*. Princeton: Princeton University Press, 1998

United Nations Development Programme. *Human Development Report 1996*. New York: Oxford University Press, 1996

van de Mheen D. *Inequalities in health: to be continued? A lifecourse perspective on socio-economic inequalities in health*. Rotterdam: Erasmus University, Rotterdam, 1998

Whelan CT. The role of social support in mediating the psychological consequences of economic stress. *Sociology of Health and Illness*, 1993; **15**:86–101

Whitehead M, Diderichsen F. International evidence on social inequalities in health. In: Drever F, Whitehead M (eds) *Health inequalities: decennial supplement*. London: The Stationery Office, 1997

WHO Regional Office for Europe. *Health 21: health for all in the 21st century*. Copenhagen: WHO Regional Office for Europe, 1998

Zoritch B, Roberts I, Oakley A. The health and welfare effects of day-care: a systematic review of randomised controlled trials. *Social Science and Medicine*, 1998; **47**:317–27

16 Do poverty alleviation programmes reduce inequities in health? The Bangladesh experience

A. Mushtaque R. Chowdhury and Abbas Bhuiya

Over the previous two decades many poverty alleviation programmes have been implemented in developing countries. Evaluation of such programmes has traditionally concentrated more on their success in increasing the income levels of participants than on the broader goals of human well-being. This chapter looks at the poverty alleviation programme of BRAC, a large non-governmental organization in Bangladesh, and, based on a scientifically-designed study, presents its impact on selected components of 'human well-being'.

The study found evidence for better child survival and nutritional status in households served by the programme. Similar evidence was also found for the programme's impact on other areas such as expenditure patterns, family planning practice, children's education, and domestic violence against women. The likely influence of 'selection bias' on the above results is also discussed.

This chapter examines a women-focused development intervention in terms of its impact on human well-being and health equity. In a country like Bangladesh, the major goal of any development intervention is the alleviation of poverty. This is not surprising as a majority of the population live in abject poverty without equitable access and entitlement to basic minimum needs. Evaluations of such programmes have traditionally looked at their success in increasing the income levels of participants. Less attention has been paid to how far these successes are translated into improvements in various aspects of human well-being.

Bangladesh

Bangladesh broke away from Pakistan in 1971 to become an independent nation. The economy was wrecked and the infrastructure normally associated with nationhood did not exist. However, over the past several years, there have been many positive changes. Between 1975 and 1992 food production almost doubled (Government of Bangladesh, 1996); life expectancy increased by 30% between 1970 and 1996; and the under-five mortality rate decreased by 55% between 1960 and 1996 (UNICEF, 1998). Bangladesh has also achieved impressive results in many other fields. Immunization coverage reached over 70% in the early 1990s from a low of 2% in 1985, although recently it has started to decline (Chowdhury *et al.*, in press). The contraceptive prevalence rate has risen to nearly 50% from under 10% in the mid-1970s, and total fertility rate has declined from over 6 in the 1970s to 3.2 in the late 1990s (UNICEF, 1998). Net enrolment in primary schools has increased to 77% and the gender gap has all but disappeared (Chowdhury *et al.*, 1999). In terms of poverty alleviation, government and non-governmental organizations (NGOs) have made significant progress: micro-credit programmes now serve nearly seven million families, more than half of the country's 12 million poor households (Abed, 1999). Based on the direct calorie intake method the percentage of poor households has declined from 63% in 1983 to 47% in 1995 (Bangladesh Bureau of Statistics, 1997).

Despite these impressive strides, Bangladesh remains one of the world's poorest nations. In the World Bank's new system of measuring the wealth of nations, Bangladesh ranks eighteenth from the bottom among 123 countries (World Bank, 1998). Per capita income has grown but at the very slow rate of only 2% a year, and is currently only US$280. This and other socio-demographic information about Bangladesh are provided in Table 16.1.

Table 16.1 Bangladesh in statistics

Population (1996)	126 million
Density (population per sq. km)	850
Human Development Index rank (1998)	147
Population growth rate (%) (1980–96)	1.9
Life expectancy (years) (1995)	
Female	57.0
Male	56.9
Infant mortality (1996)	83
Adult literacy (%) (1995)	
Female	26.1
Male	49.4
Primary school net enrolment rate (1998)	77
GNP per capita (1998)	US$280
Under-weight children under age 5 (1990–1997)	56

Source: UNDP, 1998; UNICEF, 1998; Chowdhury *et al.*, 1999

BRAC: from relief work to development and poverty alleviation

In Bangladesh the constitutional responsibility for development of the country rests with the government. However, it has not always performed this role to its full potential. This is particularly true in the area of poverty alleviation. The history of poverty alleviation efforts in Bangladesh dates back to the early days of Pakistan in the 1950s, when programmes such as the 'green revolution' and the establishment of the Bangladesh (then Pakistan) Academy of Rural Development in Comilla were initiated. However, such efforts did not make any significant dent in poverty.

The War of Liberation in 1971 raised new expectations and provided fresh impetus to create a just and poverty-free Bangladesh. The non-governmental organizations (NGOs), which were born in the aftermath of the War for relief and rehabilitation operations, started involving themselves in this task and the relatively unknown field of development. BRAC was one such organization.

BRAC was set up in 1972 as a response to humanitarian need following Independence. Its objectives at the time were reflected in its initial name: Bangladesh Rehabilitation Assistance Committee. However, it became clear early on to the leaders in BRAC that relief work was a short-term measure, given the multiple problems that the people faced. There was a shift in the objectives of the organization from addressing the 'acute crisis' of the aftermath of the War to dealing with the 'persistent crisis' of development. In keeping with this change, the organization was renamed the 'Bangladesh Rural Advancement Committee', which since 1996 has been simply known as 'BRAC'.

Over the years BRAC has grown exponentially in developmental innovation and scale. Considerable experience has been gained; some experiments were successful but others failed. Perhaps the most important lesson learned by BRAC has been that there is no fix-all strategy or blueprint for development and that only through constant learning and adaptation could it effectively serve the poor. Further details about BRAC's early experiences are available elsewhere (Chowdhury and Chowdhury, 1978; Chen, 1983; Lovell, 1992; Chowdhury and Cash, 1996; Abed and Chowdhury, 1997).

BRAC programmes today

BRAC is now the world's largest NGO in terms of the scale and diversity of its interventions. Table 16.2 presents the scale of current BRAC programmes. One of the initial activities which earned national coverage and international attention was its oral rehydration therapy (ORT) programme for diarrhoea. During the 1980s hundreds of female BRAC workers visited households in 95% of the country's villages to instruct mothers how to prepare ORT with home ingredients. ORT has now become a part of the Bangladeshi culture (Chowdhury and

Table 16.2 Some basic facts about BRAC (May 1999)

Full-time staff	23,978
Part-time staff	33,746
Participants in poverty alleviation programme	2.9 million households
Amount of loan disbursed to the poor	US$ 700 million
Percentage of loans repaid	98%
Amount saved by Village Organization members	US$ 65 million
Total primary schools run by BRAC	34,517
Total school students enrolled	1.1 million (70% girls)
Mothers taught oral rehydration for diarrhoea	13 million
Total budget (annual)	US$ 131 million
Villages with BRAC poverty alleviation programme	50,000
Number of field offices	800
Number of districts with BRAC programme	64 (out of 64)

Cash, 1993). The current health programme provides essential health services to villagers with emphasis on women's health and specific diseases such as tuberculosis, through village-based voluntary health workers (Chowdhury et al., 1997; Chowdhury, 1999).

The education programme runs over 34,000 primary schools outside the formal state system for 1.1 million pupils. Seventy per cent of the BRAC school attendees are girls and come from the poorest sections of the community, to whom the formal public sector schools are least accessible. The effectiveness of the BRAC schools in terms of dropout, attendance, achievement, and costs is very high (Chabot et al., 1993; Chowdhury et al., 1999).

The other BRAC programme, which is the main focus of the present chapter, is the Rural Development Programme (RDP). RDP is the primary poverty alleviation effort of BRAC. It is active in over 50,000 of Bangladesh's 84,000 villages and involves nearly three million poor women, representing as many families. The twin goals of BRAC, poverty alleviation and empowerment of women, are reflected in the activities and strategies of the RDP. Poverty is looked at from a holistic viewpoint; it is characterized not only in terms of insufficient income or an absence of employment opportunities but as a complex syndrome which manifests itself in many different forms. In the words of Amartya Sen (1995), 'The point is not the irrelevance of economic variables such as personal incomes, but their severe inadequacy in capturing many of the causal influences on the quality of life and the survival chances of people.'

Along with income and employment generation, BRAC helps in forming organizations of the poor, conscientization and awareness raising, gender equity, and human resource development training. The logic of these programmes is the creation of an 'enabling environment' in which the poor can participate in their own development and in improving the quality of their lives (see Fig. 16.1).

The RDP works through a process of social mobilization, delivery of inputs,

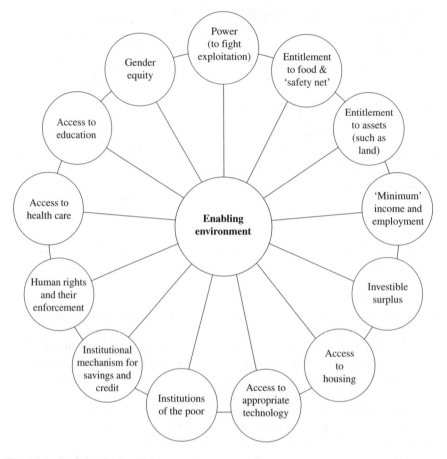

Fig. 16.1 Deficiencies leading to poverty
Source: Chowdhury and Alam, 1998

and creation of an environment of choice for the poor. Like most other poverty alleviation programmes in Bangladesh (Schuler and Hashemi, 1994; Pitt and Khandker, 1996), BRAC defines the rural poor as those having half an acre of land or less. The process of social mobilization in a village starts with the identification of those who fulfil this definition of the poor. As soon as an adequate number of eligible individuals show definite interest, an institution of the poor, called a village organization (VO), is formed. In Bangladesh about half of the households would fall into the BRAC eligibility criteria and about 30 to 40% of those eligible in the villages where BRAC has a presence have so far joined the VOs. The emphasis on gender has changed over time in BRAC: in the 1990s most VOs formed were composed of women only. A VO has 40 to 50 members, but it can start functioning with as few as 20 members.

Once a VO is established, two activities start simultaneously: a programme to raise consciousness and awareness and one for compulsory savings. Through the consciousness-raising programme, the women are made aware of the society around them; they analyse the reasons for the existing exploitative socio-economic and political system and what they could do to change it in their favour. A formal course on human rights and legal education (HRLE) is provided for members, covering constitutional and citizens' rights, and family, inheritance, and land law (Rafi *et al.*, in press). Members also participate in a compulsory savings scheme which has a minimum level of 5 Taka (10 US cents) per week. Savings are considered (by BRAC and group members) as a form of old age security.

The educational process occurs in a variety of situations: weekly and monthly meetings of the VO, training programmes at different centres outside the community, and the continuous interactions that take place between the VO members and BRAC staff, from organizing meetings to disbursement and collection of loans. In each VO, members are trained by BRAC in different trades. Thus one member may be trained as a village health worker, and another as a poultry vaccinator. These cadres cater to the need of VO members and also sell their services to other villagers for a small fee.

Within a month of formation, VO members are allowed to apply for BRAC loans on an individual basis. Three types of credit are disbursed. The members may request credit for:

- any traditional activity such as rural trading, transport (boat and rickshaw), and rice processing;
- a non-traditional activity such as grocery shop and rural restaurant management, or technology-based activity such as raising poultry, sericulture, or mechanized irrigation; or
- housing loans.

Interest on a housing loan is 10%, while for other activities it is 15%. The impressively high proportion of loans that are repaid (98%) is the result of a combination of members' consciousness, peer group pressure, and BRAC staff supervision.

An important feature of poverty alleviation activities is that an attempt is made to create a 'backward and forward linkage' for most of the technology-based activities. For example, in the case of poultry programmes, BRAC starts by providing training to women on how to rear high yielding varieties of chickens. Loans are given for operating a low-cost hatchery to supply day-old chicks to other village women. The women then rear these chicks until they start laying eggs. The eggs are then sold to the hatchery as well as to consumers. One of the major problems of poultry rearing in Bangladesh is the high mortality of the birds. The government livestock department keeps stock of vaccines but these are very much under-used. A VO member is trained to vaccinate poultry, and she is then linked to the local livestock department of the government which supplies vaccines. After receiving the vaccine, the VO member inoculates village chickens for a small fee. The woman increases her own income and ensures survival of her neighbours' chickens. Similar backward and forward linkages have been established for other programmes such as sericulture, where BRAC has established a highly successful marketing outlet for the producers through a shop-chain called *Aarong*.

Who joins BRAC?

From the beginning BRAC has recognized and taken account of the existing socio-economic stratification in the rural society and as a consequence has taken an approach that targeted only the poor and the women (Chen, 1983; Lovell, 1992). The definition of the poor (i.e. owning half an acre of land or less) was a functional one, but other characteristics, such as whether family members sold their manual labour for survival (a very low status occupation in Bangladesh), were also considered in choosing VO members. It became evident that among the 'poor' (as defined through the BRAC criteria), there were further stratifications; there were the extreme poor who belonged to households headed by a woman (where there was no male member or the male member(s) were invalids), households having neither land nor homestead, and the marginal or moderate poor who are better off than the extreme poor.

Several studies have examined the composition of the VO members in terms of their economic status, and have confirmed that the majority of the members belonged to the target group defined by BRAC. Members coming from outside the target group varied from 11% in a large population-based survey (Evans *et al.*, 1999) to 20% in a 'national' study (Mustafa *et al.*, 1996), to 29% found in a sub-district (Zaman, 1996). While Evans and colleagues used rapid rural appraisals (RRA) with 'wealth ranking', the other two studies utilized questionnaire survey methods.

There has been particular concern about the composition of the groups involved in the BRAC micro-credit based poverty alleviation programmes, specifically whether or not the poorest VO members were included. Hulme and Mosely (1996) estimated that the poorest 20% of the population were excluded from micro-credit programmes. Montgomery *et al.* (1996), in their study of the BRAC programme, estimated that 20% of the BRAC membership came from the very poor and vulnerable group, and 15% from outside the target group. Evans *et al.* (1999) developed a conceptual framework that examined the barriers to participation in micro-credit programmes. These included programme-related barriers (such as insufficient supply of micro-credit, membership requirements, peer group expectations, and institutional incentives) and client-related barriers (such as insufficient resources, ill-health or vulnerability to crisis, female head of household, lack of education, and individual and household preferences). This framework was used to analyse the BRAC programme using a large population-based survey of 24,234 households using RRA. Their conclusions were based on the data reproduced in Table 16.3. From these results they concluded that poorer households were more likely to be BRAC members compared to non-poor or less poor. They found that although the VO membership did include some people outside of the target groups, the overwhelming majority were poor as defined by BRAC and the share of the poorest of the poor in VOs was greater than their proportion of the population. As all the village poor are not included in the VO (a VO consists of 40–50 members whereas a typical village would consist of about 100 poor households), the Evans *et al.* study hypothesized a 'natural selection' mechanism through which households with more credit-worthiness ended-up being differentially enrolled as members. Rutherford (1993) in his study of the Grameen Bank in Bangladesh stressed the problem of 'self exclusion', and suggested that the ritual of membership such as rigid attendance in meetings and forced savings enhanced the 'fears and timidities' of the extreme poor, including widows and women household heads.

Impact of BRAC programmes on health and equity

The remaining parts of this chapter concentrate on the evidence of BRAC's programmes actually having an impact on welfare and health. Although BRAC works all over Bangladesh, the data for the present analysis came mostly from one sub-district called Matlab, the field station of the International Centre for Diarrhoeal Disease Research, Bangladesh (ICDDR,B), located 50 kilometres south of Dhaka city in a riverine area of Chandpur district. The ICDDR,B has maintained this surveillance area since 1963 and the many studies conducted there on demographics and action research attest to its world-wide reputation (D'Souza, 1984; van Ginneken *et al.*, 1998).

In 1992, BRAC started its Rural Development Programme in Matlab. The inputs introduced in the villages included: VO formation and organization of the poor, micro-credit, training of VO members on human and legal rights, and skills, and non-formal primary education for children. In 75 villages a total of 164 VOs were formed with 6,736 members (all women), covering over half of the

Table 16.3   BRAC VO membership status by wealth group

	Wealth group			
	1	2	3	n
VO membership (%)	11	28	61	5,535
Population (%)	24	27	49	24,234

Note: Group 1: Food secure; own >0.5 acre of land (well-off).
        Group 2: Periodic food insecurity; own <0.5 acre of land (moderate poor).
        Group 3: Chronically food insecure; own <0.5 acre of land (poorest of the poor).
Source: Evans *et al.*, 1999

villages' poor households. Since 1993 BRAC village organization members have saved over US$300,000 and the sum of US$2.8 million has been disbursed to them as loans with a 99.7% recovery rate. In addition BRAC opened 81 non-formal schools which enrolled 2,658 students. In the period up to 1998 4,098 students had completed the three-year cycle of education (70% girls) and 94% gained entry to the formal government primary schools.

Evaluation design

Given the availability of reliable individual level data, BRAC and ICDDR,B initiated a research project to examine the impact of the development-related activities on the health and well-being of the population, which became known as the BRAC-ICDDR,B Joint Research Project.

A four-cell research design was followed with villages being divided into those that had:

- only BRAC inputs;
- only ICDDR,B inputs;
- both BRAC and ICDDR,B inputs; or
- no interventions (Chowdhury *et al.*, 1995).

Except for the minimal government development programmes, which are thinly spread, no other significant development programme operated in the area (Khan *et al.*, 1997).

The data used in the present analysis came from the following sources:

- *Baseline survey.* Prior to BRAC's interventions in 1992, a survey of over 12,000 households (pop. over 60,000) in villages belonging to the above four cells collected quantitative information on assets, expenditures, education, nutritional status, health seeking behaviour, women's empowerment, family planning, and involvement with development activities.

- *Seasonal surveys.* Three rounds of seasonal surveys were carried out in a sub-sample of the baseline population in 1995–6. These collected the same information as at baseline (see above).

- *Ethnographic surveys.* Several ethnographic and other qualitative investigations were carried out using in-depth interview, focus group discussion, and observations focusing on women's status and intra-household food distribution.

- *Demographic surveillance data.* The Demographic Surveillance System (DSS) of ICDDR,B provided mortality information on all households in the villages under study. ICDDR,B routinely collects the following information on a monthly basis: births, deaths, in- and out-migration, and marriage.

- *Management information.* BRAC maintains a Management Information System (MIS) for its projects. Information pertaining to the inputs received from BRAC, such as date of joining, amount of loan received, etc., for households joining the BRAC programme was linked with the DSS information.

The concept of human well-being

A major objective of the research was to study the impact of BRAC on human well-being, which was defined as a concept with seven dimensions as shown in Fig. 16.2. Hypothetical pathways linking the BRAC programme inputs with each of the dimensions were delineated and were addressed through the research. Table 16.4 shows the conceptual framework linking the inputs with the expected impact.

In this chapter we examine the programme impact on nutritional status and mortality and relate the findings to some of the hypothetical pathways (process). The analyses compared the following three groups:

• women who joined BRAC (BRAC members);

• poor eligible women who didn't join BRAC (poor non-members); and

• non-poor women not eligible to join BRAC (non-poor non-members).

Household and individual level data have been compared between the above groups and between 1992 and 1995. Further analyses based on the four cells of the research design are currently in progress.

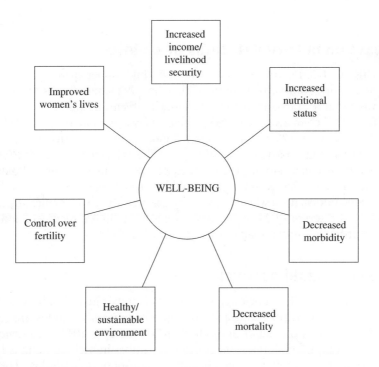

Fig. 16.2 Seven dimensions of human well-being
Source: Chowdhury *et al.*, 1995

Table 16.4   The conceptual frame linking expected impacts with inputs of BRAC in Matlab, Bangladesh

Input	Process	Health Impact
Institution building	Feeling of self-worth	Nutritional status
Children's education	Literate self and children	Intra-family food allocation
Adult's education on human and legal rights	Better skills	Fertility (level, age at marriage, birth spacing)
Training (skill & human development)	More income employment savings & assets	Morbidity (type, transmission complications, resistance to infection)
Savings and credit	Control over income assets	Mortality (level, cause)

Health services:
 • BRAC
 • ICDDR,B
   –Surveillance
   –MCH-FP
	Less hunger
	 Access to and utilization of 'modern' health care	

Source: Chowdhury *et al.*, 1995

Impact on nutritional status of children

The BRAC–ICDDR,B project collected mid–upper–arm circumference (MUAC) information at two points of time: in 1992 when the BRAC intervention was about to start and in 1995 when the intervention was about three years old. Table 16.5 compares the severe protein–energy malnutrition (PEM) (represented as MUAC < 125 mm) of children 6 months to 72 months of age according to their mothers' participation in BRAC. The prevalence of severe PEM has significantly declined among the children of BRAC member households, but there was no such change among the children of non-members.

The same information when analysed by gender showed a significantly higher prevalence of severe PEM in females among both BRAC members and poor non-members, but not among non-poor non-members.

Impact on child survival

Survival rates of children belonging to BRAC member households in comparison to poor non-member and non-poor non-member households are seen in Fig. 16.3. It shows that survival of children belonging to BRAC households is better than that for children from poor non-member households, and is in fact rather similar to survival of children from non-poor households. The pronounced survival advantage of children of poor members compared to poor

Table 16.5   Prevalence of severe PEM of children by BRAC membership status during pre (1992) and post (1995) intervention period

Malnutrition	1992 baseline poor individuals (*n*=827)	1995 BRAC Member (*n*=273)	1995 Poor non member (*n*=707)	1995 Non-poor non-members (*n*=538)	1 v. 2	1 v. 3
Severe PEM (MUAC<125 mm)	23.2	12.1	21.2	11.5	*p*<0.01	NS

Source: Khatun *et al.*, 1998*b*

non-members is seen for girls as well as boys (Fig. 16.4). It is striking that the survival advantage associated with BRAC membership among the poor was largely the result of mortality differences in the first few months of life, particularly in the neonatal period.

Food and family expenditure

The patterns in intra-family food distribution were explored through observations of a small sample of 25 households containing both girls and boys. It showed that among BRAC member households girls more commonly received equal treatment; boys were more favoured in terms of being given culturally preferred/superior parts of the fish, chicken, meat, etc. (Roy *et al.*, 1998).

In a separate assessment conducted in a larger geographic area, BRAC member households spent more overall and spent significantly more on consumption of food items than poor non-members (Table 16.6). Proportion of non-food expenditures, indicating the capacity of households to spend money

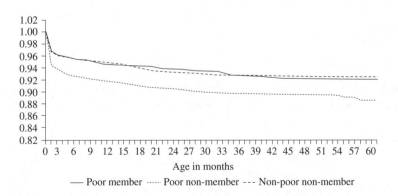

Age in months

—— Poor member ······ Poor non-member --- Non-poor non-member

Fig. 16.3   Life table probability of survival of children belonging to households of BRAC members, poor non-members, and non-poor non-members
Source: Bhuiya *et al.*, in press

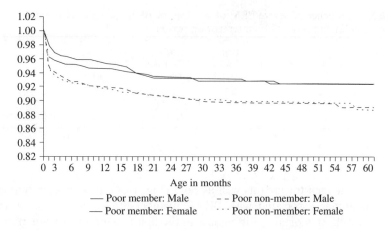

Fig. 16.4 Life table probability of survival of male and female children belonging to BRAC member, poor non-member, and non-poor non-member households

Table 16.6 Expenditure pattern of BRAC and non-BRAC sample households

	BRAC Length of membership (in months)					BRAC v. comp. (t value)
Expenditure pattern	1–11 (n=360)	12–47 (n=417)	48+ (n=295)	Total (n=1,072)	Comparison (n=223)	
Per capita monthly expenditure (Taka).	686	686	689	687	540	3.43***
% cereal to total food expenditure.	45.9	45.0	46.4	45.7	46.1	-0.26
% non-food to total expenditure.	37.9	35.4	34.2	35.9	32.4	3.57***
Per capita calorie.	2,279	2,304	2,342	2,306	2,182	3.37***

Note: *** $p<0.001$
Source: Husain, 1998

beyond food, was also greater among BRAC member households. Finally, the per capita calorie intake was also significantly higher in BRAC households.

Family planning

Table 16.7 shows that the current use of family planning methods was greater among the currently married BRAC members than among poor non-members ($p < 0.05$). BRAC members also had higher rates of use of family planning than the non-poor non-members.

Table 16.7   Current use of family planning by BRAC membership

BRAC membership	No. of respondents	Current FP use %
Member	500	57.0
Poor non-member	1,194	49.6
Non-poor non-member	1,088	51.3

Table 16.8   Distribution of children (11–15 years) achieving 'basic education' by membership status in 1992 and 1995

Sex	1992 Baseline poor individuals	1995 BRAC members	1995 Poor non-members	1995 Non-poor non-members
Girl	9.6 (188)	23.7 (152)	12.6 (340)	33.5 (337)
Boy	14.9 (215)	30.7 (163)	15.5 (330)	41.2 (381)
All	12.4 (403)	27.3 (315)	14.0 (670)	37.6 (718)

Figures within parentheses indicate the number of children.

Education

Table 16.8 shows the level of education achieved by children of 11–15 years old, at baseline in 1992 and then in 1995. Educational achievement was determined using a curriculum-independent competency test administered to children aged 11–15. A child satisfying a minimum level of competency in reading, writing, arithmetic, and life skills was considered to have 'basic education' (Chowdhury *et al.*, 1994). Educational performance improved for both member and non-member groups but the gain was much greater in the case of BRAC member households than poor non-member households and more in girls than boys.

Violence against women

The prevalence of self-reported violence against women has been studied. A total of 2,038 currently married women aged 15–55 years were interviewed with a structured questionnaire. Women were asked about occurrence of five types of violence in the previous four months:

- physical abuse;
- money taken against will;
- prevented from going to natal home;
- prevented from working outside; or
- jewellery taken against will.

In the present analysis we report only the incidence of physical violence. Table 16.9 compares the incidence of reported physical violence against women

Table 16.9 Occurrence of physical violence during last four months by BRAC membership, membership length, and membership depth, Matlab 1995

	Physical violence %
BRAC membership	
BRAC member (n=438)	8.9
Poor non-member (n=1550)	5.8
X^2 Significance	$p<.05$
Length of BRAC membership	
≤ 2 year (n=185)	10.8
2 + year (n=260)	7.3
X^2 Significance	NS
Depth of BRAC membership	
Poor non-member (n=1595)	5.6
Only savings (n=56)	5.4
Savings+credit (n=268)	11.2
Savings+credit+training (n=119)	3.4
X^2 Significance	$p<.01$

Source: Khan *et al.*, 1998

between BRAC member and non-member households. It shows a higher incidence of violence among BRAC members than among non-member households. When the incidence figures were analysed according to length and 'depth' of membership (Chen and Mahmud, 1995), however, the prevalence tended to decrease with increasing membership length. The peak in violence is reached when credit is introduced, but tapers off when other inputs, such as 'training' are offered.

Discussion

The stated objectives of BRAC are the alleviation of poverty and empowerment of the poor, particularly women, so as to reduce inequities between the rich and the poor, and between men and women. Whether existing development programmes, including those of BRAC, achieve this is a crucial question that donors, academics, and development specialists have all asked.

A large body of literature has emerged that attempts to examine the effect and impact of development interventions (Chowdhury *et al.*, 1991; Mustafa *et al.*, 1996; Pitt and Khandker, 1996; Husain, 1998). These studies usually examine how a programme delivers services, manages production, or trains participants. What is less well documented is their impact on human well-being as defined in the present study. The BRAC-ICDDR,B Joint Research Project in Matlab, Bangladesh, was designed specifically to examine such an impact.

Of the seven dimensions of human well-being identified by BRAC (Fig. 16.2), preliminary analyses relating to nutritional status and child survival have been presented. These data suggest that:

- there was a measurable improvement in terms of nutrition for the BRAC household members in comparison to a 'comparable' non-member group;
- child survival is better in BRAC households in comparison to that in poor households that did not belong to BRAC; and
- these differences in nutritional status and child survival were equally discernible for male and female members of BRAC households.

Two important questions arise. First, how can we explain these differences according to BRAC membership? Are they the result of the BRAC programmes or could they be artefacts due to selection bias in the recruitment process, whereby the 'poor' who become BRAC members are better off in a number of important ways at entry? Second, if the differences are due to BRAC programmes, what was the mechanism or pathway through which the interventions led to these improvements?

BRAC recruits poor women with a landholding of half an acre or less. Studies have documented that a certain proportion of BRAC and other NGO participants (between 11% and 29% in case of BRAC) come from a less poor group. There are several reasons why people from outside the target group are recruited. Participants may lie to field staff about their actual landholding at the time of joining or they may have improved their situation since joining. A recent study found that women who had joined BRAC for four years or more had each added ten decimals (1 acre = 100 decimals) to their landholding (Husain, 1998). The 'comparison' group selected for the present study conformed to the definition of BRAC membership. Zaman (1998) examined the background of the two groups in Matlab sub-district and found that 29% non-poor women were also VO members. When compared with members who actually conformed to the BRAC eligibility criteria (i.e. landholding of 0.5 acre or less), the comparison group had more land, assets, and number of earners in the family. Information presented in the text from other studies indicated that the majority of BRAC membership conformed to the eligibility criteria of BRAC and the share of the poorest of the poor in the village organizations was more than their proportion in the population. Nevertheless, researchers have speculated that there may still be a 'natural selection' mechanism that favours the more credit-worthy among the poor, thus allowing room for self selection (Evans et al., 1999).

Further studies to detect the possible presence of selection bias and its impact on the present results are being carried out. One analysis traced the mortality history of children belonging to BRAC and non-BRAC poor prior to 1992 when the intervention started, using the data available through the Demographic Surveillance System of ICDDR,B. Although both groups were similar prior to 1992 in mortality levels, the BRAC group children experienced a greater fall in mortality over the past seven years. Early results from an analysis of nutritional status data collected in 1992 and 1995 showed similar results. Evans et al.

(1999) noted that the women members who did not meet BRAC eligibility criteria but were inducted into VOs were the better-off poor but were not members of village élites. The mortality data presented in the text showed that the BRAC members were actually very close to the élites; even when the non-poor members were excluded from the analysis, the better performance of BRAC members persisted.

Most of the impact on mortality occurred during the neonatal period, yet most of the child survival technologies have their impact later in childhood. Something is happening to the women during pregnancy and/or during the birth process that is affecting neonates. One of the determinants could be psychological well-being. The initial analyses of a study showed that BRAC members' psychological well-being was marginally higher (Khatun *et al.*, 1998*a*). Research is under way to understand this phenomenon better.

Figure 16.2 suggested the various factors that could affect well-being. One of these was improved nutritional status. In BRAC participant households, the intra-family allocation of food is more equitable, although there is still the tendency to favour boys. The average calorie consumption is higher among BRAC participants. The per capita monthly expenditure is greater, as is the proportion of the expenditure spent on food. BRAC women were greater users of family planning methods, which may have given them a longer time between pregnancies and opportunity to participate in micro-credit financed income-generating activities. The increased violence against women that occurs in the earlier phases of the BRAC was reduced over time when credit was accompanied by other inputs such as human development and skill training. When a woman receives a loan, a new transaction and relationship emerges in her own and her extended family. A small amount of money works as a miracle in a cash-hungry society, and significantly raises the woman's power in the family (Zaman, 1998; Schuler *et al.*, 1996). Not all men are ready to accept this new power relationship and some may resort to violence to express their anger. The changes in women's economic role within the family may initially be met with resistance or resentment, and in extreme cases with violence (Khan *et al.*, 1998). Other studies have also documented reduced incidence of violence in households that are served by micro-credit programmes (Hadi, 1997). However, we also need to be somewhat cautious in accepting and interpreting this information. It may be that BRAC members, because of their increased awareness, report more details of their marital life.

Improvement in the level of basic education of children is dramatic, and more so in girls than boys. This might be expected, as BRAC schools discriminate positively in favour of girls. In recent years, there have been improvements in performance of basic education at the national level as well (Chowdhury *et al.*, 1999) and this are reflected in Matlab.

These observations provide evidence to support the following conclusions:

• poverty alleviation programmes focused on women as implemented by

BRAC are effective in improving well-being, particularly in the areas of child-hood nutrition and mortality;

• these impacts could be partially explained by other effects that take place as a result of BRAC's intervention; and

• there are indications that the BRAC programme has been successful in reducing inequity in health between the non-poor and poor.

BRAC is now one of the largest NGOs in the world. It is also one of the oldest development organizations in the developing world. BRAC's philosophy of 'learning from doing' has bestowed it with many successes. Several of its programmes have been replicated all over the country by itself and by others. For example, BRAC's non-formal primary education (NFPE) programme is being implemented by over 250 local NGOs in Bangladesh, in addition to BRAC itself. Many of the approaches and methods developed by BRAC are also now used by the government. Based on BRAC's pilot programme on nutritional supplementation in Muktagacha sub-district (Chowdhury *et al.*, 1998), the government is implementing this in 60 other sub-districts of the country with World Bank assistance. Some BRAC approaches have been adapted for use in several countries of Asia and Africa. BRAC's NFPE strategy has now been implemented, with local amendments, in Ethiopia, Uganda, Pakistan, and India (Kaur, 1997).

Acknowledgements

The BRAC-ICDDR,B Research Project is the result of the joint effort of many. Professor Demissie Habte, the former Director of ICDDR,B and Mr. F.H. Abed, the Executive Director of BRAC were the prime movers and provided all support. A large team of researchers was involved, which included Alayne Adams, Amina Mahbub, Gulrukh Selim, Hassan Zaman, M. Jahangir, Kit Vaughan, Mahmuda Khan, Maliha Mayeed, M. Mannan, Masud Rana, Masuma Khatun, Mehnaz Momen, Mohsena Khatun, M. Mohsin, Momena Islam, Monirul Khan, Syed Masud Ahmed, H. Nasreen, Parul Biswas, Rafiquddoulah, Rita Das Roy, Sabah Tarannum, Sabina Rashid, Sabrina Rasheed, Saira Ansary, Samiha Huda, Shahrier Khan, Simeen Mahmud, and Ziauddin Hyder; the large number of working papers and other papers that have come out of the project were done by them. Besides, others provided crucial support at various stages, including Aminul Alam, R. Bairagi, Ian Scott, Jane Menken, Jim Ross, John Cleland, Kim Streatfield, Lincoln Chen, Marty Chen, Patrick Vaughan, Pertti Pelto, Pierre Claquin, Richard Cash, Sadia Chowdhury, Salehuddin Ahmed, A. M. Sardar, Tim Evans, Wahiduddin Mahmud, M. Yunus, and the staff of DSS and BRAC at Matlab. Besides BRAC and ICDDR,B, various donors provided generous financial support to this project, including the Ford Foundation, Aga Khan Foundation, and the US Agency for

International Development. The authors also wish to express their special thanks to Richard Cash for his editorial help.

REFERENCES

Abed FH. *Development lecture 1999*. Amsterdam, University of Amsterdam, 1999 (unpublished)

Abed FH, Chowdhury AMR. How BRAC learned to meet rural people's needs through local action. In: Krishina A, Uphoff N, Esman M (eds) *Reasons for hope: instructive experiences in rural development*. West Hartford: Kumarian Press, 1997

Bangladesh Bureau of Statistics. *Bangladesh Household Expenditure Survey 1995–96*. Dhaka: 1997

Bhuiya A, Chowdhury AMR, Ahmed F, Adams A. *Gender and socio-economic inequality in childhood mortality in rural Bangladesh: recent trends and impact of health and poverty alleviation programmes*. Global Health Equity Initiative, New York, The Rockefeller Foundation (in press)

Chabot C, Ahmed M, Pande R, Joshi A. *Primary education for all. Learning from the BRAC experiences*. Washington DC: Academy for Educational Development, 1993

Chen MA. *A quiet revolution: women in transition in rural Bangladesh*. Rochester: Shenkman Books, 1983

Chen M, Mahmud S. *Assessing change in women's lives: a conceptual framework*. Joint Research Project working paper No. 2. Dhaka: BRAC-ICDDR,B, 1995

Chowdhury AMR. Success with the DOTS strategy. *Lancet*, 1999; **353**:1003–4

Chowdhury AMR, Alam A. BRAC's poverty alleviation efforts: a quarter century of experiences. In: Wood G, Sharif I (eds) *Who needs credit? Poverty and finance in Bangladesh*. London: Zed Books, 1998

Chowdhury AMR, Cash RA. Cultural incorporation of the ORT message. *Lancet*, 1993; **34**:1591

Chowdhury AMR, Cash RA *A simple solution: teaching millions to treat diarrhoea at home*. Dhaka: University Press Ltd., 1996

Chowdhury AMR, Mahmud M, Abed FH. Credit for the rural poor: the case of BRAC in Bangladesh. *Small enterprise development*, 1991; **2(3)**:4–13

Chowdhury AMR, Ziegahn L, Haque N, Shrestha GL, Ahmed Z. Assessing basic competences: a practical methodology. *International Review of Education*, 1994; **40**:437–54

Chowdhury AMR, Bhuiya A, Vaughan P, Adams A, Mahmud S. *Effects of socio-economic development on health status and human well-being: determining impact and exploring pathways of change*. Proposals for phase II of the BRAC-ICDDR,B Matlab joint project 1996–2000 AD. BRAC-ICDDR,B Working Paper No. 6, 1995

Chowdhury AMR, Chowdhury S, Islam MN, Islam A, Vaughan JP. Control of tuberculosis by community health workers in Bangladesh. *Lancet*, 1997; **350**:169–72

Chowdhury AMR, Mahmud Z, Chowdhury S, Hyder Z. *Muktagacha: a targeted nutrition project in Bangladesh*. Paper Prepared for the UN Food and Agricultural Organization, Rome, 1998

Chowdhury AMR, Chowdhury RK, Nath SR. *Hope not complacency: state of primary education in Bangladesh*. Dhaka: Compaign for Population Education and University Press Limited, 1999

Chowdhury AMR, Aziz, KMA, Bhuiya, A (eds). *The near miracle revisited: social science perspectives of immunization programmes in Bangladesh*. Amsterdam: University van Amsterdam (in press)

Chowdhury FI, Chowdhury AMR. Use pattern of oral contraceptives in rural Bangladesh. *Bangladesh Development Studies*, 1978 (monsoon)

D'Souza S. Small area-intensive studies for understanding morbidity process: two models from Bangladesh—the Matlab project and the Companigonj health project. In: United Nations *Data bases for mortality measurement. Papers of the Meeting of the United Nations /World Health Organization Working Group on Data Bases for Measurement of Levels, Trend and Differentials, in Mortality, Bangkok, 20–23 October 1981*. New York: United Nations Department of International Economic and Social Affairs, 1984, pp 146–58

Evans TG, Adams AM, Mohammed R, Norris AH. Demystifying participation in micro-credit; a population based analysis. *World Development*, 1999; **27**:419–30

Government of Bangladesh. *Bangladesh food and agriculture*. Country position paper. World Food Summit (Italy), Ministry of Agriculture, 1996

Hadi A. *Household violence against women in rural Bangladesh*. Watch Report No. 27. Dhaka: BRAC, 1997

Hulme D, Mosely P. *Finance against poverty*, Vol. 1. London: Routledge, 1996

Husain AMM. *Poverty alleviation and empowerment*. Dhaka: BRAC, 1998

Kaur G. *The daunting challenge*. New Delhi: Oxfam America, 1997

Khan MI, Chowdhury AMR, Bhuiya A. *An inventory of the development programmes by government and non-governmental organizations in Matlab*. Joint Research Project working paper No. 17. Dhaka, BRAC-ICDDR,B, 1997

Khan MR *et al. Domestic violence against women: does development intervention matter?* Joint Project working paper No. 28. Dhaka: BRAC-ICDDR,B, 1998

Khatun M, Wadud N, Bhuiya A, Chowdhury AMR. *Psychological well-being of rural women; developing measurement tools*. Joint Research Project working paper No. 23. Dhaka: BRAC-ICDDR,B, 1998*a*

Khatun M *et al. Women's involvement in BRAC development activities and child nutrition*. Joint Project working paper No. 30. Dhaka: BRAC-ICDDR,B, 1998*b*

Lovell CH. *Breaking the cycle of poverty: the BRAC strategy*. West Hartford: Kumarian Press, 1992

Montgomery R, Bhattacharya D, Hulme D. Credit for the poor in Bangladesh. In: Hulme D, Mosley P (eds) *Finance against poverty*, Vol. 2. London: Routledge, 1996, pp 94–176

Mustafa S, Ara I, Banu D *et al. Beacon of hope: an impact assessment study of BRAC Rural Development Programme*. Dhaka: BRAC, 1996

Pitt MM, Khandker SR. *Household and intra household impact of the Grameen Bank and similar targeted credit programs in Bangladesh*. Discussion paper 320. Washington DC: The World Bank, 1996

Rafi M, Hulme D, Chowdhury AMR. The poor and the law: BRAC's Human Rights and Legal Education Programme. *Economic and Political Weekly* (in press)

Roy RD *et al. Does involvement of women in BRAC influence sex bias in intra-household food distribution?* Joint Project working paper No. 25. Dhaka: BRAC-ICDDR,B, 1998

Rutherford S. *Alternative credit systems*. Manila: Asian Development Bank, 1993 (unpublished).

Schuler SR, Hashemi SM. Credit programs, women's empowerment, and contraceptive use in rural Bangladesh. *Studies in Family Planning*, 1994; **25**:65–76

Schuler SR, Hashemi SM, Riley AP, Akhter S. Credit programs, patriarchy and men's violence against women in rural Bangladesh. *Social Science and Medicine*, 1996; **43**:1729–42

Sen A. *Mortality as an indicator of economic success and failure*. London: London School of Economics, The Development Economics Research Programme, 1995

United Nations Development Programme. *Human Development Report*. Oxford: Oxford University Press, 1998

UNICEF. *State of the World's Children 1998*. Oxford: Oxford University Press, 1998

van Ginneken J, Bairagi R, de Francisco A, Sardar AM, Vaughan P. *Health and demographic surveillance in Matlab: past, present and future*. Special Publication No. 72. Dhaka: International Centre for Diarrhoeal Disease Research, Bangladesh, 1998

World Bank. *World Development Report 1998: knowledge for development*. New York: Oxford University Press, 1998

Zaman H. *Microcredit programmes: who participates and to what extent*. Joint Project working paper No. 12. Dhaka: BRAC-ICDDR,B, 1996

Zaman H. *The links between BRAC inputs and 'empowerment correlates' in Matlab*. Joint Research Project working paper No. 28. Dhaka, BRAC-ICDDR,B, 1998

17 Economic progress and health*

Amartya Sen

About a decade ago, I was attending a conference in Helsinki on the quality of life, when I found myself listening to a wonderfully eloquent speech by a social anthropologist of great distinction—well-known for his powerful defence of cultural relativism. Fundamental values, we were told, are typically very different in different cultures. 'For example,' said the relativist champion of Indian cultural uniqueness, 'while in the West people are worried about death, not so in India.' The temptation to jump up and record a mild dissent was strong, but I was sure that this would have appeared to be 'un-Indian' behaviour—perhaps even more shocking than the heretical belief that Indians too often worry about death. There must, I supposed, be some Indians who have never been worried about death, but I had to confess that I have not met many of them yet.

In fact, that remark made me recollect some of the earliest readings in Sanskrit I had done as a child. A particularly striking passage concerned a conversation, reported in *Brihadaranyaka Upanishad*, from around the eighth century BC, between Maitreyee and her husband Yajnavalkya. They were very learned people, but they were caught discussing a subject of rather common interest: the earning of money, a subject that has not lost any of its captivating power in nearly the last three thousand years. Interestingly, the conversation between Maitreyee and Yajnavalkya moves rapidly to a subject that is, I think, of special interest to readers of this volume, and more specifically to the subject on which I have been asked to write: 'economic progress and health'. As reported in that Sanskrit text, Maitreyee and Yajnavalkya did not linger very long on the ways and means of earning more money, and proceeded with commendable speed to a much deeper issue: *how far does wealth go to help a person get what he or she wants?* (*Brihadaranyaka Upanishad*, 1965).

Maitreyee wonders whether it could be the case that if 'the whole earth, full of wealth' were to belong to her ('just to me'), she could achieve immortality through it. 'No,' responds Yajnavalkya, 'like the life of rich people will be your

* Some of the issues investigated here are also discussed in my keynote address to the World Health Assembly (1999*b*).

life. But there is no hope of immortality by wealth.' Maitreyee remarked, 'What should I do with that by which I do not become immortal?'

Two perspectives

The rhetorical question from the learned and spirited Maitreyee has been cited again and again in Indian religious philosophy to illustrate both the limitations of the material world and the nature of the human predicament. I am too distant from other-worldly matters to be led there by Maitreyee's worldly frustration, but there is another aspect of this exchange that is of rather immediate interest to economics and to assessing the relation between economic progress, on the one hand, and health and longevity, on the other. This concerns the relation between incomes and achievements, between our economic wealth and our ability to live as long and as well as we would like. While there is a connection between opulence and the achievements, the linkage may or may not be very strong. More importantly, the force of the connection may be extremely contingent on other circumstances, including social policy, which may have a profound influence on our capabilities to live really long (without being cut off in one's prime) and to have a good and healthy life while alive (rather than a life of illness and misery)—things that would be strongly valued and desired by nearly all of us (including, I dare say, Indians).

Indeed, the gap between the two perspectives (that is, between an exclusive concentration on economic progress, and a broader focus on the lives we can lead) is not only a major issue in the conceptualization of development, it has been a crucial concern in the understanding of the nature of personal success and the requirements of a good society. As Aristotle noted at the very beginning of the *Nicomachean ethics*: 'wealth is evidently not the good we are seeking; for it is merely useful and for the sake of something else' (1980).

Deprivation of African Americans: an illustration

Even in terms of the connection between mortality and income (a subject with which Maitreyee was directly concerned), it is remarkable that the extent of deprivation for particular groups in very rich countries can be comparable to that in the so-called 'Third World'. For example, in the US, African Americans as a group have no higher—indeed have a lower—chance of reaching advanced ages than do people born in the immensely poorer economies of China or the Indian state of Kerala (or in Sri Lanka, Jamaica or Costa Rica).[1]

Figures 17.1 and 17.2 present the proportions surviving to different ages over the lives respectively of American whites, African Americans, Indians in Kerala, and the Chinese, in the early 1990s. Even though the income per capita of African Americans in the US is considerably lower than that of the American white population, they are, of course, very many times richer in income terms than the people of China or Kerala (even after correcting for cost-of-living

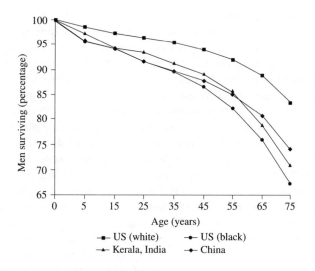

Fig. 17.1 Variations in male survival rates by region
Sources: United States, 1991–3: US Department of Health and Human Services, *Health United States 1995*, (Hyattsville, Md., National Center for Health Statistics, 1996); Kerala, 1991: Government of India, *Sample registration system: fertility and mortality indicators 1991* (New Delhi: Office of the Registrar General, 1991); China, 1992: World Health Organization, *World Health Statistics Annual 1994* (Geneva: World Health Organization, 1994)

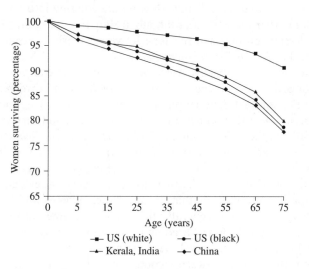

Fig. 17.2 Variations in female survival rates by region

differences). In this context, the comparison of survival prospects of African Americans *vis-à-vis* those of the very much poorer Chinese, or Indians in Kerala, is of particular interest. African Americans tend to do better in terms of survival at low age groups (especially in terms of infant mortality) *vis-à-vis* the Chinese or the Indians, but the picture changes over the years.

It turns out, in fact, that Chinese men and those in Kerala in India decisively outlive American black men in terms of surviving to older age groups. Furthermore, even African American women end up having a similar survival pattern for the higher ages as the much poorer Chinese, and decidedly lower survival rates than the even poorer Indians in Kerala. It is, of course, well-known that American blacks suffer from *relative deprivation* in terms of income per head, *vis-à-vis* American whites, but it turns out that they are also *absolutely* more deprived than the low-income Indians in Kerala (for both women and men), and the Chinese (in the case of men), in terms of living to ripe, old ages. The causal influences on these contrasts (that is, between living standards judged by income per head and those judged by the ability to survive to higher ages), which have been discussed more fully in my book *Development as freedom* (1999a), include social arrangements and community relations such as medical coverage, public health care, elementary education, law and order, and prevalence of violence, among other influences.[2]

The approach of human development

This example is striking enough, but it would be legitimate to ask how common, how widespread is such a dissonance between economic means and the human ends of good health and good living. Here we are entering into a territory that rightfully belongs to my late friend, Mahbub ul Haq, from Pakistan. Through his visionary leadership, problems of this type got very extensively explored over the last decade in the *Human Development Reports* of the United Nations Development Programme. The respective viewpoints of economic prosperity and of health and longevity can provide very contrary pictures and divergent rankings of countries. The contrast between purely economic achievement and indicators of human development (including those related to health and survival) has been well documented in the series of annual *Human Development Reports*.

How deep a contrast is this? The point is sometimes made that, while the rankings of longevity and per capita income are not congruent, nevertheless if we take the rough with the smooth, then there is plenty of evidence in inter-country comparisons to indicate that, by and large, income and life expectancy move together. From that generalization, some commentators have been tempted to take the quick step of arguing that economic progress is the real key to enhancing health and longevity. Indeed, it has been argued that it is a mistake to worry about the discord between income-achievements and survival chances since, in general, the statistical connection between them is observed to be quite close. Is this statistical point correct, and does it sustain the general inference that is being drawn?

Life expectancy and per capita GNP

The point about inter-country statistical connections, seen in isolation, is indeed correct, but we need further scrutiny of this statistical relation before it can be seen as a convincing ground for taking income to be the basic determinant of health and longevity and for dismissing the relevance of social arrangements (going beyond income-based opulence).

It is interesting, in this context, to refer to some statistical analyses presented by Sudhir Anand and Martin Ravillion (1993). On the basis of inter-country comparisons, they find that life expectancy does indeed have a significantly positive correlation with GNP per head, but that this relationship works mainly through the impact of GNP on (1) the incomes specifically of the poor; and (2) public expenditure, particularly in health care. In fact, once these two variables are included on their own in the statistical exercise, little extra explanation can be obtained from including GNP per head as an additional causal influence. Indeed, with poverty and public expenditure on health as explanatory variables on their own, the connection between GNP per head and life expectancy appears to disappear altogether.

What does this result show, if more fully vindicated by other comparisons as well? It is important to emphasize that this does not show that life expectancy is not enhanced by the growth of GNP per head, but it does indicate that the connection tends to work particularly through public expenditure on health care, and through the success of poverty removal. Much depends on how the fruits of economic growth are used. This also helps to explain why some economies, such as South Korea and Taiwan, have been able to raise life expectancy so rapidly through economic growth, while others with a similar record in economic growth have not achieved correspondingly in the field of longevity expansion.

Asian successes and recent crises

In recent years, the achievements of the East Asian economies have come under critical scrutiny—and some fire—because of the nature and severity of what is called the 'Asian economic crisis'. That crisis is indeed serious, and points to particular failures of economies that were earlier seen—mistakenly—as being comprehensively successful. This is not the place to examine the special problems and specific failures involved in the Asian economic crisis, but is occasion enough to argue that it would be an error to be dismissive about the great achievements of the East and South East Asian economies over several decades, which have transformed the lives and longevities of people in these countries.

For a variety of historical reasons, including a focus on basic education and basic health care, and early completion of effective land reforms, widespread economic participation was easier to achieve in many of the East and South East economies in a way it has not been possible in, say, Brazil or India or

Pakistan, where the creation of social opportunities has been much slower and acted as a barrier for economic development (Drèze and Sen, 1995). The expansion of social opportunities has served as facilitator of high-employment economic development and has also created favourable circumstances for reduction of mortality rates and for expansion of life expectancy. The contrast is sharp with some other high-growth countries—such as Brazil—which have had almost comparable growth of GNP per head, but also have quite a history of severe social inequality, unemployment, and neglect of public health care. The longevity achievements of these other high-growth economies have moved more slowly.

Growth-mediated and support-led progress

There are two interesting—and interrelated—contrasts here:

i) for *high economic growth economies*, the contrast between:

   a) those *with* great success in raising the length and quality of life (such as South Korea and Taiwan); and

   b) those *without* comparable success in these other fields (such as Brazil);

ii) for economies with high success in raising the length and quality of life, the contrast between:

   a) those *with* great success in high economic growth (such as South Korea and Taiwan); and

   b) those *without* much success in achieving high economic growth (such as Sri Lanka, *pre-reform* China, and the Indian state of Kerala).

I have already commented on the first contrast (between, say, South Korea and Brazil), but the second contrast too deserves policy attention. In our book, *Hunger and public action* (1989), Jean Drèze and I have distinguished between two types of successes in the rapid reduction of mortality, which we called respectively 'growth-mediated' and 'support-led' processes. The former process works *through* fast economic growth, and its success depends on the growth process being wide-based and economically broad (strong employment orientation has much to do with this), and also on the utilization of the enhanced economic prosperity to expand the relevant social services, including health care, education, and social security. In contrast with the 'growth-mediated' mechanism, the 'support-led' process does not operate through fast economic growth, but works through a programme of skilful social support of health care, education, and other relevant social arrangements. This process is well exemplified by the experiences of economies such as Sri Lanka, pre-reform China, Costa Rica, or the Indian state of Kerala, which have had very rapid reductions in mortality rates and enhancement of living conditions, without much economic growth.

Public provisioning, low incomes, and relative costs

The support-led process does not wait for dramatic increases in per capita levels of real income, and it works through priority being given to providing social services (particularly health care and basic education) that reduce mortality and enhance the quality of life. Some examples of this relationship are shown in Fig. 17.3, which presents the gross national product (GNP) per head and life expectancy at birth of six countries (China, Sri Lanka, Namibia, Brazil, South Africa, and Gabon) and one sizeable state (Kerala), with 30 million people, within a country (India).[3] Despite their very low levels of income, the people of Kerala, or China, or Sri Lanka enjoy enormously higher levels of life expectancy than do the much richer populations of Brazil, South Africa, and Namibia, not to mention Gabon. Even the direction of the inequality points the other way when we compare Kerala, China, and Sri Lanka, on one side, with Brazil, South Africa, Namibia and Gabon, on the other. Since life expectancy variations relate to a variety of social opportunities that are central to development (including epidemiological policies, health care, educational facilities, and so on), an income-centred view is in serious need of supplementation, in order to have a fuller understanding of the process of development (Sen, 1997; 1998). These contrasts are of considerable policy relevance, and bring out the importance of the 'support-led' process.[4]

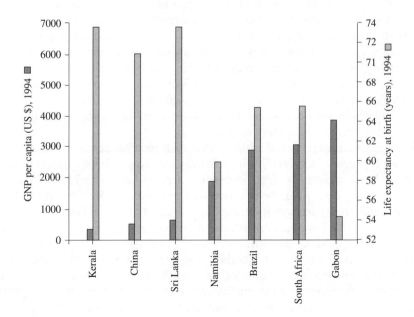

Fig. 17.3   GNP per capita (US dollars) and life expectancy at birth, 1994

Support-led processes and relative costs

Surprise may well be expressed about the possibility of financing 'support-led' processes in poor countries, since resources are surely needed to expand public services, including health care and education. In fact, the need for resources is frequently presented as an argument for postponing socially important investments until a country is already richer. Where (as the famous rhetorical questions goes) are the poor countries going to find the means for 'supporting' these services?

This is indeed a good question, but it also has a good answer, which lies very considerably in the economics of relative costs. The viability of this 'support-led' process is dependent on the fact that the relevant social services (such as health care and basic education) are very labour intensive, and thus are relatively inexpensive in poor—and low-wage—economies. A poor economy may have less money to spend on health care and education, but it also needs less money to spend to provide the same services, which would cost much more in the richer countries. Relative prices and costs are important parameters in determining what a country can afford. Given an appropriate social commitment, the need to take note of the variability of relative costs is particularly important for social services in health and education (Drèze and Sen, 1989).

Advantages of growth mediation

It is obvious that the growth-mediated process has an advantage over its support-led alternative; it may, ultimately, offer more, since there are other deprivations—other than premature mortality, or high morbidity, or illiteracy—that are very directly connected with the lowness of incomes (such as being inadequately clothed and sheltered). It is clearly better to have high income as well as high longevity (and other standard indicators of quality of life), rather than only the latter. This is a point worth emphasizing, since there is some danger of being 'over-convinced' by the statistics of life expectancy and other such basic indicators of quality of life.

For example, the fact that the Indian state of Kerala has achieved impressively high life expectancy, low fertility, high literacy, and so on, despite its low income level per head, is certainly an achievement worth celebrating and learning from. And yet, at the same time, the question remains as to why Kerala has not been able to build on its successes in human development to raise its income levels as well, which would have made its success more complete; it can scarcely serve as a 'model' case, as some have tried to claim. From a policy point of view, this requires a critical scrutiny of Kerala's economic policies regarding incentives and investments ('economic facilities', in general), despite its unusual success in raising life expectancy and the quality of life (Drèze and Sen, 1995). Support-led success does, in this sense, remain shorter in achievement than growth-mediated success, where the increase in economic opulence and the enhancement of quality of life tend to move together.

The lessons to be drawn have to be carefully scrutinized. The advantage of the growth-mediated route is clear enough. On the other hand, the success of the support-led process as a route does indicate that a country need not wait until it is much richer (through what may be a long period of economic growth) before embarking on rapid expansion of basic education and health care. The quality of life can be vastly raised, despite low incomes, through an adequate programme of social services. The fact that education and health care are also productive in raising economic growth adds to the argument for putting major emphasis on these social arrangements, without having to wait to get rich first.[5]The support-led process is a recipe for rapid achievement of higher quality of life, and this has great policy importance, but there remains an excellent case for moving on from there to broader achievements that include economic growth as well as the raising of the standard indicators of quality of life.

Life expectancy enhancement in Britain

It may be instructive, in this context, to re-examine the time-pattern of mortality reduction and of the increase of life expectancy in the advanced industrial economies. The role of public provisions and social arrangements in mortality reduction in Europe over the last three centuries has been well analysed by Robert Fogel and others (Fogel, 1986; Easterlin, 1997). The time-pattern of the expansion of life expectancy in this century itself is of particular interest, bearing in mind that at the turn of the nineteenth century, even Britain—then the leading capitalist market economy—still had a life expectancy at birth that was no higher than the average life expectancy for low-income countries today. However, longevity in Britain did rise rapidly over the twentieth century, partly influenced by strategies of social programmes. The exact time pattern of this increase is worth examining.

While there was general expansion of programmes of support of nutrition, health care, etc. in Britain throughout the twentieth century, the change was not uniformly fast over the decades. There were two periods of remarkably fast expansion of support-oriented policies in this century, which occurred during the two World Wars. Each war situation produced much greater sharing of means of survival, including health care and the limited food supply (through rationing and subsidized nutrition). During the First World War, there were remarkable developments in social attitudes about 'sharing' and public policies aimed at achieving that sharing, as has been well analysed by Jay Winter (1986). During the Second World War also, unusually supportive and shared social arrangements developed, related to the psychology of sharing in beleaguered Britain, which made these radical public arrangements for the distribution of food and health care acceptable and effective (Titmuss, 1950). Even the National Health Service was born during those war years.

How does the pattern of increase in longevity relate to the timing of expansion of health care and other social arrangements favourable to health and survival? Was there, in fact, a correspondingly faster mortality reduction in the particular periods of support-led policies in Britain? It is, in fact, confirmed by detailed nutritional studies that during the Second World War, even though the per capita availability of food fell significantly in Britain, cases of undernourishment also declined sharply, and extreme undernourishment almost wholly disappeared (Titmuss, 1950; Hammond, 1951). Mortality rates also went sharply down (except of course for war mortality itself). A similar thing had happened during the First World War (Winter, 1986).

Indeed, it is remarkable that inter-decade comparisons, based on decadal censuses, show that by a very long margin the most speedy expansion of life expectancy occurred precisely during those two 'war decades' (as shown in Fig. 17.4, which presents the increase in life expectancy in years during each of the first six decades of this century).[6] While in the other decades life expectancy rose rather moderately (between one year and four years), in each of the two war decades, they jumped up by nearly seven years.

However, we must also ask whether the greater increase in life expectancy during the war decades can be, alternatively, explained by faster economic growth over those decades? The answer seems to be in the negative. In fact, the decades of fast expansion of life expectancy happened to be periods of slow growth of gross domestic product per head, as shown in Fig. 17.5. It is, of course, possible to hypothesize that the GDP growth had its effects on life expectancy with a 'time lag' of a decade, and while this is not contradicted by Fig. 17.5 itself, it

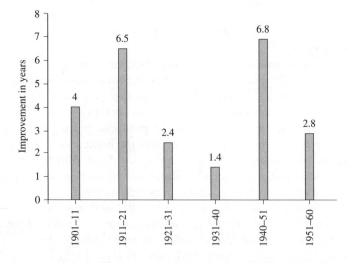

Fig. 17.4 Improvements in life expectancy in England and Wales, 1901–60

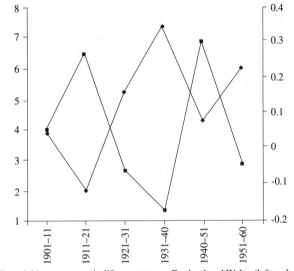

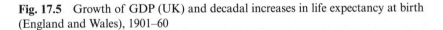

— Decadal improvement in life expectancy, England and Wales (left scale)
— Percentage decadal growth of GDP per capita in UK, 1901–1960 (right scale)

Fig. 17.5 Growth of GDP (UK) and decadal increases in life expectancy at birth (England and Wales), 1901–60

does not stand up much to other scrutiny, including the analysis of possible causal processes. A much more plausible explanation of rapid increase in British life expectancy is provided by the changes in the extent of social sharing during the war decades, and the sharp increases in public support for social services (including nutritional support and health care) that went with this. Much light is thrown on these contrasts by studies of health and other living conditions of the population through the war periods, and their connection with social and public arrangements.[7]

A concluding remark

There is indeed a close connection between economic progress and health achievement, and it would be foolish to take health to be independent of economic means. And yet, especially at the social level, the connection is weakened by two major influences. First, much depends on how the income generated by economic growth is used, in particular whether it is used to expand public services adequately and to reduce the burden of poverty. Second, even when an economy is poor, major health improvements can be achieved through using the available resources in a socially productive way.

There is much merit in economic progress, but there is also an overwhelming role for intelligent and equitable social policies. The analysis of health achievement in terms of economic causation takes us some distance, but ultimately not very far. Maitreyee and Yajnavalkya were sensible in being sceptical about the relationship between wealth and longevity. In fact, their scepticism applies not merely to the grand concern about immortality, but also to the more worldly preoccupation with postponing the evil day. There may be no wisdom in seeking permanence, but there is some permanence in seeking wisdom.

Acknowledgements

This chapter draws on the analysis presented in my recent book *Development as freedom* (1999a) and is published with kind permission of the publishers, Oxford University Press.

Notes

1.   These, and other such comparisons, are presented in my 'The economics of life and death' (1993) and 'Demography of welfare economics' (1995).

2.   See also Sen (1993) and the medical literature cited there, and also the discussion that African American men from the Harlem district of rich New York fall not only behind the Chinese or the Indians in Kerala (in terms of survival) but, by the age of 40 years or so, also behind the famished population of Bangladesh.

3.   Even though Kerala is merely a state rather than a country, nevertheless, with its population close to 30 million, it is larger than the majority of countries in the world (including, for example, Canada).

4.   See also Easterlin, 1997.

5.   The need for supplementing and supporting market-friendly policies for economic growth with a rapid expansion of the social infrastructure (such as public health care and basic education) is discussed in some detail, in the context of the Indian economy, in Drèze and Sen, 1995.

6.   The data relate to England and Wales, since the aggregate British figures could not be found. However, since England and Wales form such an overwhelmingly big part of the UK, not a great deal is lost by this restriction of coverage.

7.   See Titmuss (1950), Hammond (1951), Winter (1986) and the other works to which they refer, and also the discussion and references in Drèze and Sen (1989).

REFERENCES

Anand S, Ravillion M. Human development in poor countries: on the role of private incomes and public services. *Journal of Economic Perspectives*, 1993; **7**:133–50

Aristotle. *The Nichomachean ethics*, (revised edition). Oxford: Oxford University Press, 1980

Brihadaranyaka Upanishad. Calcutta: Advaita Ashrama, 1965, II, iv, 2–3

Drèze J, Sen A. *Hunger and public action.* Oxford: Clarendon Press, 1989, chapter 10

Drèze J, Sen A. *India: economic development and social opportunity.* New Delhi: Oxford University Press, 1995

Easterlin RA. *How beneficient is the market? A look at the modern history of mortality.* University of Southern California, 1997 (mimeograph)

Fogel RW. Nutrition and the decline in mortality since 1700: some preliminary findings. Cambridge, Massachusetts: National Bureau of Economic Research, 1986, Working Paper 1802

Hammond RJ. *History of the Second World War: food.* London: HMSO, 1951

Sen A. The economics of life and death. *Scientific American*, 1993; **268(5)**:40–7

Sen A. Demography of welfare economics. *Empirica*, 1995; **22**:1–22

Sen A. From income inequality to economic inequality. *Southern Economic Journal*, 1997; **64**:384–401

Sen A. Mortality as an indicator of economic success and failure. *Economic Journal*, 1998; **108(446)**:1–25

Sen A. *Development as freedom.* Oxford: Oxford University Press, 1999*a*

Sen A. *Health in development.* Presented at the Fifty Second World Health Assembly, Geneva, 17–15 May 1999. WHO mimeograph A52/DIV/9, 1999*b*

Titmuss RM. *History of the Second World War: problems of social policy.* London: HMSO, 1950

Winter JM. *The Great War and the British People.* London: Macmillan, 1986

Index

abortion 147
absolute scales 127–8
accidents 275
Acheson report (Independent Inquiry into
    Inequalities in Health, 1998) 3, 295
adaptation, to social/economic change 29,
    30–1, 32
adolescents
    injuries 265–8, 269–70, 275, 276
    motherhood 143
adult mortality
    infant mortality and 80–3
    life-course approaches 92–4
    poor–rich differences 223–8
    risk 210
    see also mortality
Africa
    benefit incidence studies 238–9, 240
    Eastern and Southern, see Eastern and
        Southern Africa
    poor–rich differences 224, 225, 226, 231,
        234
African Americans
    deprivation 334–6, 344
    effects of segregation 163–4
    gender differences 285
    injuries 271
    lung cancer 68
    social capital 164, 165
age group differences, injuries 268, 275
age-specific mortality, see mortality, age-
    specific
alcohol
    campaign, in Soviet Union (1985) 18, 23,
        26, 27, 31
    as cause of mortality
        in central Europe 31–2
        in former Soviet Union 23–4, 26, 29,
        31
    prohibition in India 251–2
alcohol abuse
    in developing countries 248–50
    gender differences 288
    poverty and 251–2, 255–6
    preventive strategies 258
alcohol consumption
    driving and 277, 278

family influences 167
    patterns 24, 30
alcohol-related disorders
    in former Soviet Union 21, 23
    temporal factors 60, 61
alienation 168
antenatal care 129–30
anthropometric history 37
anthropometric measures
    gender differences 288
    see also birthweight; height
anti-alcohol campaign (Soviet Union, 1985)
    18, 23, 26, 27, 31
anti-hypertensive medication 12
anxiety disorders 248
Asia
    benefit incidence studies 239, 240
    economic crisis 337–8
assets, health care claims as 184–5
associations
    promoting harm 169
    voluntary 159, 162, 170
    see also groups
attachment, parental 145, 151
Australia
    height studies 46–7, 51–3
    injuries and violence 268–9, 276
    social group differences 197, 198
auxological epidemiology 38

Baltic Republics 17, 19, 20
    validity of mortality data 21, 22
Bangladesh 14, 231, 257–8
    poverty alleviation programmes 312–32
    statistics 313
Bangladesh Academy of Rural Development
    314
Bangladesh Rehabilitation Assistance
    Committee 314
Bangladesh Rural Advancement Committee
    314
    see also BRAC
banks, local 257–8
behavioural problems 145
Belarus 17, 19, 20
benefit incidence studies 238–42, 243
binge drinking 24, 30

bipolar affective disorder 250
birth cohorts 128
birth complications, suicide and 108–9
births, attended by trained staff 218
birthweight
    in Brazil 132–3
    breast cancer and 106
    cancer and 104–5
    coronary heart disease and 98
    respiratory function and 111
Black Committee (1980) 88, 90
bladder cancer 61
blood pressure, life-course influences 97–8, 103
Boas, Franz 38
body mass index (BMI), life-course influences 98
Botswana 189
BRAC 312, 314–29
    child nutritional status 322
    child survival 322–3
    concept of human well-being 321, 326–7
    current programmes 314–18
    education 325
    evaluation design 320
    family planning 324, 325
    food and family expenditure 323–4
    historical background 314
    impact on health and equity 319–26
    membership 318–19
    violence against women 325–6
Brazil 337–8, 339
    benefit incidence studies 241, 249
    income inequalities 256
    infant and child health interventions 125–36
        population and methods 128–9
        results 129–33
    injuries 269–70
    mental health 252
    unwanted children 142
breast cancer 65
    childhood poverty/deprivation and 83
    Eastern vs Western Europe 66, 76–9
    life course influences 103–5, 106–8, 113
    risk factors 106
Britain, see United Kingdom
British 1958 birth cohort study 299
bronchitis 110
Burkina Faso 143
burns 274

Caesarean section rates 133, 134
cancer
    life-course approach 93, 94, 103–6
    temporal dimension 61
    see also neoplasms; specific types
capability, human 15
car access, women's health and 287–8

cardiovascular disease 65
    Eastern vs Western Europe 66, 74–5, 76, 77, 78
    fetal origins hypothesis 62, 74
    in former Soviet Union 22, 23–4, 25, 30
    gender differences 288, 289
    life-course influences 93, 94, 95, 96–103
    temporal dimension 61
    see also coronary heart disease; stroke
Caribbean, see Latin America/Caribbean
Caucasus Republics 18–19, 20, 21, 22
causes of health inequalities 10–12
    fundamental and proximal 90–2
    research needs 244
central Asian Republics 19–20, 21, 22
cerebrovascular disease
    in former Soviet Union 22, 27
    see also stroke
cervical cancer, Eastern vs Western Europe 66
Chadwick, Edwin 5–6, 38
chaos theory 32–3
child abuse
    in developing countries 140–1, 146–7
    potential interventions 149–51
childbearing history, breast cancer and 78–9
child health
    in Brazil 125–36
    in developing countries 137–58
        child factors 141–2
    conceptual model 139–41
    father's role 148
    maternal–child interactions 144–5
    maternal factors 142–4
    potential interventions 149–51
childhood infections 10
    coronary heart disease and 98
    interventions in developing countries 150
    respiratory function and 111–12
    stomach cancer and 74, 109
childhood injuries 265
    inequalities in occurrence 268, 269–71, 272
    policy response 275, 276
childhood social circumstances (including poverty and deprivation)
    adult mortality and 80–3
    cancer and 104–5, 107
    coronary heart disease risk and 96–7
    measures of 80, 92, 93, 96
    respiratory function and 110–11
    stomach cancer and 108–9
    stroke and 103
    suicide and 108
child labour 146
child mortality
    in former Soviet Union 29
    inequalities 221–2, 223, 224, 225, 226
    policy targets 219
    risk 210

child neglect, in developing countries 137–9,
       146–7
   conceptual model 140–1
   potential interventions 149–51
children
   disadvantaged, targeting 306
   factors affecting health 141–2
   intervention studies 297
   nutrition, *see* nutrition, childhood
   street 146
   survival rates, in Bangladesh 322–3, 327,
       328
   unwanted, *see* unwanted children
Chile 231, 252, 269–70
China 334–6, 338, 339
cholesterol, life-course influences 97
chronic illnesses, children with 146
chronic obstructive airways disease, life-course
       influences 110–12, 113
churches 169
civic culture 160, 168, 169
   in Northern and Southern US 163–4
   see also social capital
civil society organizations, injury control 276,
       277
claims, health care, *see* health care claims
Colombia 223
colon cancer 66
communicable diseases 4
   in former Soviet Union 20
   poor–rich differences 229–30
   in unwanted/neglected children 151
communication, mother–child 145
communitarianism 159
communities, personal 160
community kitchens 148
community-level inequality 213–14
community participation 186
conflict, armed, *see* war
congenital abnormalities, children with 146
consumerism 185–6
coping abilities
   in former Soviet Union 30–1, 32
   parents in developing countries 140–1
coronary heart disease (CHD) 11, 96–101
   childhood poverty/deprivation and 80, 81,
       82
   Eastern vs Western Europe 66, 74–5, 77, 78
   fetal origins hypothesis 62, 74
   in former Soviet Union 21
   gender differences 288, 289
   life-course approach 94, 96–101, 113,
       114–15
   temporal dimension 61
   vs stroke 102, 103
corporatism 169
Costa Rica 338
cost-effectiveness analysis 177

costs
   common mental disorders 255
   injuries 265
   relative, support-led progress 340
Côte d'Ivoire 231
credit scheme, in rural Bangladesh 317–18, 328
crime rate, in former Soviet Union 25
crop failure 250–1
cry, infant 145
Cuba 269–70
cultural differences, North and South US
       162–4
Czech Republic 31

data
   on health inequalities, *see* information on
       health inequalities
   on injuries 275
   missing 10
   validity, in former Soviet Union 20–2
debt
   burden, developing countries 3
   mental illness and 250–1, 252, 253
   preventive strategies 257–8
decentralization
   health care 180, 186
   occupational 169
dementia 250
demographic–epidemiological transition 231
Demographic and Health Surveys (DHS) 210,
       221, 234
Demographic Surveillance System (DSS) 320
demographic trends 303
Department for International Development
       280
depression
   in developing countries 248, 249–50
   life-course influences 109–10
   maternal 140, 143–4
   post-partum 144
   poverty and 254, 255, 256, 257
   treatment 250, 258
deprivation (and disadvantage)
   absolute 336
   African Americans 334–6, 344
   childhood, *see* childhood social
       circumstances
   cumulative exposure to 298–9
   gender differences in effects 285–6, 287
   intervention studies 296–7
   life-course approach 92–4
   mental health and 253
   pathways of 299–302
       policies targeting 305–6
   relative 161, 214, 255, 336
   tuberculosis and 69–71
descriptive studies 296–8
developed countries

injuries 264–5
perceptions of health inequalities 6–8
socio-economic gradients among women
  284–93
developing countries
  child health 137–58
  information on health inequalities 7,
    217–46
  injuries 264, 269–70
  mental health 247–62
  perceptions of health inequalities 6–8
  policy agenda 2–3
  poor–rich differences, *see* poor–rich
    differences
  poverty alleviation programmes 312
development, child, factors affecting 145,
  146–7
diabetes 27
diarrhoea
  health service use 234
  oral rehydration therapy (ORT) 314
  in unwanted/neglected children 137, 138–9,
    151
diet, *see* nutrition
difference scales 127–8
disability-adjusted life years (DALYs)
  injuries 264
  mental disorders 249, 255
disadvantage, *see* deprivation (and
  disadvantage)
discourse 181–2, 188
distance 213–14
DNA damage 104
doctors 182
domestic pathways 300–1
donors 3
  health care reform models 177, 180
  injury control role 279–80
DPT vaccine 130
drought 250–1
drowning 270–1, 274
drug dependence, gender differences 288
drug therapy, for mental illness 250, 255
drunk driving 277, 278
Durkheim, Emil 168–9

earthquake, Turkish (1999) 273
Eastern and Southern Africa (ESA)
  claiming greater equality 186
  health care reforms 177, 179–81
  "social settlement" approach 182–4
ecocide 26
ecological studies 58–9
  social capital 161–2
economic burden, *see* costs
economic change
  health effects 3–5
  reducing health inequalities and 294–5

in Soviet Union 17
economic crisis
  Asian 337–8
  in Eastern and Southern Africa 179
economic depression, height studies 52
economic development
  child health and 149
  data collection 217–18
  mental health and 253
  unequal benefits 167–8
economic growth 14, 333–45
  life expectancy and 337
  -mediated progress
    advantages 340–1
    in Britain 342–3
    vs support-led progress 338–40
economic recession
  labour market changes and 304, 305
  suicide and 110
economic status
  data sources 221
  mental health and 253
  see also income; poverty; wealth
education
  basic, impact on mortality 338, 339, 340
  programme, BRAC 315, 320, 325, 328–9
educational level
  BRAC members 325, 328
  data, for developing countries 222
  gender differences 285
  interventions to improve 306
  maternal 142–3, 150
    health service use and 235, 236
    under-five mortality and 223, 224
  mental health and 252–3, 254, 257
  mortality and 94, 95
    in former Soviet Union 24–5
  socio-economic trajectories 300
elderly 13, 219–20
employment
  maternal 144, 149
  mental health and 257
  socio-economic trajectories 299–300
  see also unemployment
empowerment, of women 315–18, 326, 328
"enabling environment" 315–18
Engels, Friedrich 91, 168
England and Wales, *see* United Kingdom
environmental degradation 26
environmental determinants of health 212
environmental factors, growth 39
epidemiological models 297–8
epidemiological studies 295, 296–8
equity of access 7, 8
  health sector reforms and 177–81
  "social settlement" approach 182–4
Estonia 17, 19
ethical issues 2

ethnic/racial differences 13
   lung cancer 68
   poor–rich mortality 231
   small-area studies 199
   social capital 164–5
   socio-economic trajectories 300
   unemployment 303
ethnographic surveys 320
Europe
   childhood injuries 270–1, 272
   Eastern and Central
      benefit incidence studies 239, 240
      mortality rates 31–2
   East–West differences
      childhood injuries 270–1, 272, 276
      mortality 63–79
   reducing health inequalities 294
evidence, for policy and interventions 13–14
exercise, life-course influences 97
explanatory studies 297–8

family
   cohesion/disruption 140, 144
   expenditure 323–4, 328
   extended 166–7
   food distribution within 144, 323–4, 328
   high-risk 142
   networks, adverse effects 165–7
   social capital within 160
family planning 324, 325, 328
farmers, suicide by 250–1
fathers
   child health and 140, 148
   interventions focusing on 151
   occupation 92, 223, 225
   social class 93, 94, 96
fees, user 178, 179–80, 186
fetal origins hypothesis 62, 74
field workers, in developing countries 137, 138–9
Finland 286–7, 304, 305
firearm control 276, 277
folic acid 23–4
food
   adulterated 91
   distribution within family 144, 323–4, 328
fostered children 147
France, height studies 42, 46, 50, 51
French paradox 61

Gabon 339
GDP per capita, *see* Gross Domestic (or
      National) Product (GDP or GNP) per
      capita
gender
   bias, in health research 283–93
   blindness, in health research 284
gender differences 13
   assumptions about 283–4

child health 141–2, 147
   food distribution 323, 328
   height 49
   injuries 268
   lung cancer 67–8
   mental disorders 252
   mortality 23, 211
   social capital 164–5
   socio-economic gradients 284–93
   socio-economic trajectories 301
   tuberculosis 70, 71
general susceptibility model 11, 88–90, 114–15
genetics 13, 39
geographical areas, small, *see* small-area analyses
geographic variations 58–87
   cause-specific mortality 60–83
   injuries and violence 270–1, 272
   mortality in former Soviet Union 25
Germany, height studies 46, 51–3
Ghana 221, 236, 237
Gini coefficient 201, 205–6
   developing countries 218
   inter-individual comparisons 213–14
Global Burden of Disease project 59, 74
Global Forum on Health Research 277
GNP per capita, *see* Gross Domestic (or
      National) Product (GDP or GNP) per
      capita
Gorbachev, M S 18
government health facilities
   differences in benefits received 238–42
   poor–rich differences in use 235–8, 243
governments
   local 169
   powerful central 168
Gross Domestic (or National) Product (GDP
      or GNP) per capita
   in Bangladesh 313
   injuries and 264–5
   life expectancy and 59, 337, 339
   vs height 42, 43
   see also income
groups
   distribution of health expectancy 210–11
   primary 160, 164–7
   secondary 160
   social, *see* social groups
   see also associations
growth
   catch-up 40
   childhood, coronary heart disease and 98
   factors affecting 39–41
   intrauterine restriction, *see* intrauterine
      growth restriction
   unwanted/neglected children 139
   velocities 38–9
   see also height
gun control 276, 277

health
    determinants, social inequalities as 212–14
    distribution 9, 201–3
    economic progress and 333–45
    objectives, setting 220
    and wealth 5–6
Health 21 strategy 294
health care claims
    definition 185
    more equal, within unequal systems 185–7
    poverty and 184–5
    relational nature 185
health care systems 12, 175–93
    in former Soviet Union 26–7
    poverty, claims and representations 184–7
    prescriptive reform models 176–7
    "social settlement" approach 182–4, 187–8
    supporting improved health 338–40
    unequalizing reforms 177–81
health expectancy
    calculation 209–10
    definition 215
    distribution
        as index of health inequality 206–9
        measurement 209–12
health inequalities
    between and within countries 58–87
    causes, *see* causes of health inequalities
    definition 195
    determinants, social group studies 197–8
    differing perceptions 6–8
    impact of health interventions 125–36
    information on, *see* information on health
        inequalities
    measurement, *see* measuring health
        inequality
    measures of, *see* measures of health
        inequality
    new approach 201–12
    options for reducing 294–311
    policy agenda 2–3
    science of 295, 296–304
health policy 54
    establishing 218–20
    health sector reforms and 176–7
    mental illness and 256–9
    poverty, inequality and 175, 187–8
health service utilization
    data, developing countries 221, 244
    poor–rich differences 234–5
health status
    data, in developing countries 221, 232, 244
    measurement 211, 232
    self-reported
        gender differences 286–7
        poor–rich differences 232–4, 243
    social group differences 197, 198
heart disease, *see* coronary heart disease

height 37
    breast cancer and 106–7
    cancer and 104, 105
    factors affecting 39–41
    industrialization and 45–54
        methodology 38–41
        temporal patterns 47–53
    stroke and 103
    urbanization and 46–7, 48–9, 52–3
    vs other measures 41–5
Helicobacter pylori infections 73–4, 109
HIV infection 20
home visits, in developing countries 137,
    138–9, 149, 151
homicide
    in former Soviet Union 22
    inequalities in occurrence 269, 270, 271
    social capital and 167
hospital services 182
    poor–rich differences 236, 239
households
    changes in composition 303–4
    surveys in Bangladesh 320
housing
    infant mortality as indicator 80, 81
    tenure, women's health and 287–8
human capital argument 6, 15
human development approach 336
human rights and legal education (HRLE) 317
Hungary 31
hunger, mental health and 252, 253
hygiene, infant mortality as indicator 80, 81
hypertension 27

income
    achievements and 334
    distribution (equality of) 11, 167–8
        changes in 303, 304
        and health 161–2
        health inequalities and 59–60, 203, 204
        height and 42
        measurement 201
        mental health and 253, 255, 256–7
        policies 308
        see also Gini coefficient
    gender differences 285
    height and 41–5
    household
        Brazilian study 129–33
        changes in 303
        in former Soviet Union 25, 29
        gender differences 286–8
    mental health and 252
    per capita, *see* Gross Domestic (or National)
        Product (GDP or GNP) per capita
    support interventions 297
Independent Inquiry into Inequalities in
    Health (Acheson report, 1998) 3, 295

index of health inequality, choosing 206–9
India 146, 238, 337–8
    deprivation in 334–6
    Kerala state 334–6, 338, 339, 340–1, 344
    mental health 249, 250–1, 257–8
    prohibition of alcohol 251–2
individual determinants of health 212
individual-mean differences (IMD) 205, 208–9
individual variation 202
Indonesia 239, 252–3
industrialization, health and 4, 37–57
    temporal patterns 47–53
    urbanization and 45–7
infanticide, female 141–2
infant mortality 12
    adult mortality and 80–3
    coronary heart disease and 97
    inequalities 221–2, 223, 224, 225, 226
    information availability 218
    policy targets 219
    rates (IMR)
        absolute vs relative gaps 127–8
        in Brazil 132–3
        in unwanted/neglected children 138–9
infants, health in Brazil 125–36
infections, childhood, see childhood infections
infectious diseases, see communicable diseases
information on health inequalities 7, 217–46
    currently available 222–42
    recent trends 220–2
    traditional neglect 217–20
injuries 12–13, 263–82
    advancing policy agenda 277–80
    classification 263–4
    evidence of effective interventions 272–4
    in former Soviet Union 21, 22–3, 30
    inequalities in occurrence 268–71
    public health burden 263–8
    reasons for limited policy response 274–7
    research needs and gaps 266–7
    see also violence
institutions
    conceptualization 181–2
    health care, "social settlement" approach
        181–4, 187–8
    legitimation 181
insulin 27
insulin-like growth factor-1 (IGF-1) 104, 107–8
insulin-like growth factor binding protein
    (IGFBP-3) 104
insulin resistance syndrome 98
inter-individual determinants of health 212–14
inter-individual differences (IID) 205–6, 208–9
internal market 177, 178–9
international agencies 3
International Campaign to Ban Landmines
    278
International Centre for Diarrhoeal Disease

Research, Bangladesh (ICDDR,B) 318,
    320, 326
International Classification of Diseases (ICD)
    21–2
interventions
    evaluative studies 296–7
    evidence for 13–14
    impact on health inequalities 125–36
    information needs 244
    injuries and violence 272–4
    unwanted/neglected children 138–9
intrauterine growth restriction
    breast cancer and 107–8
    respiratory function and 111
    stroke and 102–3
    suicide and 108–9
inverse care law 126, 133–4
Ireland, height studies 42–3

Jamaica 143
Japan
    height studies 39, 44, 46, 50–1, 54
    small-area studies 199–200
    stomach cancer 81

Kenya 183, 231
Kerala, India 334–6, 338, 339, 340–1, 344
Krygyzstan 280
Kuznet's hypothesis 231

labour, child 146
labour force turnover 25
labour market
    changes 302, 303–4
    policies 306, 307–8
    see also employment
landmines 278
latent periods 61
Latin America/Caribbean
    benefit incidence studies 239–42
    health inequalities 221, 222
    injuries 265, 269–70
    poor–rich mortality differences 224, 225,
        226
Latvia 17, 19
life-course approaches 11–12, 62, 88–124
    adult mortality 92–4
    breast cancer 103–5, 106–8, 113
    cancer 93, 94, 103–6
    coronary heart disease (CHD) 94, 96–101,
        113, 114–15
    longitudinal studies 299–302
    policy options 305–6
    respiratory function/obstructive airways
        disease 97–8, 110–12
    stomach cancer 103–4, 108–9, 113
    stroke 101–3, 113
    suicide and depression 109–10, 113

life expectancy
    in Britain 341–3
    distribution, for groups 210–11
    in former Soviet Union 5, 17–20, 30
        see also Soviet Union, former, health
        crisis
    GDP/GNP per capita and 59, 337, 339
    growth-mediated vs support-led progress
        338–40
    height and 43–5
    poor–rich differences 226–7
    small-area studies 199–201
    social capital and 161
    variation between and within countries
        62–3
life transitions, targeting critical 305–6
Lithuania 17, 19, 21–2, 30–1
living standards
    GNP as indicator 41
    height and 40–1
    increasing inequalities 302–4
    infant mortality as indicator 80, 81
    mental health and 253
    tuberculosis and 69–70
    see also social circumstances
Living Standards Measurement Studies
    (LSMS) 210, 221, 232–3
loan facilities
    access to 257–8
    in rural Bangladesh 317–18, 328
local governments 169
longitudinal studies 299–302
Longitudinal Study 107, 110
long-standing illness, limiting, gender
    differences 287–8
Lorenz curve 206
low-birthweight infants 133, 141, 143
low-income countries, see developing countries
lung cancer 10–11
    childhood poverty/deprivation and 81, 82–3
    Eastern vs Western Europe 1, 66, 67–8, 69
    in former Soviet Union 27–8
    life-course influences 113, 114–15
    temporal dimension 61
lung function, life-course influences 97–8,
    110–12

Malaysia 239, 276
malnutrition 39, 41
    in Brazil 130–2, 133
    protein–energy (PEM), in Bangladesh 322,
        323
    in unwanted/neglected children 137–8
Management Information System (MIS) 320
market mechanisms, in health care systems
    177, 178–9, 184
Marx, Karl 168, 196
maternal mortality

policy targets 219
stroke and 102
measures of health inequality 205–6
    choice of single index 206–9
        intensity of health gain/loss 207
        inter-individual vs individual-mean
        differences 208–9
        relative vs absolute inequality 206–7
    individual-mean differences (IMD) 205
    inter-individual differences (IID) 205–6
measuring health inequality 8–10, 127–8,
    194–216
    current analytical perspectives 194–201
    new approach 201–12
    operationalization 209–12
    reasons for 201–3
    small-area analyses 198–201
    social group differences 195–8
media, injury prevention 277
medical hierarchy 182
Melbourne Declaration on Injury Prevention
    276
mental disorders, common (CMD) 143
    fatherless children 148
    poverty and, see mental health, poverty and
    prevention 257–8
    public health significance 248–50
    symptoms 248
    treatability 250
    see also depression
mental health 12, 247–62
    poverty and 247, 250–9
        causal associations 253–6
        evidence for relationship 250–3
        public health policy implications 256–9
        research needed 258–9
    public health significance 248–50
    services, inadequacy 250
Mexico, small-area studies 199–201
micro-credit programme, in rural Bangladesh
    317–18, 328
mid-upper-arm circumference 322
midwives, home visits 149, 151
migrant studies 104
Moldova 17, 19, 20
Mongolia 239
mortality
    age-specific
        in former Soviet Union 29
        in poor 219–20
        poor–rich differences 223–8
        see also adult mortality; child mortality;
        infant mortality
    cause-specific
        between country differences 60–83
        gender differences 288, 289
        poor–rich differences 228–30
        in US 89–90

mortality (contd.)
    crisis, in former Soviet Union , *see* Soviet
        Union, former, health crisis
    data, in former Soviet Union 20–2
    East–West differences 63–5
    life-course approach 92–4
    mental illness and 249–50
    poor–rich differences, *see* poor–rich
        differences, mortality
    risks 210
    see also life expectancy; socio-economic
        gradients
mother–child relationship 140, 144–5
mothers
    behavioural styles 144
    clubs/groups 148
    coping abilities 140–1
    depressed 140, 143–4
    education, *see* educational level, maternal
    employment 144, 149
    factors affecting child's health 139, 142–4
    interventions focusing on 149–51
    self-esteem 139, 140, 143, 149
Mothers Against Drunk Driving 277
motor vehicle accidents, *see* road traffic
        accidents
Mozambique 179, 183
multinational corporations 279
Multiple Risk Factor Intervention Trial
        (MRFIT) 90, 99, 284

Namibia 339
National Child Development Survey (1958) 299
National Health Service (NHS)
    claiming greater equality 185–6
    "social settlement" approach 182–4
    unequalizing reforms 177, 178–9
National Rifle Association (NRA) 276
Native Americans, injuries 269
Navajo Indians, social capital 166–7
needs
    assessment, individual 186
    basic human 185, 217–18
neglect, child, *see* child neglect
neonatal services 12, 129, 133
neoplasms
    in former Soviet Union 21, 22
    poor–rich differences 229
    see also cancer
Netherlands
    height studies 42, 46, 49–50
    social group differences 197, 198
New Deal 306
Newly Independent States (NIS)
    childhood injuries 270, 272
    see also Soviet Union, former
New Zealand 294
Nigeria 146

non-communicable diseases 10–11
    poor–rich differences 229–30
    temporal dimension 60–1, 62
non-governmental organizations (NGOs) 186,
        237
    in India 251, 252
    injury control 276
    poverty alleviation programmes 314–29
nurses, home visits 149, 151
nursing 182
nutrition (and diet)
    childhood
        BRAC programme impact 322, 323, 327
        cancer and 105
        coronary heart disease and 98
        interventions 149–50
        quality of maternal care and 139, 145
    in former Soviet Union 27–8
    health and 91
    height and 39–40, 41, 53

obesity, breast cancer and 106
occupation
    current 92
    data, for developing countries 222
    father's 92, 223, 225
    gender differences 289–90
    at labour market entry 92
occupational decentralization 169
occupational exposures 211
oestrogens 108
Open Society Institute 280
oral rehydration therapy (ORT) 314
Organization for Economic Cooperation and
        Development (OECD) targets 218–19,
        220
outcomes 202, 209–10
    distribution of non-fatal 211–12

Pakistan 221, 337–8
parenthood, socio-economic trajectories 300–1
parents
    coping abilities 139–41
    relationship with child 137–8, 145
    see also fathers; mothers
Peru 137–58, 223
Philippines 239
pneumonia, in former Soviet Union 21, 24
poisoning 270–1, 274
Poland 31, 74
policy 2–3
    agenda 2–3
    evidence for 13–14
    health, *see* health policy
    reducing health inequalities 305–8
    response to injuries
        reasons for limited 274–7
        stimulating effective 277–80

poor
    age-specific mortality 219–20
    causes of poor health 91
    "enabling environment" for 315–18
    limited political influence 274
    mental illness 12
    prevention of injuries 273–4
    rural, definition in Bangladesh 316
    uptake of new interventions 126–7, 129–35
    see also deprivation; poverty
Poor Laws 5–6
poor–rich differences
    financial benefits from health services
        238–42, 243
    health service use 234–5
    interpretation 242–4
    mortality 222–32
        by cause of death 228–30
        at older ages 223–8
        time trends 231–2, 243
        at younger ages 223, 224, 225, 226
    public vs private health service use 235–8,
        243
    self-reported health status 232–4, 243
Portugal 71–2, 73, 75
poultry programmes, in rural Bangladesh
    317–18
poverty
    alleviation programmes 312–32
    childhood, *see* childhood social
        circumstances
    data, for developing countries 217–22
    and health 299
        direction of causality 5–6
        explanations for 10
    health care claims and 184–5
    health policy 187–8, 280
    height and 41–2
    increased, in UK 302–3
    line 218, 302–3
    mental health and 247, 250–9
    policy agenda 2–3
    policy targets 218–19, 220
    relative 161, 214, 255
    social capital and 166–7
    tuberculosis and 69–71
    see also deprivation; poor; poor-rich
        differences
pregnancy
    breast cancer and 106, 108
    unwanted 147
premature infants 141, 143
prevention
    injuries 273
    mental disorders 257–8
    programmes, in Brazil 129–30, 133
primary health care 129, 182
    mental disorders 258

poor–rich differences 236, 239
private sector 134, 186, 187–8
    poor–rich differences in use 235–8, 243
privatization, health care 178, 179–80
prohibition, alcohol 251–2
prostate cancer 65
    Eastern vs Western Europe 66, 76–9
protein–energy malnutrition (PEM), in
        Bangladesh 322, 323
psychiatric disorders, *see* mental disorders,
        common
psychological well-being 328
psychopharmacological therapy 250, 255
psychotherapeutic interventions 250, 255
psychotic disorders 248
public health facilities, *see* government health
        facilities
purchaser/provider split 177
Puritanism 162

racial differences, *see* ethnic/racial differences
racial segregation 161, 163–4
rank 213–14
ratio scales 127–8
rectal cancer 66
relative scales 127–8
research, gender bias in 283–93
respiratory disease
    Eastern vs Western Europe 66
    in unwanted/neglected children 137, 138
respiratory function, life-course influences
        97–8, 110–12
rich, *see* wealthy
risk 202, 209–10
risk factors, in former Soviet Union 23–4
risk-related behaviours 296
road traffic accidents 60, 248–9
    injuries related to 264–5
    prevention 274, 297
    safety programmes 276–7, 280
Roberts, Charles 38
Rockefeller Foundation 3
rural areas
    BRAC development programme 315–18
    in former Soviet Union 30
    height data 52
    mental health problems 254
    social networks/integration 166–7
Rural Development Programme (RDP), BRAC
        315–18
rural–urban residence 222
    health service use and 234–5
    injuries 270
    self-reported health status and 232–3
    under-five mortality and 223, 226
Russia 5, 17
    causes of increased mortality 22–3, 27–8,
        30, 32

Russia (contd.)
  explaining mortality upturn 28–9
  gender differences 288, 289
  injuries 268
  pattern of mortality 19, 20
  risk factors 23–4
  social and economic determinants of health 24–6
  stomach cancer 81
  validity of mortality data 21
Russian Longitudinal Monitoring Survey (RLMS) 29

safety policies 278
sanitary reform 4
sanitation
  infant mortality as indicator 80, 81
  stomach cancer and 74
savings
  mental health and 253
  scheme, in rural Bangladesh 317
scalds 274
schizophrenia 248, 250
school performance 145
  see also educational level
schools
  BRAC 315, 320
  drop-out rates 257
Schweitzer Seminars 280
science of health inequalities 295, 296–304
  case study 298–304
  descriptive studies 296–8
Scotland, see United Kingdom
security policies 278
segregation, racial 161, 163–4
selection bias 327
self-esteem
  maternal 139, 140, 143, 149
  unwanted children 147
self-harm, deliberate 249
Senegal 231
sensitive periods 39
sericulture 318
sexual abuse, child 146
siblings, number of 109
Sierra Leone 147
small-area analyses 195, 198–201
  distribution of health expectancy 210–11
smoking, tobacco 11, 67, 90
  in former Soviet Union 27–8
  life-course influences 97, 98, 103–4, 110
  maternal 111
  social patterning 68
  temporal dimension 61
social capital 60, 159–74
  adverse effects 165–7
  concept 159–60
  dialectics 162–4

ecological studies 161–2
  in former Soviet Union 25–6
  and primary groups 164–7
social change
  health effects 3–5
  reducing health inequalities and 294–5
social circumstances
  adulthood
    cancer and 105–6
    coronary heart disease and 96, 98–100
  childhood, see childhood social circumstances
  lifetime, coronary heart disease and 97–8
  tackling adverse 296–7
  see also deprivation; living standards; poverty
social class 195–6
  current 93, 94
  father's 93, 94, 96
  at labour market entry (first) 93, 94
  measurements 8
  see also socio-economic status
social epidemiology 297–8
social exclusion 184
social group differences 195–8
  comparability/generalizability of results 197
  as determinants of health 212–14
  determinants of health inequalities and 197–8
  vs individual-level inequality 203
  see also socio-economic gradients
social groups
  definition 195–7
  in developing countries 140, 148, 151
  membership of 160, 162, 170
social hierarchy 213
social integration 164–7
social marginalization 140, 141, 150
social networks (support) 160, 164–7
  changing nature 214
  in developing countries 148, 151
  harmful effects 165–7, 169
  mental health and 254
  poverty and 299
social polarization 295, 302, 303
social position 196, 255
social security
  benefits, dependency on 300, 301, 308
  systems 239
social services
  impact on mortality 338, 339, 340
  public support, in Britain 341, 343
"social settlement" approach 181–4, 187–8
social support, see social networks
socio-economic deprivation, see deprivation
socio-economic gradients 6, 62–3, 90
  in Brazil 129–35
  developing countries 222–32
  Eastern vs Western Europe 65–79
  explanatory approaches 10–12

in former Soviet Union 29
gender differences 284–93
height 41
heterogeneity 89–90
injuries and violence 268–71
interpretation 8–9
life-course approaches, *see* life-course
    approaches
measurement 8–10
vs distributional approach 9
see also poor–rich differences; social group
    differences
socio-economic status 196
and health, models of 297–9
women 284, 289
socio-economic structure
changes in 298, 302–4
national policies 307–8
socio-economic trajectories 299–302, 304
policies targeting 305–6
South Africa 276, 339
South Korea 337, 338
Soviet Union, former 5, 17–36
child injury mortality 270
health crisis 17–18, 63–4
    alternative theories 26–8
    explaining later upturn 28–9
    immediate causes 22–3
    interpretation 30–2
    methodological issues 20–2
    risk factors 23–4
    social and economic determinants 24–6
    varying patterns 18–20
history 17–18
stomach cancer 74
see also Newly Independent States; Russia
Sri Lanka 338, 339
Standard of Living debate 167–8
stature, *see* height
stomach cancer 4
childhood poverty/deprivation and 80, 81,
    82, 83
Eastern vs Western Europe 66, 72–4
life-course influences 103–4, 108–9, 113
street children 146
stress, psycho-social 11, 89, 114
in former Soviet Union 25, 26, 31
mental health and 250–1, 254–5
suicide and 110, 251
stroke 12, 24
childhood poverty/deprivation and 80, 81,
    82, 83
Eastern vs Western Europe 66, 74–5, 76, 78
fetal origins hypothesis 62, 74
life course influences 101–3, 113
substance abuse 250
suicide
anomic 168

Durkheim's view 168–9
egoistic 168
in former Soviet Union 22
global burden 264
life-course influences 109–10, 113
mental illness and 249
poverty and 250–1, 257
support-led progress
in Britain 341–2
vs economic growth mediated progress
    338–40
Sure Start programme 306
surfactant therapy 133
survey methods 7–8
Sweden 8–9, 15
height studies 46, 49
symbolism, in injury prevention 277
syndrome X 98

Taiwan 337, 338
Tanzania 183, 189, 237
taxation, progressive 308
Tocqueville, Alexis de 162, 163, 168
triglycerides, serum, life-course influences 98
trust, interpersonal 161–2
tuberculosis (TB) 20, 65
childhood poverty/deprivation and 80, 81,
    82, 83
Eastern vs Western Europe 66, 69–72
life-course influences 113
temporal dimension 70
Turkey, earthquake (1999) 273
typhoid fever 53

Uganda 231
Ukraine 17, 19, 20, 21, 27
underweight infants, in Brazil 130–2
unemployment
policies targeting 306, 307–8
suicide and 110
trends 302, 303, 304, 305
see also employment
UNICEF 280
United Kingdom (UK, including England and
    Wales, Scotland) 3, 8
changes in socio-economic structure 302–4
height studies 46, 48–9
injuries 276
life expectancy enhancement 341–3
NHS, *see* National Health Service
reducing health inequalities 294, 306, 307–8
socio-economic gradients 62, 63, 65
    gender differences 285–8
    tuberculosis mortality 70
United Nations Development Programme 336
United States (US) 7
health inequalities 62, 89–90
height studies 42, 43, 44, 46, 47–8

United States (US) (contd.)
  injuries 265, 269, 271, 275, 276
  North–South differences 162–4
  reducing health inequalities 306
  relative deprivation 334–6
  small-area studies 199–201, 210–11
  socio-economic gradients among women 285
universalism 183, 185, 186–7
unwanted children
  in developing countries 137–8, 139, 141–2,
    147
  potential interventions 149–51
urban areas
  in former Soviet Union 25
  in Northern US 163–4
  see also rural–urban residence
urbanization
  health and 45–7
  height and 46–7, 48–9, 52–3
  mental health and 254

vaccines
  coverage 130
  poultry 317–18
Venezuela 269–70
vested interests 275–6
Vietnam 221, 239
village organizations (VO) 316–18
  impact on health and equity 319–20
  membership 318–19
violence
  against women, in rural Bangladesh 325–6,
    328
  domestic 248–9, 251
  in former Soviet Union 21, 22–3, 30
  inequalities in occurrence 268–71
  injuries due to 263, 265
  public health policy 276
  see also child abuse; injuries
voluntary associations 159, 162, 170
vulnerability, gender differences 289–90

war
  in Eastern and Southern Africa 179
  in former Soviet Union 21, 22
  injuries due to 265

life expectancy trends in Britain 341–2, 343
wealth
  data sources 221
  health and 5–6
wealthy
  uptake of new interventions 126–7, 129–35
  see also poor–rich differences
Weber, Max 196
weight, at 12 months, in Brazil 130–2
welfare state services, inequalities in 308
Welfare-to-Work programmes 306, 307–8
well-being, human
  concept of 321
  impact of BRAC programmes 326–7, 328
West of Scotland Collaborative Study 92–4,
    95
  coronary heart disease 96, 97, 98, 100–1
  respiratory function 110–11
  stomach cancer 108–9
  stroke 102, 103
Whitehall studies 11, 89, 98–9, 105, 213, 284
women
  empowerment 315–18, 326, 328
  problems caused by alcoholism 251
  social classification 284, 289
  social resources/groups 148, 151, 165
  socio-economic gradients 284–93
  violence against 325–6
  see also gender; gender differences; mothers
World Bank 3, 176–7, 179, 180
  Global Road Safety initiative 276–7, 280
  information produced 218, 221
World Health Organization (WHO) 6
  country-level data 220–1, 223–30
  index of health inequality 209
  injuries and violence 276
  reducing health inequalities 294
World Wars, life expectancy trends 341–2, 343

young adults
  disadvantaged, targeting 306
  injuries 265–8, 269–70, 275, 276

Zimbabwe
  injury control 276, 277, 278
  mental health 252, 256–7